Salisbury District Hospital Library

|||||||||||||||||||||||||||||||||
T12956

WO
255
7/97.

21. AUG 97

10. SEP 97

9. 10. 97

7.11.97

01. OCT 98

5.3.99

6.4.99

6/5/99

02. SEP 99

31/8/99

3 feb 00

17. APR 01

09. DEC 02

19. MAY 06

1 9 OCT 2009

05. SEP 11

WHJ 1207

Books should be returned to the SDH Library on or before
the date stamped above unless a renewal has been arranged.

Salisbury District Hospital Library

Telephone: Salisbury (01722) 336262 extn. 4432 / 33
Out of hours answer machine in operation

Lasers in Cutaneous and Aesthetic Surgery

Lasers in Cutaneous and Aesthetic Surgery

EDITORS

Kenneth A. Arndt, MD
Professor of Dermatology
Harvard Medical School
Boston, Massachusetts

Dermatologist-in-Chief
Codirector, Joint Center for Cutaneous Laser Surgery
Beth Israel Deaconess Medical Center
Boston, Massachusetts

Jeffrey S. Dover, MD
Associate Professor of Clinical Dermatology
Harvard Medical School
Boston, Massachusetts

Codirector, Joint Center for Cutaneous Laser Surgery
Department of Dermatology
Beth Israel Deaconess Medical Center
Boston, Massachusetts

Suzanne M. Olbricht, MD
Assistant Professor of Clinical Dermatology
Harvard Medical School
Boston, Massachusetts

Director of Dermatology Surgery
Department of Dermatology
Beth Israel Deaconess Medical Center
Boston, Massachusetts

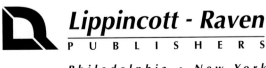
Lippincott - Raven
P U B L I S H E R S
Philadelphia • New York

Manufacturing Manager: Dennis Teston
Associate Managing Editor: Kathleen Bubbeo
Cover Designer: Karen Quigley
Production Service: Textbook Writers Associates, Inc.
Indexer: Michael Loo
Compositor: Compset Inc.
Printer: Kingsport Press

©1997, by Lippincott–Raven Publishers. All rights reserved. This book is protected by copyright. No part of it may be reproduced, stored in a retrieval system, or transmitted, in any form or by any means—electronic, mechanical, photocopy, recording, or otherwise—without the prior written consent of the publisher, except for brief quotations embodied in critical articles and reviews. For information write **Lippincott–Raven Publishers, 227 East Washington Square, Philadelphia, PA 19106-3780.**

Materials appearing in this book prepared by individuals as part of their official duties as U.S. Government employees are not covered by the above-mentioned copyright.

Printed in the United States of America

9 8 7 6 5 4 3 2 1

Library of Congress Cataloging-in-Publication Data
Lasers in cutaneous and aesthetic surgery/editors, Kenneth A. Arndt,
  Jeffrey S. Dover, Suzanne M. Olbricht.
      p.   cm.
   Includes bibliographical references and index.
   ISBN 0-316-05177-2
   1. Skin—Laser surgery. 2. Surgery, Plastic. 3. Lasers in
surgery. I. Arndt, Kenneth A., 1936–   . II. Dover, Jeffrey S.
III. Olbricht, Suzanne M.
   [DNLM: 1. Laser Surgery—methods. 2. Skin—surgery. 3. Surgery,
Plastic—methods. WO 511 L3436 1997]
RL120.L37L357 1997
617.4'77059—dc21
DNLM/DLC
for Library of Congress   97-3099
                                  CIP

Care has been taken to confirm the accuracy of the information presented and to describe generally accepted practices. However, the authors, editors, and publisher are not responsible for errors or omissions or for any consequences from application of the information in this book and make no warranty, express or implied, with respect to the contents of the publication.

The authors, editors, and publisher have exerted every effort to ensure that drug selection and dosage set forth in this text are in accordance with current recommendations and practice at the time of publication. However, in view of ongoing research, changes in government regulations, and the constant flow of information relating to drug therapy and drug reactions, the reader is urged to check the package insert for each drug for any change in indications and dosage and for added warnings and precautions. This is particularly important when the recommended agent is a new or infrequently employed drug.

Some drugs and medical devices presented in this publication have Food and Drug Administration (FDA) clearance for limited use in restricted research settings. It is the responsibility of the health care provider to ascertain the FDA status of each drug or device planned for use in their clinical practice.

To our families

Contributing Authors

R. Rox Anderson, MD *Associate Professor, Department of Dermatology, Harvard Medical School, Boston, Massachusetts; Wellman Laboratories of Photomedicine, Department of Dermatology, Massachusetts General Hospital, 50 Blossom Street, BHX 630, Boston, Massachusetts 02114–2698*

Kenneth A. Arndt, MD *Dermatologist-in-Chief, Codirector, Joint Center for Cutaneous Laser Surgery, Beth Israel Deaconess Medical Center, 330 Brookline Avenue, Boston, Massachusetts 02215*

Michael F. Becker, LICSW, BCD, PhD *Director, Services For Men and Their Relationships, 341 Marrett Road (Route 2A), Lexington, Massachusetts 02173–7036*

Michael W. Berns, PhD *Professor of Surgery, President, and Director, Beckman Laser Institute and Medical Clinic, University of California—Irvine, 1002 Health Sciences Road East, Irvine, California 92612; Professor of Surgery, University of California—Irvine, Orange, California 92613*

Donna B. C. Bourgelais *President, Medical Laser Research and Development Corporation, RR#2, Box 535, East Lebanon, Maine 04027*

Graham B. Colver, MD *Consultant Dermatologist, Chesterfield and North Derbyshire Royal Hospital, Chesterfield, S44 5BL United Kingdom*

Jeffrey S. Dover, MD *Associate Professor of Clinical Dermatology, Harvard Medical School, Boston, Massachusetts; Codirector, Joint Center for Cutaneous Laser Surgery, Beth Israel Deaconess Medical Center, 110 Francis Street, #7H, Boston, Massachusetts 02215*

Ellet H. Drake, MD *President and Medical Director, A. Ward Ford Memorial Institute, Warsaw, Wisconsin 54401; Historian, American Society for Laser Medicine and Surgery, Warsaw, Wisconsin 54401*

Gretchen Fischer Felopulos, PhD *Instructor in Psychology, Harvard Medical School, Boston, Massachusetts; Staff Psychologist, Massachusetts General Hospital, Boston, Massachusetts 02114*

Richard E. Fitzpatrick, MD *Associate Clinical Professor, Department of Medicine, Division of Dermatology, University of California—San Diego, San Diego, California 92103*

Thomas J. Flotte, MD *Associate Professor of Dermatology, Harvard Medical School, Boston, Massachusetts; Wellman Laboratories of Photomedicine, Department of Dermatology, 50 Blossom Street, BHX 630, Massachusetts General Hospital, Boston, Massachusetts 02114–2698*

Terry A. Fuller, PhD *Assistant Professor, Department of Urology, Jefferson Medical College, 1025 Walnut Street, Philadelphia, Pennsylvania 19107; President and Chief Executive Officer, Fuller Research Corporation, Inc., 944 Morgan Road, Rydal, Pennsylvania 19046*

Jerome M. Garden, MD *Associate Professor of Clinical Dermatology, Northwestern University Medical School, Tarry Building, 303 East Chicago Avenue, Chicago, Illinois 60611–3008; Divisions of Dermatology and Plastic Surgery, Children's Memorial Hospital, 2300 Children's Plaza, Chicago, Illinois 60614*

Roy G. Geronemus, MD *Clinical Associate Professor of Dermatology, New York School of Medicine; Director, Laser and Skin Surgery Center of New York, 317 East 34th Street, New York, New York 10016*

Richard O. Gregory, MD *Associate Clinical Professor of Surgery, University of South Florida, Tampa, Florida 33620*

Cynthia H. Halcin, MD *Department of Dermatology and Cutaneous Biology and Department of Biochemistry and Molecular Pharmacology, Jefferson Medical College, 233 South 10th Street, Room 450, Philadelphia, Pennsylvania 19107; Section of Molecular Medicine, Thomas Jefferson University, Philadelphia, Pennsylvania 19107*

Ulrich Hohenleutner, MD *Associate Professor and Senior Resident, Department of Dermatology, University of Regensburg, Regensburg 93053, Germany*

George J. Hruza, MD *Associate Professor of Dermatology, Otolaryngology, and Surgery, Washington University School of Medicine, 660 South Euclid Avenue, St. Louis, Missouri 63110; Director, Cutaneous Surgery Center, Barnes-Jewish Hospital, 1 Barnes Hospital Plaza, Suite 16411, St. Louis, Missouri 63110*

Alfred Intintoli *Director, Laser and Systems Development, Surgical Laser Technologies, Inc., 147 Keystone Drive, Montgomeryville, Pennsylvania 18936–9638*

Irving Itzkan, PhD *Research Associate in Dermatology, Department of Dermatology, Beth Israel Deaconess Medical Center, Boston, Massachusetts 02215*

Steven L. Jacques, PhD *Professor of Electrical Engineering, Oregon Graduate Institute; Research Associate Professor of Dermatology, Oregon Health Sciences University; Oregon Medical Laser Center, Providence St. Vincent Medical Center, 9205 SW Barnes Road, Portland, Oregon 97225*

S. Michael Kalick, PhD *Associate Professor, Psychology Department, University of Massachusetts—Boston, 100 Morrissey Boulevard, Boston, Massachusetts 02125*

Kay S. Kane, MD *Resident, Department of Dermatology, Harvard Medical School, Boston, Massachusetts 02115*

Michael Landthaler, MD *Professor and Head, Department of Dermatology, University of Regensburg, Regensburg 93053, Germany*

Margaret S. Lee *Medical Student, Class of 1998, Boston University School of Medicine, 80 East Concord Street, Box 242, Boston, Massachusetts 02118; Wellman Laboratories of Photomedicine, Department of Dermatology, Massachusetts General Hospital, 50 Blossom Street, BHX 630, Boston, Massachusetts 02114–2698*

Vicki J. Levine, MD *Department of Dermatology, New York University Medical Center, 530 First Avenue, New York, New York 10016*

Elizabeth I. McBurney, MD, *Clinical Professor of Dermatology, Tulane University School of Medicine, 1430 Tulane Avenue, New Orleans, Louisiana 70112; Clinical Professor of Dermatology, Louisiana State University School of Medicine, 1542 Tulane Avenue, New Orleans, Louisiana 70112*

Contents

Jerry L. McCullough, PhD *Professor, Department of Dermatology, College of Medicine, University of California—Irvine, 1000 Health Science Road, Med. Sci. I, C340, Irvine, California 92697–2400*

J. Stuart Nelson, MD, PhD *Associate Professor of Surgery and Dermatology and Associate Director, Beckman Laser Institute and Medical Clinic, University of California—Irvine, 1002 Health Sciences Road East, Irvine, California 92612; Associate Professor of Surgery/Dermatology, University of California Irvine Medical Center, Orange, California 92613*

Suzanne M. Olbricht, MD *Assistant Professor of Clinical Dermatology, Harvard Medical School, Boston, Massachusetts; Director of Dermatology Surgery, Department of Dermatology, Beth Israel Deaconess Medical Center, Boston, Massachusetts 02115*

Judith I. Pfister, RN, MBA *Vice President of Development, Education Design, Inc., 2170 South Parker Road, #140, Denver, Colorado 80231*

Jouni Uitto, MD, PhD *Department of Dermatology and Cutaneous Biology, Jefferson Medical College, 233 South 10th Street, Room 450, Philadelphia, Pennsylvania 19107*

Joseph T. Walsh, Jr., PhD *Associate Professor, Biomedical Bioengineering Department, Northwestern University, 2145 Sheridan Road, Evanston, Illinois 60208–3107*

Ronald G. Wheeland, MD *Professor of Dermatology, University of New Mexico, Albuquerque, New Mexico 87110*

Foreword

Lasers increasingly occupy a unique and very important position in the armament of medicine. They are the brightest known sources of light (man-made or natural) and can have extremely powerful and selective effects on biological systems. Lasers are to other sources of light as music is to noise. The uniqueness of lasers derives from a number of special properties, *viz* high intensity, coherence, collimation (which permits focusing on a spot size of one micrometer or less), extreme monochromaticity, and the ability to be delivered in very brief pulses. These collective properties can cause unique alterations of biological materials. The ability to launch high optical power into optical fibers extends the clinical applications of lasers because it permits remote delivery of precisely controlled therapeutic energy to tissue deep within the body with little or no damage to intervening structures. The precision in wavelength and control of the spatial and temporal properties of laser energy also make a number of diagnostic applications possible.

The surgical use of lasers began in the early 1960s, shortly after the first laser was invented, and now certain lasers are considered the tools of choice for various surgical procedures. For example, photocoagulation using the argon ion laser has found wide application in ophthalmology, where the transparency of the eye in the visible wavelength range permits precise focusing of the beam onto the target of interest. Conditions such as senile macular degeneration, angioproliferative retinopathy, and retinal detachment can be safely and effectively treated. CO_2 and Nd:YAG lasers are also of value in general surgery, where the ability to achieve coagulation while cutting can effect rapid hemostasis within the operative field, saving time and limiting blood loss. The speed and precision with which lasers can produce effects also make them valuable tools for ablating or removing diseased tissues. The minimal divergence of laser beams allows precise cutting or ablation of tissue with a very small spot size at any distance between the laser and tissue, allowing flexible access to operative fields.

The therapeutic uses of lasers include both surgical and nonsurgical applications, the former defined as those applications involving direct physical alteration or removal of target tissues. Nonsurgical applications include techniques such as photodynamic therapy (PDT), laser hyperthermia, and laser biostimulation. In the past, industrial demands led to development of laser systems that physicians adapted to medical use as best they could. Now, increased understanding of laser-tissue interactions favors the development of new laser systems that are specifically designed for particular medical applications.

The use of lasers in dermatology in part parallels the use of lasers in other medical specialties. Because of the ease of access to the organs of interest, laser-related research in dermatology and ophthalmology has contributed greatly to the study of laser-tissue interactions and benefited greatly by their use as diagnostic and therapeutic tools. The skin is a valuable natural laboratory for the study of laser medicine.

One of the many contributions of this book is the documentation of the "give and take" of dermatology to and from laser medicine. It was in skin that lasers found their earliest biomedical uses. Skin contains well characterized chromophores that have discrete microscopic spatial distribution. Therefore, particular cutaneous structures can be affected selectively by laser radiation. Because of the optical properties of skin and the relative thinness of the epidermis and dermis, the skin is ideally suited for therapeutic modification by laser radiation that cannot readily penetrate into deeper tissues.

It is obvious that the contributors and editors of this book are thoroughly familiar with the basic science and have the practical clinical experience required to create a readable, useful, and interesting text. Several chapters are written by the persons who made pivotal original observations described in this book. The care of skin has been permanently improved by laser technology, and this multiauthor book on cutaneous laser surgery is a practical and educational testimony to the growing impact of lasers on dermatology.

More is to come. Lasers are still underutilized in dermatology and much of medicine. Dermatologists will continue to benefit from the work outlined here and contribute broadly to health care by exploring principles of selectivity and demonstrating risks and benefits of laser medicine.

John A. Parrish, MD
Chairman, Department of Dermatology
Harvard Medical School
Massachusetts General Hospital
Boston, Massachusetts

Preface

The period that elapses between the original discovery of a new technology and its incorporation into clinical medicine is usually prolonged, but the history of lasers in medicine and surgery is strikingly different. In the relatively short time since the first ruby laser saw the light of day on July 7, 1960, to the late 1990s, lasers have become an accepted surgical modality in all specialties, are now taught in residency training programs, are a subject of questions on board examinations in many specialties, and are clearly extremely useful and unique tools for the therapy of a variety of disorders. In 1978, the Cutaneous Laser Unit, now the Joint Center for Cutaneous Laser Surgery, was founded at the Beth Israel Hospital by our late colleague Joel M. Noe, MD. This multidisciplinary, multihospital unit has been involved in ongoing studies of the effects of new and emerging laser systems on the skin, controlled trials of emerging therapies, and clinical pathologic evaluation of laser treatment techniques.

An important part of our mission has been to provide continuing medical education (CME) about lasers, and in 1979, we presented our first CME course through the Department of Continuing Education at Harvard Medical School. A book reflecting some of the information presented at these courses, *Cutaneous Laser Therapy: Principles and Methods,*[1] was published in 1983 and summarized the knowledge to date about lasers and cutaneous therapy. We subsequently saw the need for a book that described a more practical approach to the use of lasers, and in 1990, published the volume *Illustrated Cutaneous Laser Surgery: A Practitioner's Guide,*[2] which represented a "how-to" approach to therapy and provided practical information in a straightforward "cookbook approach" to laser therapy for the clinician. When we were synthesizing the material for the how-to publication, it became evident to us that the amount of new knowledge concerning laser photomedicine had increased to such an enormous extent that the availability of a more comprehensive text on all aspects of cutaneous laser surgery would be useful to complement a more practical text. This book presents an in-depth discussion of all areas of science, medicine, and psychology pertinent to the understanding of concepts necessary for the treatment of patients with cutaneous disorders that are amenable to treatment with coherent radiation. Members of our unit have written or coauthored several chapters in the book, and we have asked colleagues, both national and international, to join us in this effort to present the most up-to-date and pertinent theoretical and practical information available. This book will serve as a laser reference for dermatologists, plastic surgeons, otolaryngologists, podiatrists, and oral surgeons, as well as physicists, biomedical engineers, and biophysicists.

Kenneth A. Arndt, MD
Jeffrey S. Dover, MD
Suzanne M. Olbricht, MD

References

1. Arndt KA, Noe JM, Rosen S, eds. Cutaneous Laser Therapy: Principles and Methods. London: John Wiley and Sons, 1983.
2. Dover J, Arndt KA, Geronemus R, Noe JM, Olbricht S, Stern RS, eds. Illustrated Cutaneous Laser Surgery: A Practitioner's Guide. Norwalk, CT: Appleton and Lange, 1990.

I. General Principles of Cutaneous Laser Surgery

1 ⸺ History of Lasers in Medicine

Irving Itzkan
Ellet H. Drake

Review of the Development of Medical Lasers

At the turn of the century, scientists were faced with a dilemma related to black-body radiation, the electromagnetic energy emitted or absorbed by an object that acts as a perfect absorber. Experimentally a great deal was known about the properties of black-body radiation, in particular how the intensity of the emitted radiation varied with wavelength and with the temperature of the object. There were two theories, one that correctly predicted the behavior of black-body radiation at long wavelengths and another that correctly predicted its behavior at short wavelengths, but there was no way of reconciling the two theories with each other.

In 1905 Max Planck made the assumption that electromagnetic energy can exist only in small packets, or "quanta," and that the energy of each quantum was equal to a constant (h) multiplied by the frequency of the electromagnetic wave, or $E = h\nu$, where E is the energy, ν is the frequency, and h is what is now known as *Planck's constant*. With this one assumption he was able to derive an equation that correctly predicts all the properties of black-body radiation. These energy packets of electromagnetic radiation are now known as *photons,* and the validity of the assumption has been firmly established by the finding of its pervasive presence in a vast body of physical phenomena.

During the same period, scientists were using spectroscopes to observe the spontaneous emission of sharp spectral lines of light from excited atoms and recognizing that the emission spectrum was a unique characteristic of the emitting atom. They also observed that, when cold atoms were illuminated by light that contained many wavelengths, such as white light, they would absorb radiation from that light only at the same unique spectral lines. Niels Bohr proposed that these absorptions and emissions were related to an atomic model in which electrons orbiting the nucleus jumped from one orbit to another within the atom. The various orbits possessed different ener-

Dr. Itzkan contributed the section "Review of the Development of Medical Lasers," and Dr. Drake contributed the section "A Brief History of the American Society for Laser Medicine and Surgery."

gies, and the frequency of the light, or photon, multiplied by Planck's constant was equal to the difference in the energy of the orbits.

In 1917 Einstein realized that one could not reconcile well-known classical thermodynamics and Planck's equation using only the two effects, absorption and spontaneous emission. By postulating a third effect, stimulated emission, whereby an atom in an excited state is forced to emit its energy in the presence of a photon of the correct frequency, he could demonstrate that thermodynamics and Planck's equation are then perfectly consistent. In addition, he could derive relationships between the three effects, in that the coefficient for spontaneous emission was related to the other two by a constant which depended only on Planck's constant, the speed of light, and the third power of the wavelength.[1]

Although Einstein's work is sometimes cited as the birth of the laser, he did not discuss the nature of the stimulated photon, other than predicting that it would have the same frequency as the stimulating photon. It requires a theory of quantum electrodynamics, which includes a detailed picture of the interaction between the photons and the atoms, to be able to predict that the emitted stimulated photon is identical in phase, frequency, and direction to the stimulating photon, that is, "coherent" with it. In the 1920s Dirac published a semiclassical theory of quantum electrodynamics which, although flawed, did include coherence. A fully satisfactory theory of quantum electrodynamics was not available until the 1950s, and Feynman, Schwinger, and Tomonaga shared the Nobel prize for this work. However, in every theory proposed after Dirac's, the coherence of the emitted photon always had to be a necessary consequence of stimulated emission.

The prediction of the existence of coherent stimulated emission implied that an amplifier could be built and, by extension, an oscillator, which is an amplifier in which some of the output energy is fed back into the input to keep the process going. Amplification entails the establishment of a population inversion, in which there are more excited-state atoms waiting to be stimulated to emit photons than there are lower-state atoms waiting to absorb photons. Then one photon begets two and two begets four and the electromagnetic beam grows until the supply of excited atoms saturates.

Einstein's calculation said that atoms in an excited state decay spontaneously in a time proportional to the third power of the wavelength of the radiation emitted. Because the wavelengths of visible light are very short, the corresponding lifetimes are extremely small, and for the three decades after Dirac, the possibility of maintaining a population inversion for a long enough time to build a "light amplifier" was not given serious consideration, although stimulated emission was briefly observed during some laboratory experiments.

Shortly after World War II scientists were able to utilize in scientific research the sophisticated microwave equipment developed for wartime radar. Because microwave wavelengths are orders of magnitude longer than optical wavelengths, extremely long excited-state lifetimes exist in the microwave region of the spectrum. Charles

Townes recognized that it might be easier to maintain a population inversion in this region of the electromagnetic spectrum. He successfully operated the first MASER (an acronym standing for *m*icrowave *a*mplification by *s*timulated *e*mission of *r*adiation), using ammonia as the active medium. The success of this project caused him and others to rethink the difficulties surrounding the development of a light amplifier. In 1958 Schawlow and Townes[2] proposed the idea of building an "optical maser," which today is known as the *laser* (replacing the word *microwave* in the acronym with the word *light*). Similar work was being conducted in the Soviet Union at about the same time, led by Basov and Prokhorov.[3] All four eventually became Nobel laureates.

The race was now on to make the first laser, with hundreds of laboratories working on various systems. Townes and Schawlow worked with an electrically excited gas discharge laser. However, an optically pumped solid-state ruby system proved to be the easier laser to build, and in 1960 Maiman[4] demonstrated the first production of laser energy using a ruby crystal. Most of the lasers now used in medicine were first operated in the decade between 1960 and 1970. The first gas-discharge laser, using an infrared line at 1.15 μm in a mixture of helium and neon gases (He-Ne), was operated by Javan and colleagues[5] in 1961. The familiar visible red line of the He-Ne laser, at 633 nm, now used extensively as an aiming and alignment beam, was demonstrated by White and Rigden[6] in 1962.

The impurity neodymium in the host crystal yttrium-aluminum-garnet (Nd:YAG) was first used to produce laser energy by Geusic and colleagues[7] in 1964. Q-switching was suggested by Hellwarth[8] in 1961. Adding a Q-switch to a ruby or Nd:YAG laser enables these lasers to generate extremely intense pulses of short duration. Although the argon-ion laser was first operated in a pulsed mode by Bridges[9] in 1964, it was not until the continuous-wave version, developed by Gordon and co-workers,[10] came available that it was possible to achieve the necessary power to affect tissue.

Patel[11] first operated the CO_2 laser at the milliwatt level, but he soon discovered that this laser could produce 10 to 100 W of continuous-wave power, a power sufficient to ablate most materials, including biological tissue. The first organic dye laser was flashlamp pumped by Sorokin and Lankard[12] in 1966 with a microsecond pulsewidth. Others showed that a lot of different dyes could be used, covering all near-ultraviolet, visible, and near-infrared wavelength ranges, that the wavelengths could be tuned, and that several different pump sources could be used. The continuous-wave lasing of dyes pumped with an argon-ion laser was demonstrated by Peterson and co-workers.[13] Pumping with a nitrogen laser was demonstrated by Myer and associates.[14] Tan and colleagues[15] used a tunable laser, and Furumoto stretched the flashlamp-pump pulse to 300 μsec. Lasers are now available at all wavelengths and at many power levels. The lasing medium can be solid, liquid, or gas, and a host of waveforms are available for special applications. The only limitations today are usually cost and reliability.

Because lasers produce an intense source of radiation that can be focused and appropriately directed to a small spot, it soon became apparent to a few farsighted people that they would have applications in the field of medicine. It is not surprising that the first medical applications of lasers were in the treatment of the eye because the eye is transparent to light and ophthalmologists were already accustomed to working with light and optics. They were already reattaching detached retinas using an intense incoherent light source, so replacing this source with a laser was a logical first step. Much of the pioneer work in this regard was done by Zweng and co-workers[16] in the mid and late 1960s. Today, treatment with one of the several ophthalmic lasers available is the treatment of choice for many eye conditions.

In these early years, preliminary studies were also being carried out by Goldman and colleagues[17] and Lash and Maser[18] on the effect of some lasers on various skin lesions, because the skin was also a readily accessible target. With the advent of the continuous-wave CO_2 laser in the 1970s, with its high average power capability, the laser could be used for general surgery. This laser's ability to simultaneously cauterize while cutting makes it attractive for surgical procedures on highly vascular tissues. Neurosurgeons found the precise and noncontact nature of the tissue removal afforded by the laser very useful for working adjacent to sensitive nerve and brain tissue. More and more specific applications appeared, and in 1981 there was sufficient interest in the technology to serve as the impetus for the formation of a society, the American Society for Laser Medicine and Surgery, to meet the needs of the growing medical laser community (see the section "A Brief History of the American Society for Laser Medicine and Surgery").

In the early 1980s two important events occurred that had a bearing on the manner in which lasers were used in medicine. The first was the performance of controlled studies, such as that conducted by Noe and colleagues[19] on the use of the argon laser to treat port-wine stains, in which the tissue variables, laser variables, and end-results were carefully monitored to determine the direction future treatments would take. The other was to identify the physical, chemical, and biological properties of particular tissues, which were then used to determine the laser parameters, including the wavelength, pulse-width, and fluence, needed to achieve a desired therapeutic effect. The work of Anderson and Parrish[20] on selective photothermolysis is an example of this approach.

The rapid development in the past decade of sophisticated light applications, optics, and spectroscopy for use in many fields, including medicine, has been fueled by four key technological advances. The first of these is the laser itself. The special qualities of lasers that make the light they generate especially attractive for medical applications include their high spatial coherence, their tunability, and their ability to generate high peak and average powers. Spatial coherence is important for beam handling, shaping, and focusing, as well as for efficient coupling into optical fibers. Tunability makes it possible for the user to select optimal wavelengths for specific applications. High-power accompanying spatial coherence allows for the precise delivery of high-energy densities to selected tissue sites.

The second major technical advance that has been critical to the success of research on laser-tissue interactions and to the expansion of laser applications has been the development of low-loss optical fibers that can deliver large doses of high-intensity laser light to remote sites on and in the body. This has allowed minimally invasive treatment to be performed through endoscopes, catheters, laparoscopes, and even hypodermic needles, thereby providing an alternative to many surgical treatments in which tissue had to be cut away or removed to gain access to and reveal the surgical site. In addition to its therapeutic uses, the laser can be coupled to an optical fiber for use in the in situ diagnosis of tissue. This has been made possible by the third major advance, the development of efficient detectors and detector arrays. The advent of intensified detector arrays, particularly optical, multichannel analyzers, with high quantum efficiencies and low signal-to-noise ratios, has brought the capability for the real-time spectroscopic analysis of tissue into the medical clinic and the operating room. In many cases, it would not have been practical to accomplish the same tasks in the clinical setting using the slower, older tools. Finally, the development of high-speed, large-capacity computers for data analysis and real-time control of medical instrumentation has permitted the use of elaborate algorithms and has amplified the impact of the other technical advances already mentioned.

Not to be overlooked are the improvements in the engineering of lasers that have allowed them to be used in medical environments. Now there are reliable systems that deliver power on demand and user-friendly interfaces that free up the physician to devote all of his or her attention to the patient. Today the laser has found a niche in almost every specialty, both for treatment and for research purposes, and it continues to be a dynamic and growing field.

A Brief History of the American Society for Laser Medicine and Surgery

In March 1979 I began working with Dr. Leon Goldman to establish an American society to encourage physicians and scientists to exchange knowledge, explore new uses for present equipment, and develop new medical lasers and accessories. We invited 280 outstanding physicians and scientists from all over the world to participate in an organizational meeting held in San Diego in January 1981, and as a tribute to Dr. Goldman, the father of laser medicine in the United States, over half of them accepted our invitation and paid their own expenses to come to this meeting. The seed money necessary to establish the group was given to us by Mr. William B. Mark through the A. Ward Ford Institute. Mr. Mark died in October 1980, and each year his widow, Mrs. Carolyn Mark, presents an award in his honor to the person considered by the awards committee of the society to have made an outstanding contribution to laser medicine. The first of these awards was presented in 1982 to Dr. Goldman at the annual meeting at Hilton Head Island, South Carolina.

It was the dream of the founders that this organization be unique and include, in addition to physicians and clinicians, outstanding researchers in the areas of biophysics, biochemistry, biomedical engineering, laser biology, and laser safety. There was also a small group of people from industry included in the original charter membership. The idea was an immediate success, with membership in the society growing by approximately 40% per year during the first 8 years, as well as a steady increase in the number and size of commercial exhibits at the annual meetings. From the beginning the board established that the education of both physicians and the lay public should be a prime objective of the society and asked their Committee on Standards of Training and Practice to formulate guidelines to aid hospital and clinic staffs in the area of credentialing. At the same time, it was decided that the society would not actively participate in the credentialing process. Another committee involved with postgraduate education established other guidelines for those wishing to develop laser short courses. Their recommendations were quite specific, both with regard to the various levels of complexity and the suggested content at each level.

Honorary membership was bestowed upon selected people outside the United States who had established a worldwide reputation in the field of laser medical applications. Among these were Professor Peter Wolf Ascher, Kazuhiko Atsumi, MD, Jean-Marc Brunetaud, MD, Professor Dr. Kurt Burian, Jean-François Dumon, MD, Professor Dr. med. A. Hofstetter, Isaac Kaplan, MD, Shigenobu Mihashi, MD, Jia-Nan Qin, MD, the late Professor Carlo Sacchi, Professor Wilhelm Waidelich, N. Bloembergen, PhD, Oleg K. Skobelkin, MD, and Yi Gun Uang, MD. The International Merit Award was bestowed upon Professor Dr. med. Peter Kiefhaber of München, Germany. Other laser immortals elected to the prestigious group of Honorary Members have been Theodore H. Maiman, PhD, C. Kumar N. Patel, PhD, Arthur L. Schawlow, PhD, and Charles H. Townes, PhD. The first nurses were included in 1983, and by 1986 their number had reached a point where they were able to establish a section of the society and were granted a position on the board.

At the time the society was organized, two of its members, Drs. Billie Aronoff and Eugene Friedman, were co-editing a successful laser journal, *Lasers in Surgery and Medicine*, published by Alan R. Liss in New York. This publication has continued to be the official organ of the society. Under the recent editorship of Carmen A. Puliafito, MD, and the current editor, Robert Ossoff, DMD, MD, the journal has achieved an enviable reputation among surgical journals, in that it has been declared sixth among 84 surgical journals according to the Science Citation Index. Dr. Leon Goldman was the original editor of the society's newsletter. Among innovations introduced by Dr. Goldman was the inclusion of a job-wanted section in which resumes are printed without charge to those seeking employment regardless of whether they are society members. He also included capsule accounts of papers in the recent literature, supplying just enough information to arouse interest among readers to do additional study in that particular area. After 7 years, the editorship was taken over by Ann Siemens of the Beckman Institute and finally this responsibility was transferred to the executive secretary, Diane Geisel, at the home office in Wausau, Wisconsin, who, in addition to her other duties, publishes two excellent issues each year.

The society has continued to grow with the attendance at meetings continually exceeding 1000 and the number of commercial exhibits totaling approximately 60. An outstanding and unique feature of the annual meetings is the "Parade of Specialties," which is intended to inform members of the latest developments in specialties outside their own. The society has also served as an advisory group to the U.S. Food and Drug Administration, putting on one or more seminars each year for the benefit of the members of that agency.

The home office has remained in Wausau and now has four full-time and two half-time employees. Last year they handled 1300 applications for membership, sent out 90 course lists, fielded 60 requests for the standards of training and practice, and sent personal replies to 1600 people who sought help in reaching laser specialists in their particular medical field.

The American Society for Laser Medicine and Surgery is now 15 years old, has a total membership of 2700 in the United States and 36 in other countries, and has long since passed the 5-year mark necessary to be labeled by the American Medical Association as an "organization of medical interest." This attainment of maturity augurs the continued growth of the society and its service to those interested in the medical applications of lasers. May it also serve to constantly remind all of us of the vision, professional skill, and dedication of Dr. Leon Goldman.

References

1. Einstein A. Zur Quantentheorie der Strahlung. Physik Z 1917;18:121. (English translation in: van der Waerden BL (ed). Sources of quantum mechanics. Amsterdam: North Holland, 1967:63–77).
2. Schawlow AL, Townes CH. Infrared and optical masers. Phys Rev 1958; 112:1940.
3. Basov NG, Prokhorov AM. 3-level gas oscillator. Zh Eksp Teor Fiz 1954;27:431.
4. Maiman TH. Stimulated optical radiation in ruby. Nature 1960;187:493.
5. Javan A, Bennett WR Jr, Heriott DR. Population inversion and continuous optical maser oscillation in a gas discharge containing a He-Ne mixture. Phys Rev Lett 1961;6:106.
6. White AD, Rigden JO. Continuous gas maser operation in the visible. Proc IRE 1962;50:1796.

7. Geusic JE, Marcos HM, Van Uitert LG. Laser oscillations in Nd-doped yttrium aluminum, yttrium gallium, and gadolinium garnets. Appl Phys Lett 1964;4:182.

8. Hellwarth RW. In: Singer JR (ed): Advances in quantum electronics. New York: Columbia University Press, 1961:334.

9. Bridges WB. Laser oscillation in singly ionized argon in the visible spectrum. Appl Phys Lett 1964;4:128–130.

10. Gordon EI, Labuda EF, Bridges WB. Continuous visible laser action in singly ionized argon, krypton and xenon. Appl Phys Lett 1964;4:178–180.

11. Patel KCN. Continuous-wave laser action on vibrational-rotational transitions of CO_2. Phys Rev 1964;136A:1187.

12. Sorokin PP, Lankard JR. Stimulated emission observed from an organic dye, chloroaluminum phthalocyanine. IBM J Res Devel 1966;10:162.

13. Peterson OG, Tuccio SA, Snavely BB. CW operation of an organic dye solution laser. Appl Phys Lett 1970;14:245.

14. Myer JA, Itzkan I, Johnson CL, Kierstead E, Sharma RD. Dye laser stimulation with a pulsed N_2 laser line at 3371A. Appl Phys Lett 1970;16:3–5.

15. Tan OT, Sherwood K, Gilchrest BA. Treatment of children with port-wine stains using the flashlamp pulsed tunable dye laser. N Engl J Med 1989;320:416–421.

16. Zweng HC, Flocks M. Clinical experiences with laser photocoagulation. Fed Proc 1965;24:565–570.

17. Goldman L, Rockwell JR Jr. Laser reaction in living tissue. In: Lasers in medicine. New York: Gordon and Breach, 1971:163–185.

18. Lash H, Maser R. Paper presented at the American Society for Plastic and Reconstructive Surgery meeting, Las Vegas, Nevada, September 1972.

19. Noe JM, Barsky SH, Geer DE. Port wine stains and the response to argon laser therapy: successful treatment and the predictive role in color, age, and biopsy. Plast Reconstr Surg 1980;65:130.

20. Anderson RR, Parrish JA. Selective photothermolysis: precise microsurgery by selective absorption of pulsed radiation. Science 1983;220:524–527.

2 ___ An Introduction to Lasers

Irving Itzkan
Donna B. C. Bourgelais

Basic Laser Components

The major components common to all lasers are depicted in Figure 2-1. To generate laser output energy is first transferred from a power source, which may be electrical, optical, or chemical, to a gain medium, which may be solid, liquid, or gas. A laser is usually designated by its gain medium, that is, CO_2 laser, argon-ion laser, and so on. The energy is stored in the gain medium in the form of excited atomic or molecular energy states. The ability of the gain medium to store energy in an easily extractable form is the attribute that gives the laser the potential to achieve high output power. Photons of the correct wavelength passing through the gain medium interact with the excited-state atoms or molecules, causing the release of energy in the form of additional photons. These stimulated photons match the original photons in wavelength, phase, and direction, and hence the initial photons are amplified. This identity of photon properties with each other, or coherence, is the source of the laser's monochromaticity and ability to focus to a very small spot. The growth in the number of photons, caused by the ability of the gain medium to undergo stimulated emission, is the source of the acronym LASER: *l*ight *a*mplification by *s*timulated *e*mission of *r*adiation. A portion of these stimulated photons are extracted as laser output, and the remaining photons are fed back into the gain medium by means of an optical resonator to keep the process going. The optical resonator may consist of a full reflector and a partial reflector, as shown in Figure 2-1, or it may comprise a ring in which the amplified photons pass through a series of reflections and are returned to the input.

GAIN MEDIUM

The quantum theory of modern physics tells us that light (and in fact all electromagnetic energy) comes in discrete bundles of energy

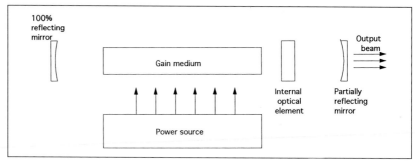

Fig. 2-1. The basic elements common to all lasers include the gain medium, optical resonator, and power source. As shown here, the optical resonator includes a 100% reflecting mirror and a partially reflecting mirror. The output beam emerges from the partially reflecting mirror. A laser is usually designated by its gain medium, for example, argon ion, CO_2, or dye.

called *photons*. Light also exhibits wavelike properties, and the energy of a photon is related to its wavelength by the equation

$$E = hc/(\lambda)$$

where:

$$h = \text{Planck's constant} = 6 \times 10^{-34} \text{ J-sec}$$
$$c = \text{speed of light} = 3 \times 10^{-8} \text{ m/sec}$$
$$(\lambda) = \text{wavelength in meters}$$
$$E = \text{energy (in joules)}$$

All emission and absorption of electromagnetic energy occurs by means of an integral number of photons, that is, there are no fractional photons.

A simplified view of an atom consists of a negatively charged cloud of electrons (Fig. 2-2) located in well-defined orbits. An atom can absorb a photon by having an electron make a rapid transition from an inner orbit to an outer orbit, but only if the photon's energy corresponds to the energy difference between the orbits. This process is called *stimulated absorption* or, more usually, just *absorption*. Similarly, an atom can emit a photon by having an electron move from an outer orbit to an inner orbit. Again, the photon's energy, and hence wavelength, corresponds to the energy difference between orbits. This process is termed *emission*. There are two kinds of emission, described in the following text.

When all electrons of an atom are in their lowest possible orbits, the atom is said to be in the ground state. Atoms with electrons in higher orbits are said to be in excited states. Excited states can be created in various ways, the most common being by means of collisions with energetic particles (electrons, atoms, ions, molecules). An atom

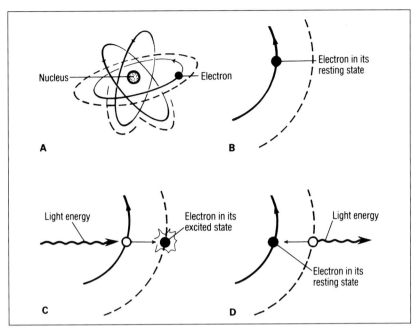

Fig. 2-2. (A and B) A highly idealized schematic of an atom with all its electrons in the resting (ground) state. (C) Light energy is absorbed by an atom, causing transition of an electron from the resting state to an excited state. (D) Energy is released as electromagnetic radiation (light) by the process of either spontaneous or stimulated emission, and the electron returns to the resting state. (Reproduced with permission from Dover JS, Arndt KA, Geronemus RG, et al. Illustrated cutaneous laser surgery: a practitioner's guide. Norwalk, CT: Appleton & Lange, 1990.)

remains in the excited state for a brief period of time, called the *life-time*, and then decays spontaneously to a lower state, in the process giving off a photon of the appropriate wavelength. This is termed *spontaneous emission*. If, however, while it is still in the excited state, it encounters a photon whose wavelength is the same as its characteristic emission wavelength, it emits a photon whose wavelength, phase, and direction exactly match those of the stimulating photon. This process is called *stimulated emission*. Normally, when a collection of atoms is in thermal equilibrium, more members of the ensemble are in the lower state than in the upper state. If a beam of photons of the appropriate wavelength passes through such an ensemble, more stimulated absorption than stimulated emission occurs and the beam is attenuated. However, if more members of an ensemble of atoms are in a particular higher excited state than in a lower state, then it is possible for the number of stimulated emissions to exceed the number of stimulated absorptions. Such an ensemble is said to be inverted, and such a population inversion offers the possibility of a net gain in identical photons. A gain medium is a medium in which a population inversion has been established.

Using a similar simplified picture, molecules can be viewed as consisting of two or more positively charged nuclei held together by a

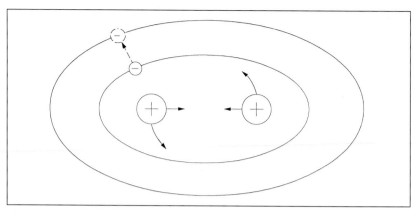

Fig. 2-3. A highly idealized schematic of a molecule containing two atoms. The positively charged nuclei are bound together by a shared orbiting electron cloud. The electrons can be excited to higher states, just as in an atom. The nuclei can also vibrate or rotate with respect to each other, providing additional spectral transitions.

shared cloud of orbiting electrons (Fig. 2-3). Again, the electrons may have higher orbits, and the same kinds of electronic transitions that occur in atoms also occur in molecules. However, molecules possess additional degrees of freedom. For example, the nuclei can vibrate relative to one another, though only at discrete frequencies, and these motions give rise to a new set of energy levels called *vibrational energy states*. The nuclei can also rotate about one another, again only at discrete frequencies, and hence there are sets of rotational energy levels. Molecular spectra consist of all three types of transitions, which can occur in combination. An energy level diagram is a symbolic representation of the energy levels of a particular atom or molecule, with the distance between levels proportional to the difference in the energy of the corresponding states. Figure 2-4 is a simplified energy level diagram for an idealized molecule, showing two electronic states and their associated vibronic and rotational sublevels.

In general, transitions between electronic states occur at wavelengths in the ultraviolet, visible, and near-infrared portions of the spectrum. Transitions between vibrational levels occur in the infrared portion of the spectrum, and transitions between rotational levels occur in the far-infrared portion of the spectrum.

Energy transitions do not occur with equal facility, however. Those that occur easily are called *allowed*, and those that occur with difficulty are called *forbidden*. There are all gradations of being forbidden or allowed, and there are also rules, called *selection rules*, that help describe this property.

The creation of a gain medium, which means establishing a population inversion between two energy levels in an ensemble of atoms or molecules, is the first requirement for making a laser.

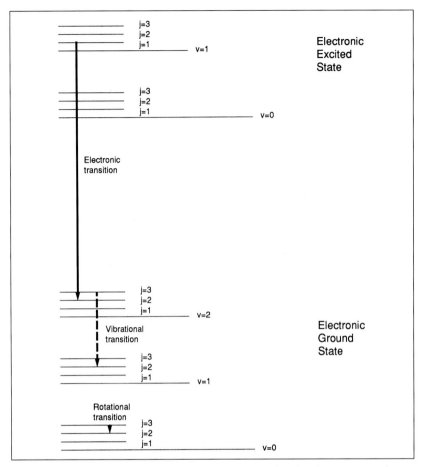

Fig. 2-4. Energy level diagram for an idealized molecule, showing two electronic states and their associated vibronic (v) and rotational (j) sublevels. The arrows represent allowed electronic, vibrational, and rotational transitions.

OPTICAL RESONATORS

An amplifier takes an input signal and generates an output signal identical to the input signal, but one that contains more power. An amplifier can be made into an oscillator, which generates a self-sustaining signal, by taking a sufficient portion of the output energy and feeding it back into the amplifier input. The remaining output energy becomes the useful output. In a laser oscillator this feedback is provided by an optical resonator, which often consists of a pair of mirrors, one of which is partially transmitting (and partially reflecting). The transmitted beam serves as the useful output, and the reflected beam is the required feedback.

Sometimes, instead of providing the feedback by means of reflection, a portion of the output is brought around the outside of the laser and back in the input. This is called a *ring resonator.*

Sometimes a slight positive curvature is added to the mirrors to confine the beam within the gain medium and limit losses due to diffraction. Such resonators are called *stable*. Conversely, resonators can be designed to accentuate the diffraction "loss," and this diffracted beam is then used as the output beam. Such resonators are called *unstable resonators*. The choice of resonator controls the "transverse modes" or spatial coherence of the laser output. As noted, spatial coherence, or as it is sometimes called, *beam quality*, is very important for focusing the laser beam.

In general, a stable resonator is useful for obtaining a highly coherent beam from lasers with comparatively low gain and a large length-to-aperture ratio, whereas unstable resonators yield the best beam quality from high-gain lasers with a smaller length-to-aperture ratio.

Often resonators are designed to provide wavelength selection or spectral narrowing. Mirror coatings are designed to reflect certain wavelengths, but not others. Dispersive elements, such as prisms, gratings, or etalons, can also be incorporated inside the resonator. Thus the optical resonator is a major factor in determining the spectral and spatial coherence of the laser.

POWER SOURCES

For electrical pumping to occur, an electric field is imposed on the gain medium. This field accelerates charged particles (either ions or electrons) that then collide with atoms or molecules; in so doing, some portion of their translational energy becomes coupled to electronic or vibrational excited states. Electrical discharges in a gas medium are continuous, pulsed, or radio frequency. In general, capacitive storage is used in pulsed pumping. Radio frequency pumping requires lower voltages than continuous or pulsed pumping, and because the radio-frequency power may itself be pulsed, this is another way of achieving pulsed operation. Examples of dc gas discharges are the argon-ion laser and some CO_2 lasers. Some CO_2 lasers are radio-frequency excited. The very smallest lasers, laser diodes, are excited by means of an electric current that flows through a semiconductor junction.

Flashlamp pumping is a common form of optical pumping. A flashlamp usually consists of a quartz tube containing a rare gas such as xenon or krypton and fitted with two electrodes, which permit a high-density electrical discharge to pass through the gas. Light from the flashlamp discharge is coupled into the gain medium with appropriate reflector elements. Ruby, dye, Nd:YAG, Ho:YAG, and Er:YAG lasers are examples of flashlamp-pumped lasers.

A hydrogen fluoride (HF) laser is an example of a chemically pumped laser. In this case, the chemical reaction between hydrogen gas and a fluorine-bearing gaseous compound produces an HF molecule in a vibrational excited state, from which laser energy is extracted.

Lasers may also be pumped by other lasers. Examples include the diode laser–pumped Nd:YAG laser and the argon-ion laser–pumped dye and titanium sapphire lasers.

Properties of Laser Light

The three unique properties of laser light that have been responsible for causing the rapid expansion of the use of lasers in medicine and surgery in recent years are spatial coherence, wavelength selection, and the pulse temporal profile, together with the fact that these properties can be achieved at substantial energy and power levels.

SPATIAL COHERENCE

Spatial coherence allows laser radiation to be focused onto a small spot. There are three advantages of such a small focal spot: (1) very high irradiance or fluence can be achieved; (2) small target volumes, such as cellular or even subcellular components, can be singled out; and (3) the beam can be coupled efficiently into fiberoptics.

As is well known, electromagnetic radiation has wave properties, which can be visualized as a series of crests and troughs. If one could view a cross-section of a laser beam (taken perpendicular to the direction of propagation) at an instant in time, one would find that at every point in that cross-section the wave is characterized by a crest, that is, the phase is constant over the cross-section. This beam would be said to have a very high degree of spatial coherence. Conversely, if in this same cross-section, one observed a significant variation in the crests and troughs, that is, the phase varied substantially over the cross section, then the beam would be said to have poor spatial coherence. The degree of spatial coherence of a laser beam is sometimes specified as "the number of times diffraction limited" (XDL). If XDL is 1, the beam can be focused to the smallest possible spot allowed by wave optics. The diameter of the smallest spot is $2.4(\lambda)F\#$, where (λ) is the wavelength of the light and $F\#$ is the "speed" of the focusing lens, defined by the focal length divided by the beam diameter. Because the spot area varies with the square of the beam diameter, irradiance varies inversely with the square of XDL. For example, if a laser beam is 10 XDL, the achievable irradiance is 1/100th that which could be obtained from a diffraction-limited beam. Thus this is an important laser system specification.

There may also be an intensity variation over the cross-section of the beam, but this is much less important than the phase profile in terms of focusing properties. A common specification for the laser beam profile is "TEM 00." This implies that, over a cross-section, the phase is constant and the intensity distribution is gaussian. Such a beam is sometimes said to be nearly diffraction limited.

Another advantage of good spatial coherence is that radiation can be propagated over long distances without appreciable spreading, though this is generally more useful in star wars or surveying applications than in medical and surgical applications. Most laser beams can be transmitted to different operating suites by means of fiberoptics. However, there are no commercially available fibers that can adequately transmit some wavelengths, such as that produced by the CO_2 laser. In this case, the beam may be piped between rooms using turning mirrors, and the attendant ability to propagate long distances without spreading is an important advantage. Similarly, alignment lasers rely on this property.

The spread of a laser beam as it propagates through space is termed *divergence,* and it is most often composed of two parts: a correctable part, which can be eliminated through the use of appropriate lenses or mirrors, or both, and an inherently uncorrectable part. The latter is directly related to the spatial coherence just discussed. A diffraction-limited beam provides the smallest focal spot and has the smallest uncorrectable divergence.

A laser operator working with a laser delivery system that provides a divergent beam may utilize the divergence to control the irradiance incident on the tissue being treated by adjusting the distance between the tissue and the output aperture of the delivery system.

WAVELENGTH SELECTION

Another important attribute of laser radiation of value for clinical uses is that a wavelength (and hence laser medium) can be chosen that is absorbed selectively by a specific target within a larger volume of tissue. The light may be absorbed by either endogenous or exogenous chromophores. An example of the use of endogenous chromophores is the treatment of a port-wine stain with 577-nm radiation, which is selectively absorbed in the vasculature, sparing the surrounding, highly transparent tissue. An example of the use of exogenous chromophores is photodynamic therapy, in which neoplastic tissue is tagged with an absorbing, phototoxic substance, such as hematoporphyrin derivative, and then irradiated with light in the pump band for that phototoxic substance.

In other situations, high absorption of a wavelength by tissue is desired, in particular for tissue ablation. The Er:YAG laser, which emits a 2.94-μm wavelength that is the most strongly absorbed by water, is capable of such ablation.

A wavelength may also be chosen that is poorly absorbed. Such a wavelength penetrates deep into tissue and is also effective for producing volumetric hyperthermia. Such deep penetration is desired in the treatment of cavernous hemangiomas, and an Nd:YAG laser emits such a wavelength.

In general, biological action spectra are broad, that is, they cover a range of wavelengths of tens of nanometers. Although laser radiation may be obtained with extremely narrow spectra, this is usually not a requirement. The property of a very narrow linewidth is known as *spectral coherence,* which should not be confused with spatial coherence discussed earlier. Spectral coherence is often not of relevance to surgical applications, although it may be of much use in the diagnosis of diseases using spectroscopic techniques.

Some lasers, such as the argon-ion laser, produce multiple lines distributed over a broad spectrum. If all of these lines fall within the desired biological action spectrum, it may be possible to use the laser in a multiline mode of operation, in which laser radiation is obtained on all of these lines simultaneously. If not, it may be necessary to select only certain lines. Ophthalmologists, for example, use only the green line of the argon-ion laser for panretinal photocoagulation, using laser systems that eliminate the blue laser lines.

In dye laser radiation, usually a broad spectral band is emitted near the peak of the emission curves for the specific dye being used. This emission may be narrowed through the use of appropriate laser optics. It can also be tuned, using a grating or other dispersive element in the laser resonator. Different dyes may be used to access very wide ranges of wavelengths. Commercial units are available that, with two or three sets of optics and a few dyes, can provide essentially all of the visible region of the spectrum and some of the near-infrared region.

PULSE TEMPORAL PROFILE

The third characteristic of laser systems that must be selected with the application in mind is the temporal profile, or pulse shape. The various options are depicted in Figure 2-5. A continuous-wave (cw) laser is capable of being on all the time. It may, however, be shuttered, in which case a shutter, usually a mechanical one, is opened to allow a burst of energy to pass through. The laser energy may also be chopped, producing a repetitive chain of shuttered pulses. Pulsed lasers, by their inherent nature, provide bursts of power in the 1- to 300-μsec range. In some cases, the power rises smoothly to a peak and then falls off; in other cases, it consists of a train of random peaks inside a rising and falling envelope, referred to as *spiking.* Pulsed lasers may be Q-switched, in which case the energy is stored internally during most of the natural pulse time and then emitted in an intense spike of much shorter duration at what would have been the end of the pulse. Continuous-wave lasers may also be repetitively Q-switched, thereby producing a train of spikes. Mode locking is another way of producing a train of spikes. Both continuous-wave and pulsed lasers can be mode locked. In general, mode-locked pulse trains are higher in frequency than pulse trains produced by Q-switching a continuous-wave laser. Thus there is a vast array of temporal profiles that can be accessed. The choice of profile is determined by the tissue effect one wants to achieve.

Examples of medical applications in which the temporal pulse shape is important include photocoagulation, thermal ablation, and

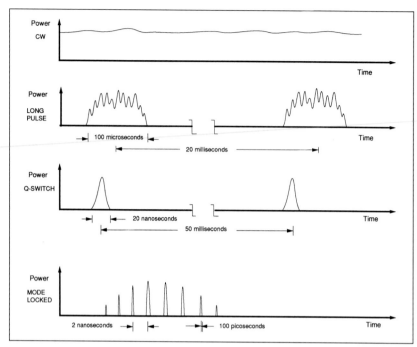

Fig. 2-5.   Laser temporal power profiles. The pulsewidths and interpulse spacings indicated are typical but vary with the type of laser. (*CW* = continuous wave.)

photoacoustic generation. Thermal diffusion times are important for photocoagulation. During and after laser irradiation, heat diffuses from absorbing targets into surrounding tissue. If one wishes to minimize damage to the tissue surrounding the absorbing chromophore, laser irradiation times should be short. For example, the diffusion length associated with 1 msec is approximately 30 μm. The thermal diffusion length varies as the square root of the pulse time.

For laser ablation, which is used in tissue removal, shorter pulses may be more effective, up to an intensity so high that a laser-generated plasma is formed. In some cases, a longer pulse time, which accomplishes less efficient tissue removal, is more desirable in order to achieve hemostasis by means of lateral thermal diffusion.

Photoacoustic generation, the phenomenon exploited in laser lithotripsy, requires pulses on the order of a microsecond in duration. Photodisruption, which is used for posterior capsulotomies, requires pulses on the order of 10 nsec or less. Both of these uses require the production of a laser-generated plasma.

Energy and Power Considerations

The effect of laser radiation on tissue is governed by five parameters relating to energy or power. These are energy, fluence, energy density, power, and irradiance. The relative importance of each of these depends on the intended effect. Energy, usually measured in joules, is proportional to the total number of photons incident on the target. Both the energy per pulse and the total energy, which is the sum of energy over all the pulses, may be important. The energy per unit area is fluence, which is usually specified in joules per square centimeter. Energy density is the energy deposited per unit of volume, given in joules per cubic centimeter, and is dependent on the incident fluence, tissue-scattering parameters, and absorption coefficient. In addition to the fluence delivered in a single pulse and the integrated value of fluence summed up over many pulses, variations in the spatial distribution are important. Power is the energy delivered per unit time and is usually measured in joules per second, or watts. In this regard, both the time-averaged value and the peak value may be important. Irradiance is the power per unit area, normally reported in watts per square centimeter, and again both the peak and time-averaged values as well as the spatial and temporal distributions may be important.

As an example of the relative importance of the five parameters, in photoradiation therapy the intended effect is to kill malignant cells by direct photochemical means or by destruction of the tumor vasculature. In either case the important parameter, within typical operating bounds, is the total number of photons incident on each targeted cell, or the energy density. In laser therapies in which fluence is the dominant parameter, there is a low threshold of fluence, below which no therapeutic effects are obtained. An example of this is the treatment of port-wine stains, which involves the use of either argon-ion or dye lasers. In typical treatment regimens, approximately 7 J/cm^2 is delivered to the lesion. At levels significantly below this, no lightening of the lesion occurs. There is also an upper limit to fluence, in that excessive fluence can result in nonselective thermal damage.

If hyperthermia is the desired effect, the dominant parameter is generally power. It involves the delivery of laser power by means of a fiberoptic to a diffusing tip placed within the body of a tumor. Because the objective is to raise the tissue to a temperature adequate to kill malignant cells, sufficient power must be delivered to achieve this temperature.

In most laser tissue ablation techniques, the crater depth is dependent on the fluence delivered. The total tissue volume removed is a function of the energy delivered.

As mentioned earlier, in both photodisruption (posterior capsulotomy) and lithotripsy, a plasma is formed at the surface of the target tissue and tissue damage results from the ensuing shock wave. Minimal irradiance is required to create a plasma.

Lasers in Medical Use

A wide range of lasers are currently used for medical applications. These include the CO_2, argon-ion, Nd:YAG, KTP, excimer, dye, erbium, holmium, hydrogen fluoride, diode, and ruby lasers.

CO_2 lasers are typically used for ablative therapies or surgery, because the CO_2 wavelength is strongly and nonselectively absorbed in tissue. Continuous-wave or shuttered CO_2 lasers are generally effective for cutting, with the hemostasis provided by the thermal sealing of blood vessels in the target tissue. There are many reports of post-procedural pain being reduced after CO_2 laser surgery as compared with the pain after conventional scalpel removal. This may be due to the sealing of both vasculature and lymphatics, with an attendant reduction in tissue edema. The superpulse CO_2 laser is a pulsed laser with a pulse time too short for thermal-diffusion hemostasis to occur, but it is very effective in tissue removal and leaves minimal if any char. Sharp-pulsed CO_2 lasers with pulse durations less than 1 msec can remove epidermis and dermis with little surrounding thermal damage and are used for resurfacing procedures. Low-dose cw CO_2 laser energy can be used for the removal of superficial hyperpigmented lesions such as actinic lentigines or café au lait spots.

The gain medium in a CO_2 laser is a gas composed of carbon dioxide, nitrogen, and helium. Some lasers are sealed systems, and some require a continuous gas flow from a high-pressure cylinder. As mentioned earlier, electrical excitation of the medium may be continuous, pulsed, or radio frequency. The most common wavelength for CO_2 laser emission is at 10.6 μm, although a multiplicity of lines from 9.4 to 10.6 μm up may be obtained using a grating. CO_2 laser delivery is generally accomplished by means of articulated arms or rigid endoscopes, although flexible waveguides have recently come available that can be used for this purpose. These are bulky, however, compared with the silica-core fibers used for visible-wavelength radiation.

Argon-ion lasers use argon gas as the gain medium, pumped by an electrical discharge. It has multiple emission lines available in the blue-green portion of the spectrum, with the principal lines at 488 and 514 nm. These systems are always sealed, and they are among the oldest medical lasers. Krypton lasers are closely related to argon-ion lasers and are similar in manufacture, except that the gas and resonator optics are different. Krypton has a strong line at 647 nm.

The gain media solid-state lasers consist of impurity atoms in crystalline hosts. In the most common of these, neodymium is used as the impurity and yttrium-aluminum-garnet as the crystalline host; this is the Nd:YAG laser. The gain medium is optically pumped using either flashlamps or diode lasers. Nd:YAG has two important emission lines, one at 1.06 μm and the other at 1.3 μm. Usually, different resonator optics are required for the two different lines. The 1.06-μm line penetrates more deeply into body tissue. Commercial units are available that operate as cw, pulsed, Q-switched, or mode locked. This laser can be frequency doubled to a wavelength of 532 nm using a KTP crystal. The resulting laser is sometimes referred to as a *KTP laser.* All of the wavelengths available with this laser are well transmitted by silica-core fibers.

Another impurity that may be used with the YAG crystalline host is erbium, which lases at 2.94 μm, near the peak of the water-absorption band. Thus it is an excellent laser for tissue ablation, but unfortunately, the wavelength is slightly beyond the working range of commercially available silica fibers. However, promising work is being done at several centers to develop fibers with a high transmission capability in this portion of the spectrum. When such fibers are perfected, the resulting laser will be an effective laser for surgery. Holmium in a YAG crystalline host lases at a wavelength of 2.1 μm. The water absorption at this wavelength is higher than that at the Nd:YAG wavelength but lower than that at the Er:YAG wavelength. Systems using Ho:YAG and silica-fiber delivery systems are being investigated for surgical applications.

The gain medium of the ruby laser consists of a chromium impurity in a sapphire host. Ruby lasers are flashlamp pumped and may be Q-switched. One of the earliest lasers developed, this was also one of the first to be used in medical research. Its wavelength of 694 nm penetrates deep into tissue, making it unsuitable for applications such as tissue ablation. It has recently been used with great success in the removal of tattoos. The high-power short pulse disrupts the tattoo pigment, making it more susceptible to macrophage scavenging. The alexandrite, Q-switched Nd:YAG, and frequency-doubled Q-switched Nd:YAG lasers have also proved useful in tattoo removal. Results vary from one pigment to the next, with different laser wavelengths yielding better results, depending on the pigment.

Excimer lasers use a gaseous gain medium containing halide and a rare gas, such as xenon fluoride (XeF, 351-nm wavelength), xenon chloride (XeCl, 308-nm wavelength), krypton fluoride (KrF, 248-nm wavelength), and argon fluoride (ArF, 198-nm wavelength). The gain medium is usually pumped by a pulsed electrical discharge. The laser pulse times range from 10 to 100 nsec. Very sharp, char-free cuts are obtained with these lasers. Excimer lasers are used for corneal refiguring and ablative angioplasty.

The gain medium for dye lasers is a liquid solvent containing a fluorescent dye. This is most often a flowing system, which permits the rapid removal of waste heat from the lasing volume. The power pump sources used include flashlamps and other lasers, either continuous-wave or pulsed. Different dye and solvent combinations are used to obtain lasing in different portions of the spectrum. Dispersive elements can be used that allow tunability or spectral narrowing. Pulsed dye lasers are used in the treatment of cutaneous vascular lesions such as port-wine stains and in lithotripsy.

Copper vapor (511- and 578-nm wavelengths) and gold vapor (628-nm wavelength) lasers have as their gain medium a metal vapor created by electrical discharge heating. The optical output consists of a train of 10- to 20-nsec pulses delivered at a 5- to 20-kHz repetition rate. These are currently being used in some research applications;

in particular the gold vapor laser is being used in photodynamic therapy utilizing hematoporphyrin derivative.

Suggested Reading

General Textbooks on Lasers
1. Katzir A. Lasers and optical fibers in medicine. New York: Academic, 1993.
2. Lengyel BA. Introduction to laser physics. New York: Wiley, 1966.
3. Sliney D, Trokel SL. Medical lasers and their safe use. New York: Springer-Verlag, 1993.
4. Siegman A. Lasers. Sausalito, CA:University Science Books, 1986.
5. Verdeyen JT. Laser electronics. Prentice Hall, 1981.
6. Young M. Optics and lasers. New York: Springer-Verlag, 1984.

Reference Handbooks
7. Hecht J. The laser guidebook (2nd ed). Summit, PA: TAB Books, 1992.
8. Koechner W. Solid-state laser engineering. New York: Springer-Verlag, 1976.
9. Weber M, ed. CRC handbook of laser science and technology, Vols 1–4. Boca Raton, FL: CRC Press.

3 _____ Laser-Tissue Interactions in Dermatology

R. Rox Anderson

It is common knowledge that lasers produce intense beams of light that are capable of cutting, welding, or exploding target materials by heating them rapidly. In dermatology, sudden, destructive heating plays a central role in all of the surgical laser uses. However, an array of versatile and essentially unique treatments have been developed to achieve this common end, all of which depend on the occurrence of interesting physical and chemical interactions with living tissue. Laser technology has now reached a point where we routinely use high-energy laser pulses to accomplish treatments that were impossible 10 years ago. This chapter emphasizes the fundamental mechanisms of laser surgery as they apply to dermatologic uses, including practical consequences and questions yet to be answered.

ELECTROMAGNETIC RADIATION

Electromagnetic radiation (EMR) is a fundamental form of energy that exhibits both wave properties, because of an alternating electric and magnetic field, and particle properties, because the energy is carried in quanta known as *photons*. Long-wavelength photons carry less energy than short-wavelength photons, as expressed by Planck's law. The EMR spectrum is diagrammed in Figure 3-1. Starting from the long-wavelength, low-photon-energy end of the spectrum, EMR includes radio waves, microwaves, infrared radiation, visible light, ultraviolet radiation, and x rays.

Whenever a photon is absorbed, some movement or separation of charged matter occurs and the photon ceases to exist. The energy carried by the photon causes the absorbing molecule, called a *chromophore*, to become excited. Absorption and excitation are necessary for all photobiologic effects and laser-tissue interactions to occur. The

This chapter was adapted from Anderson RR. Laser tissue interactions. In: Goldman MP, Fitzpatrick RE, eds. Cutaneous laser surgery. 1994. St. Louis: Mosby–Year Book, 1994.

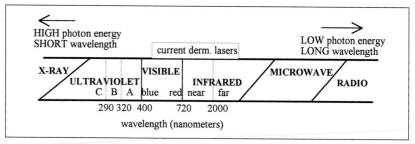

Fig. 3-1.   The continuous spectrum of electromagnetic radiation. (Reproduced with permission from Goldman MP, Fitzpatrick RE. Cutaneous laser surgery. St. Louis: Mosby–Year Book, 1994.)

quantum energy carried by each photon must be equal to an allowed transition in the molecular structure of the chromophore. Therefore the absorption of EMR is a wavelength-dependent process, with effects related to the photon energy. In the x-ray and short-wavelength ultraviolet (UV) region of the spectrum, the photon energy is high enough to strip electrons away from molecules, hence the term *ionizing radiation.* UV, visible, and near-infrared wavelengths correspond to transitions between electron-bonding orbitals in molecules. The excited states produced by UV, visible, and near-infrared light within the chromophores often undergo reactions, called *photochemical reactions.* In general, however, most of the energy absorbed at any EMR wavelength ends up as heat. The quantum energy of far-infrared radiation corresponds to vibrational and rotational modes in molecules. Far-infrared radiation, such as that emitted by a surgical CO_2 laser, therefore directly causes kinetic excitation (heat).

EMR is measured in units that constitute an important part of the understanding of laser-tissue interactions. *Energy* is measured in joules. The amount of energy delivered per unit of area is the *fluence,* sometimes called the *exposure dose,* and is usually given in joules per square centimeter. The rate at which energy is delivered is called *power,* measured in watts. By definition, 1 W equals 1 J/sec. The power delivered per unit of area is therefore the rate of energy delivered per the amount of skin surface and is called the *irradiance,* usually given in watts per square centimeter (W/cm²). The duration of laser exposure (called the *pulsewidth* for pulsed lasers) is extremely important because this sets the time over which energy is delivered. The fluence delivered to skin by a pulse is equal to the irradiance times the pulsewidth, or *J/cm² = W/cm² × seconds.* Laser exposures used in dermatology range from seconds to nanoseconds (10^{-9} seconds). The *beam geometry* is also important. For example, the exposure spot size can greatly affect the intensity of laser light and its depth of penetration into the skin. It may also matter whether the incident light is convergent, divergent, or diffuse; whether the irradiance is uniform over the exposure area; and whether the light is delivered through air or some other external medium.

Before discussing laser-tissue interactions in detail, however, the optics of human skin are reviewed first because they determine the penetration, absorption, and internal dosimetry of laser light in skin.

Skin Optics

Two fundamental processes govern all interactions of light with matter. These are *absorption* and *scattering*. When absorbed, the photon surrenders its energy to the chromophore molecule. The excited chromophore may undergo a photochemical reaction or reemit the energy in the form of light (e.g., fluorescence) but almost always dissipates most of the energy as heat. Chromophore molecules exhibit characteristic bands of absorption around certain wavelengths.

The absorption spectra of major skin chromophores dominate most laser-tissue interactions in dermatology. For any material, including tissue, the *absorption coefficient* is defined as the probability per unit of path length that a photon at a particular wavelength will be absorbed. The absorption coefficient is therefore rendered in units of 1/distance and is sometimes designated as μ_a, given in units of cm^{-1}. The degree of absorption depends on the concentration of chromophores present. Skin has interesting pigments and distinct microscopic structures that have different absorption spectra.[1,2] Absorption coefficients for major skin chromophores at typical concentrations as they appear in skin are shown in Figure 3-2. Ironically, the curve for melanin is least well known, despite the fact that it is the only skin chromophore whose major function appears to be that of a pigment. In this figure it can be seen that melanin, which is normally present in epidermis and hair follicles but not in the dermis, absorbs broadly across the optical spectrum. In contrast, blood absorption is dominated by oxyhemoglobin and reduced hemoglobin, which exhibit strong bands in the UV, blue, green, and yellow region of the spectrum. The 577-nm (yellow) absorption band of oxyhemoglobin has been chosen for the selective photothermolysis of superficial microvessels[3] but is certainly not the only band that could be used for this.[4] Despite the high absorption by blood in the blue region (420 nm), limited penetration due to absorption and scattering and interference by epidermal melanin absorption make this region less desirable. It is theoretically possible that near-infrared pulses within the broad oxyhemoglobin band beyond 900 nm would both work well and penetrate much more deeply, but this has not been attempted yet.

Scattering occurs when the photon changes its direction of propagation. All light returning from skin is scattered light. As light strikes the skin surface, about 5% is reflected because of the sudden change in the refractive index between air (1.0) and the stratum corneum (1.55) (regular reflectance). Once inside skin, the remaining 95% of the light is either absorbed or scattered by molecules, particles, and structures in the tissue. Scattering by large particles is rather wavelength

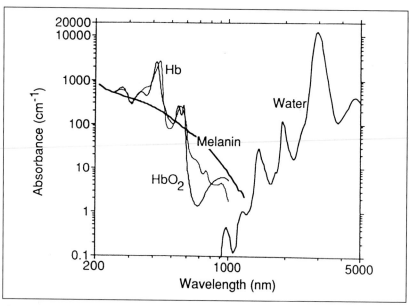

Fig. 3-2.   Absorption spectra of the major skin pigments at the concentrations for which they typically occur. Across the range of racial skin colors, melanin absorption varies by two orders of magnitude. The melanin absorption shown corresponds approximately to epidermal absorption in a darkly pigmented Caucasian. The absorption coefficient of single melanosomes is unknown. (Figure courtesy S. Prahl, PhD, and reproduced with permission from Goldman MP, Fitzpatrick RE. Cutaneous laser surgery. St. Louis: Mosby–Year Book, 1994.)

independent, as illustrated by white and gray colors in clouds. In contrast, the scattering of shorter-wavelength radiation is much stronger in the presence of particles smaller than the wavelength of light, that is, those less than a few hundred nanometers in diameter. For example, the sky is blue because molecular scattering is stronger at shorter wavelengths.

Absorption is the dominant process in normal epidermis over most of the optical spectrum. For wavelengths of from 320 to 1200 nm, absorption by melanin dominates epidermal optical properties, depending on the skin type. The transmission of Caucasian epidermis increases steadily from about 50% at a wavelength of 400 nm (blue) to 90% at a wavelength of 1200 nm. In contrast, the epidermis of a dark black person transmits less than 20% throughout the visible spectrum but rises to 90% by 1200 nm.[5] There are no skin types that fall into the infrared region beyond 1200 nm, and epidermal transmission at 1200 nm and longer wavelengths depends on its thickness and water content but not on its pigmentation. Melanin in both the epidermis (as in café au lait macules and lentigines) and the dermis (as in nevus of Ota) is an important target chromophore for laser selective photothermolysis.

Optical penetration into the dermis is affected by the strong, wavelength-dependent scattering produced by collagen fibers. Dermal scattering varies approximately with $1/\lambda^2$, where λ is the wavelength, but is less wavelength dependent in the near-infrared region. However, there are essentially no reliable in vivo measurements of optical penetration in human skin. The absorption coefficient of dermis other than that of its blood vessels is very low throughout the visible and near-infrared region of the spectrum. The absorption coefficient of dermis is less than about 1 cm^{-1} in most of the visible spectrum and decreases to less than 0.1 cm^{-1} in the near-infrared region between water absorption bands. In contrast, blood has extremely strong absorption in the blue, green, and yellow wavelengths of the visible spectrum and a weak but significant absorption band in the 800- to 1000-nm region, as shown in Figure 3-2.

Optical penetration into skin is governed by a combination of absorption and scattering. Both tend to be stronger at shorter wavelengths, from the UV through the near-infrared region. In general, therefore, the depth of penetration into skin gradually increases as the wavelengths increase over a very broad spectrum. However, the strong, narrow absorption bands of hemoglobin are such that 532-nm radiation probably penetrates live dermis deeper than 577-nm radiation, which is at one of the oxyhemoglobin maxima. The 650- to 1200-nm, red and near-infrared region is deeply penetrating (millimeters) and is the region for which photodynamic therapy drugs are being developed for cancer treatment. The most penetrating wavelength is about 1100 nm, and the least penetrating wavelengths are in the far-UV (protein absorption) and far-infrared (water absorption) region. For example, the 193-nm excimer laser radiation penetrates only a fraction of a micrometer into the stratum corneum. The surgically popular CO$_2$ laser, with a wavelength of 10.6 μm (10,600 nm), penetrates only about 20 μm into water and is therefore excellent for vaporization and cutting. Table 3-1 gives the approximate optical penetration depths in Caucasian (fair) skin of many laser wavelengths of current interest in dermatology, along with the dominant skin chromophores at each laser wavelength. It also gives the depth of penetration of a wide incident beam. When the beam radius is less than or approximately equal to the penetration depth, the intensity within the skin decreases more rapidly with depth, because of the beam broadening resulting from optical scattering to the sides. It should be borne in mind, however, that one is rarely treating normal skin and that optical penetration is frequently less in vascular or pigmented skin lesions.

The exposure spot size also affects the loss of intensity with increasing depth into skin; this occurs as a result of the optical scattering that takes place as the beam penetrates the dermis and occurs in a wavelength-dependent manner. For example, spot sizes (diameters) equal to or less than about 3 mm would likely suffer a significant loss of intensity at 1064 nm. In essence, the spot size affects optical penetration

Table 3-1. Approximate optical penetration
in normal fair caucasian skin* for a wide incident beam

Wavelength (nm)	Laser	≈50% Penetration depth (μm)	Chromophores
193	Excimer	0.5	Protein
355	Tripled neodymium	80	Melanin
488	Argon-ion	200	Melanin, blood
514	Argon-ion, dye	300	Melanin, blood
532	Doubled neodymium	400	Melanin, blood
577	Pulsed dye	400	Blood, melanin
585	Pulsed dye	600	Blood, melanin
694	Ruby	1200	Melanin
760	Alexandrite	1300	Melanin
1060	Nd:YAG	1600	Blood, melanin
2100	Holmium	200	Water
2940	Erbium	1	Water
10,600	CO_2	20	Water

*Compiled from in vivo and in vitro data.
Source: Reproduced with permission from Goldman MP, Fitzpatrick RE. Cutaneous laser surgery. St. Louis: Mosby–Year Book, 1994.

whenever the exposure spot radius is equal to or less than the distance for which light is free to diffuse within the tissue. However, another factor is the forward-directed nature of scattering in dermis (anisotropy of scattering), which is also wavelength dependent. Because accurate, direct measurements of fluence or irradiance profiles inside skin have never been done for any spot size, however, the table contains approximations gleaned from a combination of in vitro measurements and mathematical models for skin optics.

PHOTOCHEMISTRY AND PHOTODYNAMIC THERAPY

Life on earth, the formation of most skin cancers, vitamin D production, and vision would all be impossible were it not for photochemical interactions. Of the various medical specialties, dermatology makes the most use of such interactions, in the form of UV phototherapy, the use of photosensitizers such as psoralens, and the treatment of photodermatoses such as porphyria and xeroderma pigmentosa.

Photosensitizers activated by deeply penetrating red and near-infrared light have been developed for photodynamic therapy of tumors.[6] Although lasers have been used lately for photodynamic therapy, they are not essential, especially for dermatologic uses. There is now a major emphasis on the development of new drugs with varying photochemical mechanisms that can localize to different tissues and be administered by different routes. Drugs currently being tested for this purpose include porphyrin derivatives, porphyrin precursors (aminolevulinic acid), phthalocyanines, and chlorins, all of which are oxygen-dependent photosensitizers. They primarily work by transferring energy to molecular oxygen, which produces singlet oxygen, a potent oxidizer. These drugs will probably have a broader use in dermatology than that initially anticipated,[7] and this will be described more fully in another chapter.

Thermal Laser-Skin Interactions

As mentioned earlier, almost all laser applications in dermatology rely on the heating of tissue as the basis for their therapeutic effect. In contrast to photochemical reactions, heating does not require any particular photon energy. Therefore, the absorption of any wavelength of EMR can and does cause heating. The consequences of laser-induced heating cover a wide range of effects, including gentle, highly selective effects, gross coagulation necrosis, submicroscopic explosions, and the wholesale vaporization of skin.

Temperature expresses the average kinetic excitation of molecules—in essence, the amount of vibration, rotation, and other molecular motion. As temperature increases, the large, specially configured molecules necessary for life are literally shaken open. Most proteins, DNA, RNA, membranes, and their structures start to unwind or melt, or both, at temperatures ranging from 40° to 100°C. Because the tertiary structure (molecular shape) is necessary for biologic activity, the result is a loss of function, referred to as *denaturation*. At the high concentrations of macromolecules present in tissue, the unfolded molecules also become entangled with each other and the tissue becomes coagulated. The most familiar example of denaturation and coagulation is the cooking of *egg white*.

Thermal denaturation is both temperature and time dependent and is crudely described in tissue by a classical thermodynamics (Arrhenius) model.[8,9] The rate of thermal denaturation for most proteins increases exponentially with increases in temperature above a certain region, such that thermal denaturation tends to have a thresholdlike behavior. For a given heating time, there is usually a narrow temperature region above which biologically significant denaturation occurs. For most proteins, one must increase the temperature about 10° to 20°C for every decade of decrease in the heating time to achieve the same amount of thermal coagulation.

Thermal coagulation causes cell necrosis, hemostasis, "welding," and a gross alteration in the extracellular matrix at specific temperature–heating time combinations. Surprisingly little is known about tissue responses to specific thermal transitions in the major molecules and cell types in skin. With the exception of prolonged heating in the 40° to 45°C region used for tumor hyperthermia treatment, little is also known about the cellular effects of brief, high-temperature hyperthermia. Gross thermal coagulation of the dermis constitutes a burn, and it is well worth remembering that the performance of laser surgery consists mainly in controlling where and how much heat injury occurs. The relatively low power continuous-wave lasers such as the CO_2 and argon-ion laser and the quasi–continuous-wave (rapid-pulsed) lasers such as the copper vapor and KTP lasers usually cause a well-controlled, superficial, partial-thickness burn. In contrast, pulsed yellow-dye lasers designed for selective photothermolysis of microvascular lesions selectively coagulate microvessels.

Selective photothermolysis is a term coined by Dr. Parrish and myself[10] over 14 years ago to describe the sequence of light-heat-ruin that occurs at microscopic sites, such as blood vessels, pigmented cells, and tattoo ink particles, which selectively absorb light pulses. Selective photothermolysis is qualitatively different from gross thermal injury and is like a "magic bullet" in its ability to target certain structures. Short pulses are necessary to deposit energy in the targets before they can cool off, thus achieving extreme, localized heating of the targets. Thermal coagulation or thermally mediated mechanical damage, or both, are involved, depending on the rate of energy deposition in the targets. This technique led to the development of a new generation of dermatologic lasers that cause much less scarring, and these are discussed in detail here.

Mechanical injury, sometimes misnamed "photoacoustic injury," occurs as the result of the rapid heating produced by high-energy, short-pulse lasers. The rate of local heating can be so severe that structures are torn apart by *shock waves* (a highly destructive supersonic pressure wave), *cavitation* (the sudden expansion and collapse of a steam bubble), or rapid *thermal expansion.* Terms such as *fracture, rupture,* or *explosion* are appropriately used in reference to these processes, even though they occur on a microscopic scale. Mechanical damage plays a central, positive role in the tattoo removal achieved by selective photothermolysis using high-energy, submicrosecond lasers. However, mechanical damage can also be an unwanted side effect, such as in the form of the bleeding caused by pulsed yellow-dye lasers and the ejection of tissue fragments caused by high-energy, Q-switched laser pulses.

THERMAL INJURY TO CELLS

Most human cells can withstand prolonged exposure to a temperature of 40°C. At 45°C, cultured human fibroblasts have been observed to be destroyed after about 20 minutes of exposure. However, the same cells can withstand a temperature of more than 100°C if exposed to it for only 10^{-3} seconds.[11] Thus, it is not the temperature per se but a combination of the local temperature and the heating time that determines whether cells in the skin are injured. This is presumably because thermal denaturation is a rate-dependent process, as described earlier. This behavior has an important bearing on the cell injury that occurs in the setting of selective photothermolysis, during which extreme temperatures are present in target sites, such as microvessels, for a very short duration. Essentially nothing is known about the temperature-time relationships pertaining to vascular cell lethality in the millisecond heating-time domain produced during the pulsed yellow-dye laser treatment of port-wine stains (PWSs).

Nature provides an intriguing example of maximal thermal adaptation, in that some thermophilic bacteria can survive and reproduce at 80° to 90°C but not at our body temperature. These organisms possess specialized proteins and a unique cell membrane structure. It is known that thermal cell killing involves irreversible protein denaturation. About fifty years ago, Henriques[12] determined the time-temperature behavior for the coagulation necrosis of animal epidermis, which was described using an Arrhenius integral model. All cells have mechanisms for removing denatured proteins, provided the cell is still viable. The induction of heat-shock proteins is a ubiquitous phenomenon that occurs in diploid cells and that appears to confer resistance to further thermal injury. Heat-shocked keratinocytes are thermotolerant,[13] but the molecular mechanisms underlying induced thermotolerance remain obscure. Heat-shock proteins are induced by laser exposures, and a heat-shock response has been shown to protect human fibroblasts to a modest degree against CO_2 laser–induced thermal injury.[11]

EXTRACELLULAR MATRIX THERMAL EFFECTS

In contrast to the epidermis, connective tissues such as dermis are dominantly composed of extracellular structural proteins such as collagen and elastin and of glycosaminoglycans. Elastin survives boiling for hours with no apparent change. However, type I collagen fibers, which is the major type of collagen fiber in dermis, have a sharp melting transition point between about 65° and 70°C, depending to some extent on the amount of cross-linking. The melting of collagen fibers causes impressive, immediate shrinkage of the tissue that can be seen easily during procedures such as CO_2 laser resurfacing. This transition appears to pose an absolute limitation for the bulk dermal temperature, beyond which scarring is highly likely. If the entire collagen-based scaffolding of the dermis is destroyed, it is likely that nothing short of complete tissue remodeling will allow healing. In contrast to diffuse coagulation injury, selective photothermolysis can produce high temperatures in structures or individual cells with little risk of scarring, because gross dermal heating is minimized. The bulk dermal temperature rise after a single 6-J/cm² pulse at 585 nm is probably about 15°C.[3,14]

VAPORIZATION, ABLATION, AND CHARRING

The boiling temperature of water at 1 atmosphere pressure is 100°C. However, lasers and electrosurgical tools usually vaporize tissue well above this temperature, because (1) higher pressures are present, especially with pulsed lasers, (2) water is superheated before it is vaporized, and (3) with continuous-wave (cw) lasers the surface layer becomes desiccated and charred (carbonized), reaching temperatures of several hundred degrees Celsius.

High-energy pulsed and cw lasers can differ greatly in their ability to ablate tissue and cause residual thermal damage. For example, CO_2 lasers are available both in cw and in so-called superpulsed modes. A CO_2 laser used in a cw mode at modest powers for vaporization causes charring. Because of heat conduction, the residual thermal coagulation injury occurs to a depth of about 1 mm, despite the 20-μm shallow penetration depth of CO_2 laser radiation. The charring occurs because of the extreme heating of desiccated tissue, which then carbonizes. Thus, the tissue bed remaining after cw CO_2 laser vaporization is typically coagulated to a depth of about 1 mm, desiccated, and charred. In contrast, appropriately short (less than 10^{-3} seconds), energetic (greater than 5 J/cm^2) pulses of CO_2 laser radiation remove tissue with greater efficiency but with less thermal damage (about 50–100 μm of residual coagulation) and no charring.[15]

These two basically different modes of tissue ablation, however, *are not unique to either.* That is, a tightly focused cw CO_2 or other laser that is scanned rapidly enough along the target tissue can produce the intense, short-exposure-time conditions needed to produce pulsed laser ablation effects. Conversely, a short-pulsed CO_2 laser, if operated at a subablative pulse fluence (e.g., less than about 1 J/cm^2 per pulse) at repetition rates of less than about 100 Hz, can produce the deeper injury and charring associated with cw laser effects. Therefore, despite the convenience of labeling laser vaporization as pulsed or cw, a more precise understanding of the dynamics of each is clearly necessary. The following paragraphs attempt to provide this.

Water requires about 2300 J/cm^3 of energy for it to vaporize. Tissue is removed efficiently, with minimal thermal injury and no charring, if the entire heat of vaporization is delivered to the most superficial layer possible, that is, the layer about equal to the optical penetration depth, during a time equal to or less than the thermal relaxation time (the time it takes for significant cooling to occur) for this superficial heated layer. Thus, the thinnest layer possible (for a given wavelength) is endowed with all the energy it needs to vaporize, before much heat is transferred to the underlying tissue. Under these conditions, the layer suddenly vaporizes away, leaving behind a residual thermally injured layer only about two to four times the optical penetration depth. Because the laser energy is switched off before desiccation occurs, charring does not occur. In contrast, if energy is delivered for a much longer time, the attendant thermal conduction causes an increase in the depth of injury, decreases ablation efficiency, allows desiccation during the laser exposure, and may allow charring to occur.

These principles are illustrated quantitatively in the context of the important practical example of the CO_2 laser. The laser energy deposited per unit of volume (E_v) is equal to:

$$E_v = E\mu_a \qquad\qquad \text{Eq. 1}$$

where E = the local fluence (J/cm^2) and μ_a = the tissue's absorption coefficient (in centimeters^{-1}), defined earlier.

Setting E_v = 2500 J/cm^3 to account for the heat of vaporization for water plus the energy required to bring the tissue to 100°C closely approximates the energy requirement for the removal of tissue. Solving for E, the applied fluence needs to be E = (2500)/μ_a, in joules per square centimeter. The value of μ_a at the CO_2 laser wavelength of 10,600 nm is about 500 cm^{-1}, which yields E = 5 J/cm^2 as the necessary pulse fluence to achieve the ablation of skin tissue.

To limit thermal injury, this 5 J/cm^2 must be delivered before the superficially heated layer has time to cool. The penetration depth of CO_2 laser radiation is $1/\mu_a$, or about 20 μm, and the thermal relaxation time (τ_r) for a layer of thickness (d) is about:

$$\tau_r \approx d^2/4\kappa \qquad\qquad \text{Eq. 2}$$

where κ = thermal diffusivity $\approx 1.3 \times 10^{-3}$ cm^2/sec.

Thus, the thermal relaxation time for the pulsed CO_2 laser–heated, 20-μm superficial layer is: $\tau_r \approx d^2/4\kappa \approx (2 \times 10^{-3}$ cm)$^2 \div [(4 \times 1.3 \times 10^{-3}$) cm^2/sec] = 0.8 $\times 10^{-3}$ seconds. In effect, using the CO_2 laser wavelength, the necessary 5 J/cm^2 fluence must be delivered in at most 0.8 msec to minimize injury to the underlying tissue. When this is done, each exposure pulse should remove about one optical penetration depth (20 μm) of tissue and leave two to four times the optical penetration depth, that is, about 40 to 80 μm of residual thermally damaged tissue. It is this layer of thermally damaged tissue that is responsible for producing hemostasis, or the lack thereof, and also for effecting wound healing.[16]

As noted earlier, it is important not to become dogmatic about pulsed versus cw laser effects, in that pulsed lasers can be made to mimic cw laser effects by means of rapid, low-energy pulsing, and cw lasers can to some extent mimic pulsed laser effects. The same analysis can be used to find the conditions under which a cw CO_2 laser can operate in a focused, scanning mode to mimic the pulsed CO_2 laser effects. The high irradiance and short exposure time needed for pulsed laser ablation can be achieved by tightly focusing and automatically scanning a cw laser beam. No matter how it is done, the task of making a CO_2 laser remove tissue with maximum efficiency and minimum thermal injury requires the delivery of at least 5 J/cm^2 of fluence in at most 0.8 msec, which requires an irradiance of at least 6250 W/cm^2. Because lasers can be easily focused to extremely small spots (e.g., less than 0.1 mm), even a 10-W cw CO_2 laser can achieve this irradiance in a small focal spot. Once focused this tightly, automated scanning is needed to deliver the proper exposure ("dwell") time, which is simply equal to the spot diameter divided by the scan velocity.

From the foregoing example, it is apparent that both the fluence needed for ablation and the depth of residual injury depend on the penetration depth, $1/\mu_a$. This holds true for other infrared lasers and governs the development and also the utility of new infrared lasers in medicine. The *holmium* laser output of nearly 2000 nm, with an absorption coefficient of 50 cm[-1] and a penetration depth of about 200 μm, requires a fluence of about 50 J/cm² (ten times that of the CO_2 laser), removes about 200 μm per "pulse," and leaves behind about 400 to 800 μm of thermally coagulated tissue, when delivered in less than about 80 msec. The holmium laser is being developed mainly because it is fiberoptic compatible and thus can be used for endoscopic procedures, and also because it produces excellent hemostasis. A holmium laser is generally a poor choice for tasks requiring extremely high-precision, low-injury ablation, however.

The 2.9-nm wavelength of the *erbium* laser is very strongly absorbed by water, and this laser is capable of extremely high precision, superficial ablation. With an absorption coefficient of about 10,000 cm[-1] in skin, a mere 0.25 J/cm² of fluence is required for tissue removal (1/20th that of the CO_2 laser), but it must be delivered in a few microseconds or less to remove just 1 μm of tissue per pulse, leaving the minuscule residual injury depth of only 2 to 4 μm. Short-pulsed erbium lasers are therefore capable of ablating only one or two cell layers at a time, with very minimal residual injury. This is excellent for extremely fine ablation, but this laser is a poor choice when hemostasis is needed. However, hemostasis can be achieved (and thermal injury increased intentionally) by using longer pulses, which allows more thermal conduction to occur. Erbium or other lasers operating near the 3000-nm water-absorption band should therefore be versatile tools for ablation; however, they have not yet been developed for dermatologic uses.

Excimer laser pulses, at a wavelength of 193 nm, have been shown to remove tissue by a combination of thermal and photochemical ablation.[17] At this wavelength the absorption coefficient is about 12,000 cm[-1] in skin, similar to the absorption coefficient for the erbium laser wavelength. However, the photon energy is sufficient to break chemical bonds in polymers, such that tissue is removed not only through the thermal vaporization of tissue water but also through the photochemical breakage of large macromolecules. To date, excimer laser ablation has not been used for dermatologic purposes, other than the experimental removal of stratum corneum.[18] However, because of the precision with which the excimer laser can ablate the cornea, this laser is being developed for the correction of visual refraction.[19] The same 193-nm wavelength, when used for the ablation of skin, produces shock waves that disrupt and injure cells well into the epidermis and upper dermis.[20]

SELECTIVE PHOTOTHERMOLYSIS

Selective photothermolysis has changed the scope of the uses of lasers in dermatology over the decade since its development.[10] *It is by far the most precise use of heat in medicine.*

Light deposits energy only at sites of absorption. Heat is created at wavelengths that penetrate into skin and are preferentially absorbed by chromophoric structures, such as blood vessels or melanin-containing cells. As soon as the heat is created, however, it begins to dissipate as the result of conduction and radiative transfer. Thus, the competition between active heating and passive cooling determines how hot the targets become. The most selective target heating is achieved when the energy is deposited at faster than the rate of cooling of the target structures.

Three basic elements are necessary to achieve selective photothermolysis: (1) a wavelength that reaches and is preferentially absorbed by the desired target structures, (2) an exposure duration less than or equal to the time necessary for cooling of the target structures, and (3) sufficient fluence to produce a damaging temperature in the target structures. When these criteria are met, exquisitely selective injury occurs in thousands of microscopic targets, without the need to aim the laser at each one. The effect is equivalent to the legendary magic bullets that seek out only the desired target. Selective photothermolysis makes use of a variety of thermally mediated damage mechanisms, including thermal denaturation, mechanical damage resulting from rapid thermal expansion or phase changes (cavitation), and pyrolysis (changes in the primary chemical structure).

A useful construct is the *thermal relaxation time,* mentioned earlier. When the laser exposure duration is less than the thermal relaxation time, maximal thermal confinement occurs because the target cannot then get rid of its heat during the laser exposure. Many processes are involved in cooling, including convection, radiation, and conduction. Of these, thermal conduction is the one that dominates the cooling of microscopic structures in skin. However, microscale radiational cooling in tissue has never been thoroughly examined and in theory may be of importance for very small targets at high temperatures, such as tattoo ink particles or melanin granules.

It is common experience that smaller objects cool more quickly than larger objects. For example, a cup of tea cools faster than a hot bath, even though both involve hot water in a porcelain container. More precisely, the thermal relaxation time for heat conduction is proportional to the square of size (see Eq. 2). That is, for any given material and shape, an object half the size will cool in one fourth the time and an object one tenth the size will cool in one hundredth the time. This behavior is important in optimizing the pulse duration or the exposure duration for the selective photothermolysis of blood vessels. Blood vessels vary in size, from capillaries, which have thermal relaxation times of tens of microseconds, to venules and arterioles, which have thermal relaxation times of hundreds of microseconds, to the large venules of adult PWSs, which have thermal relaxation times of tens to hundreds of milliseconds. This means that there are vessels in a typical adult PWS with thermal relaxation times ranging over three orders of magnitude, and thus it is ludicrous to attempt to define "the" thermal relaxation time for vessels.

It is theoretically possible to select the target size by picking the pulse or exposure duration appropriately. In a typical PWS, the ectatic vessels are the targets, and it is their thermal relaxation time that should not be exceeded (e.g., up to about 5–10 msec). When the pulse duration exceeds a target's thermal relaxation time, heating of the target becomes inefficient. Therefore, it is theoretically possible to select for larger-vessel damage by choosing laser exposures that exceed the thermal relaxation times of capillaries, yet are less than the thermal relaxation times of the target PWS vessels. Capillaries are relatively spared by pulses of at least several hundred microseconds, because they cool significantly during the delivery of laser energy. This concept has not yet been explored in the setting of dermatologic laser applications, however.

The thermal relaxation time is also related to the shape of the target, because of the differences in the volume and surface area of the target. For a given thickness, spheres cool faster than cylinders, which cool faster than planes.[5] All three are relevant to dermatology, in that melanosomes are elliptical, vessels are cylindrical, and tissue layers are planar. A material property called *thermal diffusivity* (κ), mentioned earlier, expresses the ability of heat to diffuse and is equal to the ratio between heat conductivity and specific heat capacity. Thermal properties for soft tissues other than fat are dominated by their high water content. The thermal diffusivity for water, 1.3×10^{-3} cm^2/sec, is approximately the same as that for most soft tissues, as used in the earlier example describing laser tissue vaporization.

For most tissue targets, a simple rule of thumb that can be used to estimate thermal relaxation times is as follows: the thermal relaxation time in seconds is about equal to the square of the target dimension in millimeters. Thus, a 0.5-μm melanosome (5×10^{-4} mm) should cool in about 25×10^{-8} seconds, or 250 nsec, whereas a 0.1-mm PWS vessel should cool in about 10^{-2} seconds, or 10 msec. The natural variation in the sizes of biologic targets means that there is an even greater variation in thermal relaxation times, such that more precise calculations, though certainly possible, are usually unnecessary.

MICROVASCULAR INTERACTIONS OF SELECTIVE PHOTOTHERMOLYSIS

Many details of the laser-tissue interactions that occur during selective photothermolysis in dermatology are poorly understood, but the observations made to date have served as the basis for a good conceptual understanding of the process. The visible laser pulse effects on microvessels are the best studied. These were studied during the development of the pulsed yellow-dye lasers used for treating PWSs in children. Indeed, the histology of pediatric PWSs was used to define the task of this laser,[8,21] and this laser works very well for this purpose. The same laser can be used for the treatment of adult PWSs, telangiectases, and other microvascular lesions, but different laser parameters may be better for some of these lesions, as discussed later.

In general, an "ideal" set of laser parameters are not the only ones that can be used effectively in particular settings. That is, an experienced laser surgeon can often achieve good results with a less-than-ideal tool, and conversely, bad results are certainly possible even when an ideal laser is used. As an example of this, selective photothermolysis with a long-pulsed (300–500 μsec), flashlamp-pumped, tunable dye laser near a wavelength of 585 nm has now become the strongly preferred method for treating pediatric PWSs because of the very low risk of scarring when it is used in single pulses at 6 to 8 J/cm² of fluence.[22] However, the present generation of these lasers is still far from ideal, both in terms of the interactions with skin vessels and the clinical results.

In the first version of selective photothermolysis,[3] a 1-msec, 577-nm pulse of at least 2 J/cm² was predicted on theoretical grounds to be ideal. Initially such long pulses were not available at this wavelength, so a 0.3- to 1-μsec pulsed dye laser (1/1000th the ideal pulse duration) was tested at 577 nm in normal skin. However, this was noted to cause histologically selective injury to dermal vessels that included extensive hemorrhage.[23,24] The temperatures and fluences needed to produce this damage, seen grossly as purpura, were consistent with those causing the mechanical rupture of vessels resulting from the vaporization of blood.[25] In an attempt to minimize vaporization injury and maximize the thermal coagulation of vessels, the pulse duration was lengthened. Garden and associates[26] studied the effect of the pulse duration and noted that hemorrhage was significantly less in normal human skin when pulses longer than 20 μsec were used, and that, in accordance with theory, the fluence required for vascular damage increased with pulse duration.

A 400-μsec, 577-nm pulsed dye laser was constructed, tested clinically on PWSs, and noted to work well,[27] with a low risk of scarring, even in children.[28] A longer, approximately twice-as-penetrating wavelength was shown to be capable of similar vascular selectivity, but at a greater depth of effect,[29] and a wavelength of 585 nm was subsequently used clinically.[30] At present, a 585-nm, 400-μsec laser pulse delivered at 6 to 8 J/cm² of fluence in single, nonoverlapping pulses, to exposure spots 5 mm in diameter, is widely considered to be the standard approach to treatment. Histologically, this produces selective intravascular and perivascular coagulation necrosis, with epidermal injury in dark skin types.[31] Hypopigmentation is a frequent and usually transient side effect, as is postinflammatory hyperpigmentation.[32] This laser produces transiently disfiguring purpura as the result of hemorrhage and a delayed vasculitis, presumably because of its still shorter-than-ideal pulse duration. In addition, six or more treatments are usually needed to remove PWSs and, for unknown reasons, some PWSs cannot be removed by this method.

An ideal set of laser-pulse parameters for the treatment of PWSs has never been tested. Recently, a longer pulse width dye laser has become available (1.5 ms), which may prove to be superior to the 0.4-ms devices. The best pulse duration for pediatric PWSs is probably in the region of 1 to 5 msec and may be longer for adult PWSs, which in general contain larger vessels.

With regard to wavelength, the small improvement in the optical penetration depth between a wavelength of 577 and 585 nm could be improved further by using still longer wavelengths, with little loss in selectivity. Although the study leading to the choice of the 585-nm wavelength[29] was well performed, it was intrinsically flawed, in that fixed fluences at various wavelengths were compared with regard to the histologic depth of injury in dermal vessels in an animal model. However, as the absorption coefficient of blood decreases with increasing wavelengths beyond 577 nm, greater local fluence is required to achieve the same thermal excitation at any given vessel site. By comparing a limited and fixed fluence range, the ability to selectively damage vessels seemed to simply disappear at longer wavelengths. The inappropriate conclusion was therefore reached that longer wavelengths were ineffective in causing highly selective microvascular injury.

However, with higher incident fluences, selective microvascular injury can be obtained well into the penetrating, visible red wavelengths of 600 nm and beyond.[33] Vessel-selective injury is not completely lost until the absorption coefficient of venous blood approaches that of the surrounding dermis, which does not occur throughout the entire red/near-infrared region. The major fundamental limitation to using red laser pulses for PWS treatment is the absorption of the radiation by epidermal melanin, which varies widely with skin type. In fact, the 694-nm Q-switched ruby laser is highly selective in causing damage to melanized cells alone.[34] Despite this, long-pulse, higher-fluence red (i.e., 600–650 nm) laser pulses might work well for treating PWSs or telangiectases. At the longer pulse durations appropriate for PWS treatment, pigment cell injury is minimized.[35] In a small comparative clinical trial, 600-nm pulsed dye laser exposures were found to work well for treating microvascular lesions.[36]

Another important issue is the number of pulses delivered to a single skin site. With each laser pulse, the pigmented target sites experience a thermal cycle of heating and cooling. However, if hemorrhage is caused by the first laser pulse for the treatment of microvessels, subsequent laser pulses can cause widespread dermal injury simply because the target chromophore is then no longer confined to blood vessels. However, the Arrhenius model suggested that thermal injury is cumulative over time; therefore, in theory, it was realized that multiple, lower-fluence pulses, which do not cause hemorrhage, might be used to produce a cumulative, selective, "gentler," and more complete damage to microvessels. This proved to clearly be the case, and this technique now offers a wholly new approach to the delivery of selective photothermolysis. Using 585-nm, 160-µsec dye laser pulses delivered at 0.5 Hz, Troccoli and colleagues[37] reported that the threshold fluence for hemorrhage in 50-µm-diameter hamster cheek pouch venules was 6 J/cm², but only half of the vessels were closed (thrombosed). In contrast, using 10 to 100 pulses at fluences of 2 to 4 J/cm², vessel closure was achieved consistently without hemorrhage. These findings indicate that one reason PWSs require so many treatments is that the probability for irreversible vessel damage is far less than unity for single-pulse exposures within the tolerated fluence range. PWSs may respond more rapidly, or even to a single treatment, if multiple lower-fluence pulses are delivered at an average irradiance (pulse fluence × repetition rate), which does not cause gross thermal injury.

PIGMENTED LESION REMOVAL BY SELECTIVE PHOTOTHERMOLYSIS

Melanin is normally present only in the epidermis and hair follicles, which are impressively capable of regeneration. Therefore, almost any laser with sufficient power, if used skillfully, can remove benign pigmented lesions of the epidermis; this includes CO_2 lasers, which heat the skin nonselectively through absorption of the radiation by water.[38] Indeed, almost every dermatologic laser currently on the market has been shown to remove lentigines effectively, without scarring. However, a more precise interaction occurs with selective photothermolysis. Electron microscopy showed the selective rupture of skin melanosomes produced by 351-nm, submicrosecond excimer laser pulses of only about 0.1 J/cm².[10] At fluences that cause damage to melanocytes and pigmented keratinocytes, epidermal Langerhans cells apparently escape injury.[39]

Melanosomes are the fundamental site for melanin synthesis and occur in the form of 0.5 to 1 µm oblong organelles. They exist in melanocytes in various stages of pigmentation and are bound to cytoskeletal proteins in the cytoplasm. Upon transfer to keratinocytes, they appear in membrane-limited phagosomes. In Caucasians, the melanosomes are smaller and packaged in groups within keratinocyte phagosomes.[40] As noted earlier, the thermal relaxation time of melanosomes is unknown but probably lies in the region of 250 to 1000 nsec, depending on their size. The wavelengths absorbed by melanin extend from the deep UV region through the visible region and well into the near-infrared region of the spectrum (see Fig. 3-1). Across this broad spectrum, optical penetration into skin increases from several micrometers to several millimeters. One would therefore expect melanosomes and the pigmented cells containing them to be affected at different depths across this broad spectrum.

Melanosomes rupture in a manner consistent with that proposed in the basic theory of selective photothermolysis. The rupture of melanosomes is independent of pulse duration below 100 nsec, including even picosecond- (10^{-12} sec) and femtosecond- (10^{-15} sec) domain pulses.[35] This indicates that optical absorption by melanin may not be saturable, that is, even terawatt per square centimeter intensities are absorbed the same as lower-intensity pulses, a situation that is highly unusual for organic chromophores. The wavelength dependence for melanosome rupture in guinea pig epidermis is quantitatively consistent with the absorption spectrum of melanin.[41] At longer wavelengths, leukotrichia was observed after hair regrowth in pigmented guinea pigs following the administration of Q-switched laser pulses. The wavelength dependence for leukotrichia was consistent with the increased penetration depth of red and near-infrared radiation compared with the penetration depth of green or UV-argon laser pulses.[41] Melanocytes were found to be permanently absent from the hair follicles of guinea pig skin after Q-switched ruby laser irradiation.[42] However, leukotrichia has not been observed to occur in human skin in the thousands of patients who have undergone high-fluence treatments with this laser system to remove tattoos. This may be due to the increased depth of human hair follicles or to a fundamental difference in the follicular pigmentation between guinea pig and human skin.

The rupture of melanosomes is a submicroscopic, mechanical form of damage. Local pressure waves or deformations beyond the elastic limits, or both conditions, probably account for the killing of pigmented cells.[43] At sublethal fluences, pulses appear to stimulate melanogenesis by means of unknown mechanisms. Shorter-wavelength pulses well below the threshold for melanosome rupture appear to cause melanocyte stimulation in guinea pigs that is histologically apparent days after exposure.[44]

Grossly the immediate effect of submicrosecond near-UV, visible, or near-infrared laser pulses in pigmented skin is "immediate whitening." This response correlates very well with the melanosome rupture seen on electron micrographs[35] and is therefore presumably a direct consequence of melanosome rupture. A nearly identical, but deeper, whitening occurs in tattoos exposed to Q-switched laser radiation; like melanosomes, tattoos consist of insoluble, submicrometer-sized, intracellular pigmented granules. Although the exact cause of the immediate whitening is unknown, it is almost certainly related to the formation of gas bubbles that intensely scatter light. Over several to tens of minutes, these bubbles then dissolve and the skin color returns to normal or nearly normal. A common misconception is that these bubbles are steam. Although the vaporization of water to form steam creates transient vapor cavities, to truly constitute only steam (water vapor) these bubbles must collapse to zero volume within microseconds. The residual gas bubbles must therefore contain some other gas. Regardless of its cause, *immediate whitening offers a clinically useful immediate end-point* which apparently relates directly to melanosome or tattoo ink rupture produced by Q-switched laser pulses.

Clinically, selective photothermolysis has not been effective for the eradication of dermal melasma, postinflammatory hyperpigmentation, or drug-induced hyperpigmentation.[45,46] However, it is highly useful for the removal of epidermal and dermal lesions in which cellular pigmentation itself is the cause. These include lentigines, café au lait macules (which exhibit a high rate of recurrence), nevus spilus, Becker's nevi, blue nevi, and nevus of Ota. Currently, probably the best combination of selectivity, depth of penetration, and broadest effectiveness in the removal of pigmented lesions is that offered by the Q-switched ruby laser at 694 nm, or the practically equivalent Q-switched alexandrite laser at 760 nm. However, there are two commercial short-pulsed green lasers that are also effective for the treatment of epidermal lesions; these are the 510-nm, 300-nsec pulsed green-dye laser and the 532-nm, Q-switched, frequency-doubled Nd:YAG laser.

TATTOO REMOVAL BY SELECTIVE PHOTOTHERMOLYSIS

Remarkably little is known about the mechanisms by which selective photothermolysis removes tattoos, aside from the fact that it works. Tattoos mainly consist of intracellular, submicrometer-sized, insoluble ink particles that have been ingested by phagocytic skin cells after intradermal injection. They are contained in the phagolysosomes of these phagocytic cells—the fibroblasts, macrophages, and mast cells. The stability and longevity of most tattoos show that many phagocytic skin cells do not "traffic" or migrate widely, though tattoos do become less distinct over decades. A great variety of inks are used in professional tattoos, and they mainly consist of insoluble metal salts, oxides, or organic complexes. The substances used to make amateur tattoos are almost always carbon in some form—india ink (amorphous carbon), graphite, or ash.

Conventional tattoo treatments, including surgical excision, dermabrasion, salabrasion, and CO_2 laser vaporization, are grossly destructive, however. It was Goldman[47] who was the first to note that tattoos were responsive to pulsed laser treatment, using normal-mode ruby laser pulses, and this treatment was later used widely in Japan. Afterward it was reported that tattoos could be successfully removed without tissue removal using Q-switched ruby laser pulses.[48,49] A dose-response and histologic study was subsequently performed, and the findings led to widespread interest in Q-switched ruby lasers in the United States,[50] followed by further ultrastructural studies of the response.[51] It is now apparent that the Q-switched ruby laser is a generally effective and relatively well tolerated means of removing black, blue-black, and green tattoos. However, multiple treatments are required at fluences ranging from 4 to 10 J/cm², depending on the skin type and response. Typically, four to six treatments given at 1-month intervals are needed for the removal of amateur tattoos and six to eight such treatments are needed for the removal of professional tattoos, although the individual response is extremely variable. The risk of scarring for the series of treatments is about 5% to 10%,[52] though over a fourth of patients show transient textural changes.[53] The Q-switched ruby laser causes blistering and hypopigmentation in most patients and permanent depigmentation in about 1% to 3%.[53]

As already noted, the mechanisms involved in tattoo removal are largely unknown. Electron micrographs do indicate that, after treatment with a Q-switched ruby laser, the average ink particle is fractured into 10 to 100 smaller fragments, which are extracellular in location, presumably as the result of being released when the phagocytic cells that contain them rupture. Local collagen denaturation marking thermal coagulation injury is occasionally seen but does not appear to be central to ink removal. Rephagocytosed, laser-altered ink particles can be found weeks after treatment and are occasionally obvious histologically despite nearly complete removal of the tattoo clinically. It is clear that much of the ink, although apparently removed from the skin, is not removed from the body, because the lymph nodes draining the tattooed skin of all persons with tattoos who undergo such treatment are pigmented with tattoo ink. It is likely that this is the fate of most of the ink after laser treatment. Lightening of the tattoo occurs gradually about 1 week after each treatment and may go on for months. Occasionally, it is clear that ink is present in the scale-crust that forms after epidermal injury and sheds 1 to 2 weeks after treatment, but it is equally apparent that tattoos are removed in cases in which no scale-crust forms. These collective observations[50,51] strongly indicate, but do not prove, that the primary effects are (1) the fragmentation of ink particles, (2) their release into the extracellular dermal space, (3) partial elimination of ink in a scale-crust, if present, (4) probably greater elimination into the lymphatics, and (5) rephagocytosis of laser-altered, residual tattoo ink particles.

Irreversible laser-induced photochemical changes can occur in tattoo inks, especially those used in cosmetic skin-colored tattoos.[54] Such photochemical changes may conceivably affect the removal of some kinds of tattoo ink. All of the pulsed lasers used for tattoo removal occasionally cause irreversible, immediate darkening of the tattoos, which may be temporarily obscured in part by the immediate whitening reaction, discussed earlier. It is therefore prudent to test a small area of cosmetic, red, or white tattoos to see whether immediate darkening occurs, especially because, in some cases, the darkened ink cannot be removed by subsequent laser treatments and this then adds to the disfigurement. The mechanism of tattoo ink darkening is not known but probably involves the reduction of ferric oxide (rust color) to ferrous oxide (black). Pure ferric oxide, which is present in many cosmetic tattoos, has been observed in in vitro conditions to be easily converted in this manner by Q-switched laser pulses. However, titanium oxides and other compounds are also present and appear to darken as well.

Results from a side-by-side comparison study of Q-switched ruby (694-nm, 40-nsec) and Q-switched Nd:YAG (1064-nm, 30-nsec) laser pulses at equal fluences (2–6 J/cm^2) and delivered to equal exposure spot sizes (5 mm) were reported by DeCoste and Anderson.[55] They noted that the efficacy of each in the removal of black ink was equal at equal fluences and that there was a significant dose-response relationship. However, in contrast to the Q-switched ruby laser, the Q-switched Nd:YAG laser was incapable of lightening green ink tattoos but produced no blistering, hypopigmentation, or textural changes. The currently available commercial Q-switched ruby and Nd:YAG lasers operate at shorter pulse durations (26 and 12 nsec, respectively) than those used by DeCoste and Anderson, and the Q-switched Nd:YAG laser is typically used with a smaller (2 or 3 mm) exposure spot diameter because of its limited pulse energy. A recent side-by-side comparison of these two lasers reported on by Levine and Geronemus[56] showed that the Q-switched ruby laser was better at lightening black ink and also that the incidence of textural change was lower in patients so treated. Because higher fluences and smaller exposure spot diameters were used with the Nd:YAG laser in this study, this means that different wavelengths, spot sizes, fluences, and pulse durations were being simultaneously compared, and it is therefore unclear which factors are most important. Taken together with DeCoste and Anderson's study, however, it does appear that the exposure spot size is a very important factor. This is consistent with the skin optics behavior of red and near-infrared wavelength pulses, especially in targets deep within the dermis.

Other available lasers known to work in the selective photothermolysis of tattoos are the 760-nm, 75- to 100-nsec Q-switched alexandrite laser; the 532-nm, 10-nsec, frequency-doubled, Q-switched Nd:YAG laser; and the 510-nm, 300-nsec, short-pulsed dye laser. It is clear that, in general, results are better for colored tattoos when the laser wavelength is well absorbed by the particular ink. For example, the alexandrite, ruby, and infrared Nd:YAG lasers only occasionally remove bright red inks, which can usually be subsequently removed in only a few treatments with either of the green pulsed lasers.

Physicians interested in providing this kind of treatment have every right to be confused. There has been an impressive rush of lasers to the marketplace by laser manufacturers, resulting in the availability of lasers capable of a range of wavelengths and pulse durations, chosen on the basis of "well-educated guesses" and sometimes promoted on the same basis. Essentially no controlled studies have been done with the goal to enhance our understanding of and lead to the optimization of tattoo removal. Of major importance, the nature of pulsewidth dependence is unknown, though strong arguments can be made for radically shortening the pulsewidth, if mechanical fracture of the ink particles is the goal. In a manner somewhat analogous to the concept of thermal confinement, inertial confinement can be achieved if the laser pulse is delivered within the time in which pressure can be relieved from the ink particles. The inertial confinement time is arrived at simply by dividing the particle diameter by the speed of sound, which for tattoo ink particles is about 1 nsec. It may therefore be that all of the laser pulses used now are too long. Significant details about wavelength-dependent effects are unknown. The chemical identity of most tattoo inks and the way in which they are affected by high-intensity laser pulses are also unknown, as are the physical mechanisms underlying ink particle and phagocyte cell rupture. More importantly, the latter have never been linked with clinical response. Is a laser-induced plasma involved? Must the ink particles be fractured? Is it the ink, or the cells containing it, that are the targets? How is the ink removed, and where does it go? What role, if any, does phagocytosis by different cell types play in the retention of ink after treatment, and how can this be optimized? It is hoped that a chapter on this topic 5 years from now will have more information on this than this one does.

HAIR REMOVAL BY SELECTIVE PHOTOTHERMOLYSIS

Hair removal with lasers is a recently rediscovered application that has great market potential. Outrageous claims, wishful conclusions based on results from anecdotal or uncontrolled studies, and zealous marketing schemes are common among those with a commercial interest in selling light sources and among practitioners eager to provide an expensive new treatment. Popular magazines and other media often mislead public opinion by portraying lasers as nearly magical tools. Despite the hype, it is clear that lasers offer a new method of hair removal, in addition to the conventional methods of shaving, wax epilation, mechanical epilation, and electrolysis.

There are several settings in which permanent hair removal is desired. Hypertrichosis is a common inherited trait for both men and women. In particular, coarse dark hair is easily seen in fair-skinned individuals. Women with polycystic ovary disorder or androgen excess develop hirsutism. Surgical reconstruction with hair-bearing skin grafts is another situation in which removal of coarse, terminal hair is desired. The human hair follicle is a complex structure derived from both epidermal and dermal components. The hair shaft is produced by outward growth of rapidly dividing matrix cells located at the base of the hair follicle, 2 to 7 mm below the skin surface. At this depth, only red and near-infrared wavelengths are useful. The matrix is heavily pigmented (leading to a pigmented hair). In general, the concentration of melanin in the hair is greater in the matrix than in the overlying epidermis. The matrix is supplied by a neurovascular tuft of dermis called the *papilla*. At the beginning of each anagen (growth) phase in the hair growth cycle, stem cells from a region near the insertion of the arrector pili muscle (about 1.5 mm below the surface) proliferate and differentiate to form the matrix. This stem cell region is called the *bulge*, because in mice it appears as a distinct bulge in the follicular epithelium. At the end of the anagen phase, the matrix and lower portion of the follicle degenerate by apoptosis, and the follicle enters a resting phase called *telogen*. Telogen may last from a few weeks to more than a year, depending on the body site. In sites with short hair (i.e., legs), the anagen phase is brief and the telogen phase tends to be longer. In contrast, on the scalp, the anagen phase lasts for years and telogen is relatively brief. The bulge and the papilla appear to be important targets for laser-induced permanent hair removal, but their relative importance is unknown.

Two versions of selective photothermolysis have been attempted for hair removal based on two different target chromophores: melanin and a carbon-containing cream. Ruby lasers have long been known to cause selective injury to pigmented hair follicles. As described above, light at 694 nm is very selectively absorbed by melanin and penetrates deeply into dermis. The Q-switched ruby laser (short pulsewidth) causes damage specifically to pigmented cells, without destroying the ability of follicles to produce a hair shaft.[42] With longer pulses, heat flow during the laser pulse causes more widespread damage to hair follicles and requires higher fluences to compensate for the greater heated volume. Grossman recently reported selective injury and prolonged hair removal by 0.3-ms, 694-nm ruby laser pulses delivered at fluences of 30 to 60 J/cm^2, in a 6- to 8-mm spot size.[57] In this study, fair-skinned volunteers with brown or black hair on the back or thighs were treated with a range of fluences in sites that were either shaved or wax-epilated prior to treatment. Histology showed thermal injury confined to the follicular epithelium and immediately adjacent dermis. At 1 and 3 months after a single treatment, a hair count revealed that there was significant hair loss compared with both control shaved and control wax-epilated sites. Therefore, a biological effect was produced that retarded or eliminated hair growth. Six months after a single treatment, only the shaved sites treated at the highest fluence had significant hair loss, and the control sites all had completely regrown hair. This suggests that the pigmented hair shaft itself acted as a chromophore to enhance injury in the follicles. Two years after a single treatment, 2 of the 12 subjects still have alopecia in the treatment sites (C. Dierickx and M. Grossman, unpublished observation). Side effects were minimal, consisting of transient erythema, edema, focal epidermal injury, and transient pigmentation changes; there was no scarring. Long-pulsewidth ruby laser pulses at high fluence produce selective injury to human hair follicles, prolonged hair growth delay, and in some people permanent hair loss after a single treatment.

Ironically, the only approach now cleared by the FDA and marketed for hair removal in the United States has not been shown to work. In this method, a suspension of amorphous carbon particles is applied to the skin after wax epilation of the hair, followed by 1064-nm Q-switched, Nd:YAG laser-pulse exposures at fluences of about 2 to 5 J/cm^2. The carbon, which is physically similar to that in a tattoo, supplies an exogenous chromophore that is intended to penetrate the hair follicle and produce selective local absorption of light. As with tattoos, Q-switched pulses produce injury to cells in the immediate vicinity of the carbon particles. However, it is unknown whether this produces a significant biologic effect on hair follicles. Physically, it is unlikely that necrosis of either the bulge or papilla can be achieved using short pulses absorbed by carbon particles that are confined to the central space of the hair follicles. Goldberg[58] reported complete or nearly complete hair regrowth after a series of treatments, on a time course similar to that following wax epilation alone. Because the technique is a combination of wax epilation and laser treatment, the role of the laser remains unclear until quantitative measurements are performed of hair regrowth in wax-epilated versus wax-epilated followed by carbon plus laser treatment sites.

Summary

The use of lasers in dermatology has grown at a steady pace, largely as the result of a better understanding and manipulation of the underlying laser-tissue interactions. This trend will continue apace with the increase in the high-technology options that can be integrated with lasers, including light sources that can replace lasers but using similar principles. Leon Goldman, who was the first to use a laser as a surgical tool and has been doing so ever since, kindly warns us: "If you don't need a laser, don't use one." This timeless advice emphasizes that a practical understanding of laser-tissue interactions is more important than the gizmos themselves, no matter how fancy they are.

References

1. Anderson RR, Parrish JA. The optics of human skin. J Invest Dermatol 1981;77:13–19.
2. Van Gemert JMC, Jacques SL, Stereborg HJCM, Star WM. Skin optics. IEEE Trans Biomed Eng 1990;36:1146–1154.
3. Anderson RR, Parrish JA. Microvasculature can be selectively damaged using dye lasers: a basic theory and experimental evidence in human skin. Lasers Surg Med 1981;1:263–266.
4. Van Gemert JMC, Henning JPC. A model approach to laser coagulation of dermal vascular lesions. Arch Dermatol Res 1981;270:429–433.
5. Everett MA, Yeargers E, Sayre RM, Olsen RM. Penetration of epidermis by ultraviolet rays. Photochem Photobiol 1966;5:533.
6. Henderson BW, Dougherty TJ, eds. Photodynamic therapy: basic principles and clinical applications. New York: Marcel Dekker, 1992.
7. Lui H, Anderson RR. Photodynamic therapy in dermatology: recent developments. Dermatol Clinics 1993;11:1–13.
8. Birngruber R. Thermal modelling in biological tissues. In: Hillencamp F, Pratesi R, Sacci CA, eds. Lasers in biology and medicine. New York: Plenum, 1979.

9. Welch AJ. The thermal response of laser irradiated tissue. IEEE J Quant Electron 1984;QE-20:1471–1481.
10. Anderson RR, Parrish JA. Selective photothermolysis: precise microsurgery by selective absorption of pulsed radiation. Science 1983;220: 524–527.
11. Polla BS, Anderson RR. Thermal injury by laser pulses: protection by heat shock despite failure to induce heat-shock response. Lasers Surg Med 1987;7:398–404.
12. Henriques FC. Studies of thermal injury. Arch Pathol 1947;43:489–502.
13. Maytin EV, Wimberley JM, Anderson RR. Thermotolerance and the heat shock response in normal human keratinocytes in culture. J Invest Dermatol 1990;95:635–642.
14. Jacques SL, Nelson JS, Wright WH, Milner TE. Pulsed photothermal radiometry in port-wine lesions. Appl Optics 1993;32:2439–2446.
15. Walsh JT Jr, Flotte TH, Anderson RR, Deutsch TF. Pulsed CO_2 laser tissue ablation: effect of tissue type and pulse duration on thermal damage. Lasers Surg Med 1988;8:108–118.
16. Green HA, Bua D, Anderson R, Nishioka N. Burn depth estimation using indocyanine green fluorescence. Arch Dermatol 1992;128:43–49.
17. Srinivasan R. Ablation of polymers and biological tissue by ultraviolet lasers. Science 1986;234:559–565.
18. Jacques SL, McAuliffe DJ, Blank IH, Parrish JA. Controlled removal of human stratum corneum by pulsed laser. J Invest Dermatol 1987;88: 88–92.
19. Trokel SL, Srinivasan R, Braren B. Excimer laser surgery of the cornea. Am J Ophthalmol 1983;96:710–716.
20. Watenabe S, Flotte JF, McAuliffe DJ, Jacques SL. Putative photoacoustic damage in skin induced by pulsed ArF excimer laser. J Invest Dermatol 1988;90:761.
21. Barsky SH, Rosen S, Geer DE, Noe JM. The nature and evolution of portwine stains: a computer-assisted study. J Invest Dermatol 1976;74: 154–157.
22. Garden JM, Polla LL, Tan OT. The treatment of port wine stains by the pulsed dye laser: analysis of pulse duration and long-term therapy. Arch Dermatol 1990;124:889.
23. Greenwald J, Rosen S, Anderson RR et al. Comparative histologic studies of the tunable dye (at 577 nm) laser and argon laser: the specific vascular effects of the dye laser. J Invest Dermatol 1981;77:305–310.
24. Anderson RR, Jaenicke KF, Parrish JA. Mechanisms of selective vascular changes caused by dye lasers. Lasers Surg Med 1983;3:211–215.
25. Paul BS, Anderson RR, Jarve J, Parrish JA. The effect of temperature and other factors on selective microvascular damage caused by pulsed dye laser. J Invest Dermatol 1983;81:333–336.
26. Garden JM, Tan OT, Kershmann R et al. Effect of dye laser pulse duration on selective cutaneous vascular injury. J Invest Dermatol 1986;87: 653–657.
27. Morelli JG, Tan OT, Garden J et al. Tunable dye laser (577 nm) treatment of port wine stains. Lasers Surg Med 1986;6:94–99.
28. Tan OT, Sherwood K, Gilchrest BA. Treatment of children with portwine stains using the flashlamp-pulsed tunable dye laser. N Engl J Med 1989;320:416–420.
29. Tan OT, Murray S, Kurban AK. Action spectrum of vascular specific injury using pulsed irradiation. J Invest Dermatol 1989;92:868–872.

30. Tan OT, Morrison P, Kurban AK. 585 nm for the treatment of port-wine stains. Plast Reconstr Surg 1990;86:1112–1117.
31. Tong AKF, Tan OT, Boll J, Parrish JA, Murphy GF. Ultrastructure: effects of melanin pigment on target specificity using a pulsed dye laser (577 nm). J Invest Dermatol 1987;88:747–752.
32. Reyes BA, Geronemus R. Treatment of port-wine stains during childhood with the flashlamp pumped pulsed dye laser. J Am Acad Dermatol 1990;23:1142.
33. Levins PC, Grevelink JM, Anderson RR. Action spectrum of immediate and delayed purpura in human skin using a tunable pulsed dye laser. J Invest Dermatol 1991;96:588.
34. Polla LL, Margolis RJ, Dover JS et al. Melanosomes are a primary target of Q-switched ruby laser irradiation in guinea pig skin. J Invest Dermatol 1987;89:281–286.
35. Watanabe S, Anderson RR, Brorson S et al. Comparative studies of femtosecond to microsecond laser pulses on selective pigmented cell injury in skin. Photochem Photobiol 1991;53:757–762.
36. Rispler J, Neister SE. Coaxial flashlamp dye laser in clinical use. Lasers Surg Med 1991;3[suppl]:281.
37. Troccoli J, Roider J, Anderson RR. Multiple-pulse photocoagulation of blood vessels with a 585 nm tunable dye laser. Lasers Surg Med 1992; 4[suppl]:3.
38. Dover JS, Smaoller BR, Stern RS, Rosen S, Arndt KA. Low-fluence carbon dioxide laser irradiation of lentigines. Arch Dermatol 1988;124: 1219–1224.
39. Murphy GF, Shepard RS, Paul BS et al. Organelle-specific injury to melanin-containing cells in human skin by pulsed laser irradiation. Lab Invest 1983;49:680–685.
40. Szabo G et al. Racial differences in the fate of melanosomes in human epidermis. Nature 1969;222:1081–1083.
41. Anderson RR, Margolis RJ, Watenabe S et al. Selective photothermolysis of cutaneous pigmentation by Q-switched Nd:YAG laser pulses at 1064, 532, and 355 nm. J Invest Dermatol 1989;93:28–32.
42. Dover JS, Margolis RJ, Polla LL et al. Pigmented guinea pig skin irradiated with Q-switched ruby laser pulses: morphologic and histologic findings. Arch Dermatol 1989;125:43–49.
43. Ara G, Anderson RR, Mandel KG, Ottesen M, Oseroff AR. Irradiation of pigmented melanoma cells with high intensity pulsed radiation generates acoustic waves and kills cells. Lasers Surg Med 1990;10:52–59.
44. Margolis RJ, Dover JS, Polla LL et al. Visible action spectrum for melanin-specific selective photothermolysis. Lasers Surg Med 1989;9:389–397.
45. Geronemus R. Q-switched ruby laser therapy of nevus of Ota. Arch Dermatol 1992;128:1618–1622.
46. Taylor CR, Flotte T, Michaud N, Jimbow K, Anderson RR. Q-switched ruby laser (QSRL) irradiation of benign pigmented lesions: dermal vs. epidermal. Laser Surg Med 1991;11[suppl 3]:65.
47. Goldman L, Blaney DUJ, Kindel DJ et al. Pathology of the effect of the laser beam on the skin. Nature 1963;197:912.
48. Laub DR, Yules RB, Arras M et al. Preliminary histopathological observation of Q-switched ruby laser radiation on dermal tattoo pigment in man. J Surg Res 1968;5:220.
49. Reid WH, McLeod PJ, Ritchie A et al. Q-switched ruby laser treatment of black tattoos. Br J Plast Surg 1983;36:455–459.

50. Taylor CR, Gange RW, Dover JS et al. Treatment of tattoos by Q-switched ruby laser: a dose-response study. Arch Dermatol 1990;126: 893–899.
51. Taylor CR, Anderson RR, Gange RW, Michaud NA, Flotte TJ. Light and electron microscopic analysis of tattoos treated by Q-switched ruby laser. J Invest Dermatol 1991;97:131–136.
52. Levins PC, Grevelink JM, Anderson RR. Q-switched ruby laser treatment of tattoos. Lasers Surg Med 1991;3[suppl]:63.
53. Grevelink JM, Casparian JM, Gonzalez R et al. Undesirable effects associated with treatment of tattoos and pigmented lesions with the Q-switched lasers at 1064 nm and 694 nm—the MGH experience. Lasers Surg Med 1993;5[suppl]:270.
54. Anderson RR, Geronemus R, Kilmer SL, Farinelli WA, Fitzpatrick RE. Cosmetic tattoo ink darkening: a complication of Q-switched and pulsed laser treatment. Arch Dermatol 1993;129:1010–1014.
55. DeCoste SD, Anderson RR. Comparison of Q-switched ruby and Q-switched Nd:YAG laser treatment of tattoos. Lasers Surg Med 1991;3 [suppl]:64.
56. Levine V, Geronemus R. Tattoo removal with the Q-switched ruby and the Nd:YAG laser: a comparative study. Lasers Surg Med 1993;5[suppl] 260.
57. Grossman MC, Wimberly J, Dwyer P et al. PDT for hirsutism. Lasers Surg Med 1995;7[suppl]:44.
58. Goldberg D. Topical solution-assisted laser hair removal. Lasers Surg Med 1995;7[suppl]:47.

4 ____ Laser Instrumentation

Terry A. Fuller
Alfred Intintoli

The surgical laser is a powerful instrument that has, with time, proved invaluable to medicine. As the base of technology has expanded, almost every type of laser (alexandrite, argon, CO_2, diode, dye, erbium, excimer, frequency-doubled Nd:YAG, holmium, krypton, metal vapor, Nd:YAG, and ruby) has found applications in medicine.

The first operational laser was developed in 1960 by Maiman.[1] His work was based on Albert Einstein's description of stimulated emission of radiation and Townes and Schawlow's work in optical masers. In this laser, a pulsed helical lamp was used to excite a synthetic ruby crystal, producing a concentrated beam of red light. In 1963 Zwang and Peabody, both of whom were ophthalmologists, were the first to use the laser as a surgical instrument. The red beam (694 nm) can pass undisturbed through the transparent ocular media, producing a therapeutic thermal effect at target lesions in the heavily pigmented retina. This simple application elegantly demonstrated the value of lasers in medicine, proving that potent and accurate treatments can be developed that minimally disrupt surrounding healthy tissue.

During the subsequent three decades, tremendous technological advances were made in the field of laser medicine. New wavelengths, sophisticated delivery methods, and more powerful, compact, and reliable laser systems had the effect of transforming the surgical laser from an experimental device into a standard feature in the practice of medicine. Regardless of these changes, however, certain basic constraints define the surgical utility of a given laser. Engineering and design factors determine how practical the system is and which parts of the body energy can be applied to. The physical characteristics of the light-tissue interaction determine the type of therapeutic effects achieved (e.g., vaporization, coagulation).

Numerous lasers use light energy to create principally mechanical or acoustical tissue effects. Other lasers interact with exogenous drugs to produce therapeutic results. Most surgical lasers, however, cause specific thermal effects on targeted tissue. They work through the transformation of light energy into thermal energy. Depending on the temperature at a given point within a volume of tissue, this thermal energy is capable of coagulating, vaporizing, or ablating.

Some tissue effect parameters cannot be controlled, such as the optical characteristics of the target tissue (which dictate the degree of light absorption, or scatter), its thermal conductivity, and the presence of circulating or overlying fluid. Other factors can be controlled, such as the laser power and wavelength, pulse duration and repetition rate, and certain aspects of the delivery system.

The absorption coefficient, α, and the Rayleigh scatter (λ^{-4}) help to define the depth of penetration of a particular wavelength of light into tissue. With high values of α, as occur in the CO_2 laser, energy is readily absorbed by a shallow volume of tissue, which rapidly converts this energy to heat, resulting in very high temperatures. For low values of α, as occur in the noncontact, continuous-wave (cw) Nd:YAG laser, energy is not absorbed as well, producing a more gradual temperature increase distributed throughout a larger, deeper volume. Rayleigh scattering is inversely proportional to the fourth power of the wavelength and is much more pronounced at short wavelengths than at long wavelengths. The scatter at 1064 nm (Nd:YAG laser) is significant and is responsible for large lesions. At 10,600 nm (CO_2 laser), scatter is virtually not present, resulting in lesions about the size of the incident laser beam. Certain qualities of the delivery system can modulate these interactions and, to some degree, uncouple the tissue effect from strict dependence on the laser wavelength.

Laser and delivery systems available today reflect the constant advances being made through research and engineering. The performances and clinical applications of each of these vary, and these are briefly reviewed here for each.

Lasers

CO_2 LASER

The CO_2 laser was developed by C. K. N. Patel[2] at Bell Laboratories in 1964 and for many years was the most widely used laser in medicine. It involves the combination of CO_2, helium, and nitrogen gases in a sealed tube and uses them as the excitation medium. In the past the active medium was stimulated longitudinally by high-voltage direct current, producing up to 100 W of cw output at a wavelength (far-infrared) of 10,600 nm. Because this beam is invisible, a low-power red (633 nm) helium-neon laser beam is aligned coincident with the treatment beam to assist in aiming. Currently a radio-frequency discharge transverse to the tube axis permits the electronic control of the laser output and allows the user to operate in a pulsed mode. Although the electronics necessary for this approach can be more expensive and complex, the system operates at a lower voltage and uses simpler, less costly tubes. The sealed gas tube needs to be replaced occasionally, and the aiming beam needs to be realigned periodically, but otherwise the CO_2 laser is a comparatively simple, efficient, and dependable instrument.

CO_2 laser light is extremely well absorbed by water, which is ubiquitous in all organs, including skin. As a result, 90% of the energy dissipates in the first 0.1 mm of skin, using a 0.2-second exposure time and a 1-mm spot size. Historically the CO_2 laser has been used as a cw laser. Pulsed CO_2 laser technology has gained popularity for cutaneous applications.

Once CO_2 laser light impacts skin, it produces several changes. If the temperature of skin is brought no higher than 45°C for 20 minutes or no higher than 90°C for less than 1 msec, only reversible damage is done. There is, however, a threshold for irreversible damage at approximately 60°C. Type I collagen melts when exposed to this temperature for more than 1 second. DNA melts at 75°C. Tissue vaporizes at 100°C and above 300°C carbonization is frequent (Anderson, verbal communication). When CO_2 laser light impacts skin, vaporization occurs centrally, surrounding which is a zone of irreversible thermal damage and necrosis, which in turn is surrounded by a zone of reversible thermal damage. As a focused beam, the CO_2 laser light generates very high power densities, which cut tissue. Defocusing the beam increases the spot size and decreases the power density, such that the tissue temperatures are lower and the tissue is vaporized rather than excised. Although the cw CO_2 laser can be used to vaporize thin layers of skin, the residual thermal damage is between 50 and 600 μm in depth. By using short pulses of CO_2 laser light, thin layers of skin can be ablated with a much smaller zone of thermal damage, on the order of 20 to 100 μm deep. Data indicate that, as long as the pulse duration of short-pulse CO_2 laser light is less than 1 msec at fluences above the ablation threshold of skin, which is 2 to 5 J/cm^2, a significant portion of the impacted tissue is ablated or vaporized and a very thin layer of residual thermal damage is left behind.

There are several devices currently approved by the U.S. Food and Drug Administration and being marketed in the United States for skin resurfacing. Two are true pulsed CO_2 lasers: the Coherent Ultrapulse 100-W laser, which produces fluences per pulse of up to 500 mJ at a pulse duration ranging from 600 μsec to 1 msec. Tissue Technologies makes a 60-μsec, pulsed CO_2 laser that generates fluences above the ablation threshold of skin. Several superpulsed CO_2 lasers that produce individual pulses or a train of CO_2 laser pulses are being marketed for laser skin resurfacing. They remove less tissue per pulse than the pulsed CO_2 lasers and leave behind a wider zone of thermal damage. Sharplan produces a cw CO_2 laser (Silktouch) that is scanned through a computer-driven mechanical device that is affixed to the handpiece of the CO_2 laser. This device scans a 0.2-mm spot in a helical pattern from 2 to 9 mm at a constant velocity so that no individual spot within the helix is hit more than once and the dwell time on any individual spot is less than 1 msec. The skin perceives a CO_2 laser light pulse above the ablation threshold, and as a result, this clever device is able to ablate thin layers of skin with a narrow zone of thermal damage.

Far-infrared light does not transmit through quartz, glass, or other materials transparent to visible light that are commonly used as light guides in flexible endoscopic delivery devices. The CO_2 laser beam must, however, be delivered as a free beam or through rigid endoscopes and mirrored, jointed articulated arms. Semiflexible waveguides have been developed, but it is unlikely that they will rival quartz optical fibers in terms of flexibility and size, though some progress has been made in this regard.

CO_2 lasers range in size and power, from small units delivering 40 W or less of power, which is suitable for use in a physician's office or clinic, to more substantial hospital units ranging up to 100 W in power. CO_2 lasers are used almost exclusively in open surgical operations and rigid endoscopy procedures, as in the treatment of cervical dysplasia.

ARGON-ION AND KRYPTON-ION LASERS

The introduction of a practical cw argon-ion gas laser in 1966 marked, in many respects, the true beginning of the surgical laser revolution. Operating in the blue-green region of the visible spectrum (488–514 nm), the argon laser possesses one of the lowest absorption coefficients for water. However, its beam is preferentially absorbed by tissue pigments such as hemoglobin and melanin. The argon-ion laser quickly replaced the ruby laser for retinal laser therapy and has since been approved for other ophthalmic applications.

The active medium for the argon-ion and krypton-ion lasers is a rare gas that has had an electron, or electrons, removed to form a positive ion. The positive ions are excited by a high-current discharge, producing laser emissions in the near-infrared, visible, and ultraviolet regions of the spectrum.

Compared with the CO_2 laser, the argon-ion and krypton-ion lasers offer a mixture of advantages and drawbacks. With regard to the former, the visible argon and krypton beams do not require a separate, coincident aiming beam. Because the beam can pass through quartz optical fibers, the argon-ion and krypton-ion lasers can be used with operating microscopes and slit lamps and the radiation can be delivered to virtually every part of the body accessible with current endoscopic devices. On the other hand, gaseous ion lasers are inherently inefficient. A very high input power (8–26 kW) is required to generate comparatively low light output (argon, 3–5 W; krypton, 0.75 W). Cooling devices consist of forced air for lower-power units and water cooling for higher-power units, making units with an output of more than 20 W prohibitively unwieldy. In addition, the life of a tube is several thousand hours and replacements are about one third the total cost of the system.

FREQUENCY-DOUBLED ND:YAG AND ND:YAG LASERS

Lasers employing a neodymium-doped crystal of yttrium-aluminum-garnet (Nd:YAG) were introduced in 1963.[3] These lasers require a visible aiming beam because they typically emit light at 1064 nm, in the near-infrared region of the spectrum. This wavelength can be transmitted through quartz optical fibers and is more highly scattered and less rapidly absorbed in tissue than green laser light is. These solid-state lasers are reliable and relatively efficient. Commercial units require 120 volts at 20 amps (single phase) to deliver power up to 40 W and 220 volts at 30 amps (single phase) to attain powers of 100 W. Technological improvements made within the past several years have made it possible to produce portable models measuring approximately 20 inches (50 cm) square and 35 inches (87.5 cm) high and weighing under 300 pounds (135 kg).

Because of its low absorption coefficient and less dependence on tissue pigmentation for its effect, the Nd:YAG laser beam (at 1064 nm) penetrates 5 to 7 mm into most tissue. This makes it a powerful coagulating device for use at sites of active bleeding or for the relatively imprecise ablation of vascular tissue. Used in its conventional, noncontact mode, the 1064-nm beam cannot, however, be used for accurate cutting, though the introduction of contact laser delivery devices has made it possible to slightly modify the Nd:YAG photothermal effect.

In addition to the cw mode, the Nd:YAG laser beam can be delivered in short, high-power pulses or the laser can be used in a special mode called *Q-switching*. The pulse-pumped, Q-switched Nd:YAG laser delivers 10- to 12-nsec pulses at peak power levels, measured in gigawatts. These intensities do not create a thermal effect but do ionize atoms, creating an explosive shock wave that photodisrupts adjacent structures upon their collapse. These pulse-pumped, Q-switched lasers are commonly used by ophthalmologists to rupture the posterior capsule of the eye, which sometimes opacifies after cataract extraction. Q-switched Nd:YAG lasers are also used in the treatment of cutaneous pigmented lesions and tattoos.

The frequency-doubled Nd:YAG (or KTP) laser emits a 532-nm green beam, which is comparable to the argon beam in terms of the therapeutic effect. Technologically, however, the KTP laser is entirely different. Rather than a gas, it employs a crystal of potassium titanyl phosphate (KTP) to double the frequency of the 1064-nm Nd:YAG beam. The fact that it is a solid-state laser renders it significantly more efficient and reliable than argon, though its surgical performance is essentially the same and available power levels are currently limited to about 30 W.

The green light of the argon-ion and KTP laser passes through water and transparent media. It is scattered and absorbed within a depth of 1 to 2 mm in average tissue, though this varies considerably depending on the pigmentation. These lasers can create sufficiently high power densities to cut adequately in vascular tissue, but they do not provide efficient hemostasis. In avascular tissue, however, the green beam has very good shallow hemostatic capabilities.

The Nd:YAG laser can also operate at 1319 or 1444 nm when the strongest emission at 1064 nm is suppressed. Both are pulse-pumped with a flashlamp and produce long pulsewidths of 250 to 650 μsec. Their output is in the near-infrared region of the spectrum and is invisible, thus a coincident aiming beam is required. These systems are capable of producing average powers of 30 W; however, their efficiencies are lower than 1064 nm and they require higher input powers (i.e., three-phase, 208 volts, 30 amps). Cooling is provided by a closed-circuit water system, with forced air used to control the water temperature. These systems tend to be larger and heavier (e.g., 450 pounds [202.5 kg]) than conventional 1064-nm systems.

Both 1319- and 1444-nm beams are readily absorbed by water and therefore require the use of low-water (OH$^-$)–content quartz fiberoptics to deliver the pulsed energy to the target tissue. Compared with the 1064-nm beam, the 1319-nm beam provides better vaporization as the result of its relative reduction in tissue penetration, while still achieving good coagulation. The 1444-nm beam is excellent for vaporization because of its shallow (0.4-mm) penetration of tissue, though this results in minimal to no coagulation. The combination of the long pulse length and shallow penetration depth can prevent damage to adjacent tissue because the thermal energy is then diffused away from the ablation site. The 1319-nm beam is well suited to a wide variety of general surgical applications. The 1444-nm beam, which is identical in its therapeutic effect to that of a holmium laser, with a 2127-nm beam, should prove readily acceptable for arthroscopic (avascular) procedures.

HOLMIUM LASER

The holmium laser was recently introduced commercially and has gained immediate popularity for use in orthopedic procedures and other applications requiring the vaporization of avascular tissue. This solid-state laser emits light at 2127 nm and can be delivered through low-water-content quartz fibers. The holmium laser beam is highly absorbed by water and vaporizes with a 0.4-mm tissue penetration, identical to that of the 1444-nm beam. As a result of the shallow penetration, minimal to no coagulation is possible. Deep-tissue necrosis is minimized by the combination of the short pulse length and shallow penetration depth.

The active medium of this laser is a YAG crystal doped with holmium, erbium, and thulium. The crystal is excited by a pulsed flashlamp and produces long pulsewidths of 250 to 400 μsec. Its output is in the mid-infrared spectrum and is invisible, thus a coincident aiming beam is required. The holmium laser is capable of producing average powers of 30 W, but its efficiencies are low and it requires high input powers. Cooling is provided by a closed-circuit water system with forced air. The present system is large, heavy (i.e., 600 pounds [270 kg]), and costly. Its efficacy is being investigated in a variety of medical applications beyond orthopedics, and it has already been approved for use in peripheral angioplasty procedures.

ERBIUM LASER

The erbium laser, operating at a wavelength of 2940 nm, has the potential to be the best device for tissue vaporization. The active medium of this solid-state laser is a YAG crystal doped with erbium. The crystal is excited by a pulsed flashlamp and produces long pulsewidths of 0.1 to 4 msec. If the laser is Q-switched, pulses as short as 50 nsec can be generated. Its output is in the mid-infrared region of the spectrum and is invisible, thus a coincident aiming beam is required. The erbium laser is capable of producing average powers of 5 W. Cooling is provided by a closed-circuit water system with forced air.

Investigators are studying the erbium laser's efficacy in a variety of medical settings, including soft and hard dental surgery and intraocular microsurgery. The absorption of its beam by water is the highest of that for any commercially available laser, producing coagulation of tissue to a depth of 25 μm. Because of the shallow penetration, hemostasis is not practical, however. Adjacent tissue necrosis is eliminated by the combination of short pulse length and shallow penetration depth, resulting in precise tissue cutting.

A 2940-nm beam cannot pass through the standard silica materials commonly used as light guides in flexible endoscopic delivery devices. Because of this, the erbium laser beam must be delivered as a free beam or through rigid endoscopes and mirrored, jointed, articulated arms. Semiflexible infrared fibers have been developed, but they are made of toxic materials, and it is unlikely that they will equal quartz optical fibers in terms of flexibility and durability. The lack of a good flexible delivery system has seriously impaired the marketability of this laser, but its potential has nonetheless fueled continued research and development.

RUBY LASER

The ruby laser was the first operational laser. This solid-state laser emits light at 694 nm. The active medium of this laser is a sapphire crystal doped with chromium. The crystal is excited by a pulsed flashlamp and Q-switched to produce short pulsewidths of 25 nsec. Its output in the red region of the spectrum is visible, so no aiming beam is required. The ruby laser typically produces 2 J of energy per pulse at a repetition rate of 1 Hz. Efficiencies are low, however, and high-input powers are required. Cooling is provided by a closed-circuit water system with an integrated chiller to control the water temperature. Like the holmium laser, this system is large, heavy (i.e., 500 pounds [225 kg]), and costly.

Standard silica materials, which are commonly used as light guides in flexible endoscopic delivery devices, can transmit the 694-nm beam. However, the ruby laser beam's high peak power density (irradiance) exceeds the damage threshold of the silica material. Because of this, mirrored, jointed, articulated arms must be used. The 694-nm beam is not well absorbed by water, though its absorption by melanin is nearly four times greater than that of the 1064-nm beam. Additionally, the green, blue, and black pigments of tattoos readily absorb the 694-nm beam. These qualities, together with the combination of its short pulse length (25 nsec) and deep penetration (>1 mm), make the ruby laser well suited to the removal of tattoos and epidermal and dermal pigmented lesions.

METAL VAPOR LASER

The copper vapor laser was introduced in 1966 by W. T. Walter and colleagues at TRG Inc. The active medium is created by heating a neutral metal beyond its vapor point and exciting the metal ions with a fast (pulsed) electric discharge. The wavelength emitted is dependent on the metal used.

The gold vapor laser, emitting at 628 nm, is useful for the photoradiation and photodynamic therapy of cancer. The copper vapor laser, at 511 and 578 nm, is finding applications in dermatology. Both the 511- and 578-nm beams operate simultaneously, however, and have to be separated before delivery. The 511-nm beam is well absorbed by melanin and is best suited to the treatment of epidermal pigmented lesions. The 578-nm laser output is well absorbed by hemoglobin and is used in the treatment of vascular lesions.

Very high temperatures are required to vaporize the metals. This entails heating the laser tube for 45 minutes before lasing. The pulsewidths of the laser output are less than 100 nsec, with repetition rates of 4 to 15 kHz. At these fast repetition rates, the laser output appears to be a continuous wave. Pulse energies vary from 1 to 20 mJ. These lasers' overall electrical efficiencies are low (Cu, 0.2%–1.0%; Au, 0.1%–0.2%), however, and they require high-input powers. These systems also tend to be large, and frequent maintenance is required, especially to replenish the metals.

ALEXANDRITE LASERS

The year 1979 brought J. Walling's discovery that the solid-state alexandrite laser is more efficient and tunable at longer wavelengths (720–800 nm) than at 680 nm. The alexandrite laser has chromium-doped chrysoberyl as its active medium. The solid-state crystal can be pumped by a pulsed flashlamp or cw arc lamp. What is unusual about it, however, is that, as the system temperature rises, the laser output increases. The laser is adequately efficient (1% overall), requiring only 220 volts at 30 amps. Cooling is provided by a closed-circuit water system with forced air. Like the Nd:YAG laser (1064 nm), this system is compact, measuring 33 inches (82.5 cm) wide, 22 inches (55 cm) deep, and 38 inches (95 cm) high and weighing less than 350 pounds (157.5 kg).

The fundamental wavelength of the alexandrite laser is 755 nm. Its output in the red region of the spectrum is past the limit of visibility, and thus an aiming beam is required. When pulse pumped, the energy ranges from 1 to 3 J with pulsewidths of 100 to 400 μsec. If Q-switched, the energy output varies from 0.1 to 0.5 J with pulsewidths of 30 to 250 nsec. The average power of the fundamental output could equal 20 W. Frequency doubling results in laser outputs tunable from 360 to 400 nm.

The advantages of the alexandrite laser are that it is absorbed by pigments (blue and black) in tattoos, less absorbed by melanin, and minimally absorbed by hemoglobin. These factors, along with its pulsewidth and tissue penetration, enable the alexandrite laser to be used in tattoo removal and in the treatment of benign pigmented lesions. Its delivery system does not require an articulated arm and permits the use of a flexible light guide. Clinical studies are currently being conducted on the efficacy of the alexandrite laser in the fragmentation of urinary and biliary calculi (stones).

DYE LASERS

Dye lasers, first developed at IBM Laboratories in 1966, offer the unique advantage of allowing operators to tune the wavelength over a considerable range to obtain the absorption coefficient and tissue interaction best suited to the particular application.

Dye lasers operate using an organic fluorescent material that is dissolved in a solvent and optically pumped using a pulsed flashlamp, argon, or other laser. Continuous-wave and pulsed dye lasers, emitting wavelengths between 400 and 1000 nm, have proved extremely useful in ophthalmology for the accurate treatment of macular lesions. They are also of great value in dermatology for the treatment of vascular and pigmented lesions of the epidermis. In addition, their photoacoustic effect also makes them effective in the fragmentation of urinary and biliary stones. Dye lasers have been used to help sort cells and in the application of photodynamic therapy for cancer treatment. Dye lasers are highly inefficient generators of optical power. They require considerable electrical power, and the hazardous, costly dye is consumed rapidly. Dye lasers are also relatively large and expensive, but their adjustable wavelengths are of benefit in certain applications.

DIODE LASERS

Diode lasers are semiconductor devices that were developed in 1972. These devices fall into several distinct groups. The groups of most significance to the medical history are the GaAs and GaAlAs devices (780 to 870 nm) and, most recently, the InGaAlP and InGaP types (630 to 700 nm). The light output is generated when electric current is passed through the diode. Individual diodes emit light from the edge of a wafer or from their surface. Multiple-diode lasers grown in linear and two-dimensional arrays are being used in the pumping of solid-state lasers (e.g., Nd:YAG) in the place of flashlamps. The advantage of these lasers is the improved electrical efficiency of the overall laser system, but this is outweighed by the present high cost of the diodes. By coupling laser diode power directly to fiberoptic delivery devices, it is possible to get a power of 10 W from an individual diode array and of 25 W from groups of diodes. These long-lived systems are extremely small and portable and require no maintenance or water cooling. The only disadvantage to the high-powered diode laser is its expense. Currently, commercial laser diode–based instruments are available for photodynamic therapy and ophthalmic applications. There are also ones to directly replace cw Nd:YAG (1064 nm) lasers operating to 60 W.

EXCIMER LASERS

The name *excimer* comes from "excited dimer" and refers to a group of lasers with high peak powers (nanosecond pulsewidths) and emissions in the ultraviolet or near-ultraviolet region of the spectrum. The most important excimers make use of rare gas halides (i.e., ArF, 193 nm; KrF, 249 nm; XeF, 350 nm; XeCl, 308 nm; KrCl, 222 nm).

The active medium of the excimer lasers requires three flowing gases: an inert buffer (He or Ne), an active rare gas (Ar, Kr, Xe), and a halogen (Cl or Fl). A repetitively pulsed electric discharge excites the active medium to produce the laser output, with the gas life expectancy dependent on the number of pulses. A vacuum pump is needed to remove the spent gases, which are hazardous and costly to replenish. The electrical efficiency of these lasers is relatively good (e.g., KrF laser, 1.5% to 2.0%), and most systems use 120 volts at 10 amps. The laser is typically cooled with a closed-circuit water system with forced air to control the water temperature. As a medical device, the excimer laser is still evolving. Tremendous interest has been focused on its ability to sculpt the surface of the cornea (ArF laser, 193 nm), thereby correcting refractive errors in vision, and to remove plaque from clogged arteries (XeCl laser, 308 nm) (angioplasty).

Delivery Devices

ARTICULATED ARM

An articulated arm is a precision assembly of hollow tubes, mirrors, and joints. It permits the delivery of a light beam, through simple reflection, from the laser head to the operating site. The beam emerging from the distal end of the arm retains the same spatial and temporal characteristics of the original laser beam and can be focused or defocused by lenses to produce the spot size and resulting power density appropriate for a particular application.

The articulated arm is widely used for CO_2 lasers, whose infrared beam cannot pass through flexible quartz fiberoptics. Though these devices make the laser considerably more versatile, the complex mechanical joints render them cumbersome. Rough treatment of the delicate mirrors, or poor maintenance, can lead to degradation of the beam quality. Moreover, if a second laser beam is employed for aiming (as in the CO_2 laser), it is possible for the two beams to be misaligned, resulting in inaccurate targeting of the treatment beam.

MICROMANIPULATORS

Many applications of laser energy require or benefit from manipulation of the laser beam through an optomechanical mechanism. Such a device, referred to as a *micromanipulator* or *joystick,* is generally used with a surgical microscope. As the joystick is manipulated the laser beam is moved around the surgical site while in direct magnified view of the surgeon. The motion of the beam can be controlled directly by the surgeon or directly by a computer. Computer or microprocessor control permits the surgeon to simply outline an area for treatment, and then the computer scans the beam within the outlined area.

SCANNERS

With the advent of the scanner, an accurate and repeatable microprocessor-controlled delivery of pulsed or cw laser output was possible, circumventing the problems posed by inconsistent freehand methods. The scanner's nonaligned treatment pattern allows the thermal energy in adjacent tissue to cool adequately between pulses of laser energy. The scanner has proved of value to both dermatologists and plastic surgeons.

FIBEROPTICS

The most common and convenient way of delivering laser energy to tissue is through flexible optical fibers. They can be used with micromanipulators or handpieces or can be passed through most standard operating endoscopes. Fiberoptics are composed of two or more concentrically arranged optical materials, and light is carried along the length of the fiber by total internal reflection.

Surgical fiberoptics are relatively inexpensive and are far more convenient than articulated arms. They can carry power from any cw laser that operates in the visible or near-infrared regions of the spectrum. Disposable fibers and fibers with integrated specialized handpieces have now largely replaced reusable fibers, which required periodic recleaving or polishing of the distal quartz surface.

Once light is captured in the fiber, it is transmitted the length of the device, so that there is no alignment problem with aiming and treatment beams. On the other hand, the beam does lose coherence as it passes down the fiber, resulting in a slightly divergent beam and increased spot size at the treatment site. Lenses and contact probes can be used to focus this emergent beam.

ENDOSCOPIC DEVICES

In the beginning, endoscopy was an exclusively diagnostic technique, though early in the 20th century limited therapeutic procedures were carried out using this technology. Over the past decade, small-incision endoscopic surgery has revolutionized the treatment of numerous diseases. This is attributable to the simultaneous development of practical laser systems (capable of vaporizing and coagulating via flexible fiberoptics) and the achievement of technological advances in high-resolution charge-coupled device (CCD) cameras; endoscopic ligating, suturing, and clipping devices; safer electrosurgery instruments; flexible endoscopes; and an expanding array of fine manipulating instruments. Though lasers do not deserve sole credit for this revolution, and are not the appropriate endoscopic treatment modality in all settings, the ability to cut or ablate tissue endoscopically with simultaneous hemostasis has largely eliminated one of the most problematic aspects of small-incision surgery.

CONTACT ND:YAG LASER

The ultimate concern in laser surgery is the tissue effect. Photothermal lasers produce their surgical effect through the transformation of light energy into heat, usually as a result of light energy being absorbed by tissue. When affixed to the distal end of a fiberoptic, contact laser probes can alter the optical, mechanical, and thermodynamic properties of the delivery device.

Whereas light emerges from a fiberoptic as a slightly divergent beam, it refracts within a contact tip. Depending on such factors as the angle of convergence and the size and shape of the distal face, the beam can be emitted as a divergent or convergent beam or it can be laterally radiated from the sides of the contact tip. Contact probes are made of durable, rigid materials with high melting points. They can be used mechanically and brought in contact with tissue, unlike a bare fiberoptic that can break or melt easily. A 2.5-mm-diameter cylindrical probe can provide a surface area to tamponade a bleeding vessel, together with a laser power density suitable for coagulation. A contact laser scalpel, tapered to 0.2 mm in diameter, can provide the small spot size and high-power density needed for fine incision with minimal coagulation.

The most important property of contact laser probes is the manner in which they titrate the light and thermal energy that emerges from the delivery device. Rather than delivering a beam of pure light energy that is converted to heat entirely within the tissue, special absorbant coatings and surfaces on the contact laser probes can transform a predetermined portion of the light energy into heat at the probe's surface. This modifies the surface temperature and tissue temperature gradient to suit the surgical need. Therefore, rather than selecting a laser type according to the absorption coefficient that produces the desired effect in the tissue, one can choose the contact laser probe or scalpel that creates the appropriate temperature gradient.

Contact laser probes can be employed with any cw laser operating in the visible or near-infrared regions of the spectrum. One cannot, however, increase the penetration of a laser beam with a relatively high absorption coefficient, such as the green light lasers. Though a contact probe will enable them to cut well, it cannot increase their capacity for deep coagulation. With longer-wavelength lasers, such as the diode or Nd:YAG, it is possible to use the full penetration or, when deep thermal effects are not wanted, to reduce penetration by transforming more light energy into heat at the probe surface. In this way, a single laser can be made to mimic the tissue effects of many lasers of different wavelengths, while adding optical and mechanical features not available with a simple fiberoptic device.

References

1. Maiman TH. Stimulated optical radiation in ruby. Nature 1960;187:493–494.
2. Patel CKN, McFarlane RA, Faust WL. Selective excitation through vibrational energy transfer and optical maser action in N_2-CO_2. Phys Rev 1964; 13:617–619.
3. Johnson LF. Optical maser characteristics of rare-earth ions in crystals. J Appl Physics 1963;34:897–909.

Bibliography

Hecht J. The laser guidebook. Blue Ridge Summit, PA: TAB Books, 1992.

II. Laser Modalities and Selection

5 ——— Continuous-Wave and Quasi–Continuous-Wave Lasers

Vicki J. Levine
Margaret S. Lee
Roy G. Geronemus
Kenneth A. Arndt

The discussion in this chapter focuses on continuous-wave and pulse-train lasers emitting beams in the visible region of the spectrum and used in the treatment of cutaneous disorders. These lasers include the argon laser, whose principal wavelengths are 488 and 514 nm; the continuous-wave argon-pumped dye laser, most often used at wavelengths of from 577 to 585 nm; the krypton laser, with wavelengths of 520 and 568 nm; the two lasers whose train of pulses are interpreted by tissue as continuous-wave radiation, the copper vapor and copper bromide, used at a wavelength of 511 nm for pigmented lesions and a wavelength of 578 nm for vascular lesions, and the KTP laser, which emits radiation at 532 nm. Robotic optical scanners and automated robotized handpieces, which may be used with all of these lasers, are also described.

The Argon Laser

HISTORY

The argon laser was the first laser to be widely used in clinical practice, and its history, design, and physics are discussed here in detail. Thirty years after Albert Einstein postulated that stimulated emission of radiation was possible, C. H. Townes, in 1954, announced the creation of the first working laser, which produced microwaves from ammonia molecules. Six years later, J. P. Gordon and colleagues[1] operated the first visible light laser. Just 6 months after T. H. Maiman reported his success with the ruby crystal laser,[2] Javan, Bennett, and Herriot[3] reported their operation of the first gas laser, a helium-neon laser. After this, the discovery of the other laser emission wavelengths and the development of laser applications progressed rapidly. By 1965, a thousand different laser wavelengths had been observed, including argon laser wavelengths.[4] For a decade (1975–1985), the argon laser became the most well known and most widely used laser in medicine.

In 1964, W. B. Bridges[5] operated and fully described the first argon laser, a pulsed ion laser. Convert, Armande, and Martinot-

Lagarde,[6] of France, unexpectedly discovered a blue argon laser line while using argon to buffer a mercury vapor discharge, and they published a paper about it, which appeared 9 days before Bridges' paper did. However, because they did not know where the blue line came from, credit for the argon laser is rightfully given to Bridges. His laser consisted of a fused quartz discharge tube, approximately 1 m long and 4 mm in diameter, with Brewster angle windows and filled with either pure argon or with neon or helium added as a buffer gas, maintained at a pressure of a few millimeters of mercury for argon and 200 mm Hg for the buffer gas. He used different dielectric-coated or aluminized mirrors to obtain ten different wavelength outputs, the strongest of which were 488 and 514.5 nm. The total average output power was between 0.2 and 0.5 mW, and the peak output power was between 0.4 to 1.0 W. In his paper Bridges provides a table giving the measured laser wavelengths, the tentative energy level assignments, and the estimated gains. It is likely, however, that several researchers began studying argon at the same time, because argon was so commonly used in experiments to buffer mercury.[7]

A few weeks after Bridges' paper appeared, W. R. Bennett, Jr., and associates[8] published a paper describing the quasi–continuous-wave operation of seven argon lines, in which they reported power outputs of 1 W at 488 nm and about 10 W at 514.5 nm. In the same issue of the journal, immediately before Bennett's article, E. I. Gordon, E. F. Labuda, and W. B. Bridges reported on the fully continuous-wave argon laser operation of all ten of the wavelengths described in his paper. At a wavelength of 488 nm they obtained an approximate output power of 1.5 mW with a DC discharge current of 6 amp and at a pressure of 0.45 mm Hg. They found that relatively high currents and pressure are required to obtain highly charged particle densities within the laser cavity. The paper also included data on the threshold current and showed the dependence of output power on the discharge current. Gordon and associates[9] also were the first to use a reflecting prism to single out a particular wavelength and were able to do this even at high currents.

In 1965 and thereafter these men continued to make contributions to our understanding of the performance of the argon-ion laser. Labuda, Gordon, and R. C. Miller discovered that, by using an axial magnetic field with high currents, low pressure, and large-diameter tubes or by using metal-walled discharge vessels, the problem of high-energy ions bombarding—and thereby decomposing—the quartz discharge tubes was solved. An axial magnetic field also increases the density of the charged particles, thus increasing the output power available and decreasing the output power dependence on the tube diameter. The metal-wall discharge vessel is able to conduct away generated heat, and it does not decompose and contaminate the laser discharge because ionized metal particles are deposited elsewhere on the tube wall; thus, the wall thickness remains acceptably constant for a much longer time than that of the quartz tubes. Eventually, however, the walls do erode and metal is deposited at the anode and cathode ends. Limits on the length of metal tubing that worked optimally were overcome by assembling several metal discharge tubes or disks connected by ceramic insulator sections and sealing them within a vacuum envelope.[10]

Further work on inert gas lasers led to a great increase in their power, efficiency, and practicality. In addition, many innovative medical laser applications available today were made possible as the result of the development of specialized light delivery systems and energy production or emission control systems.

PRESENT DESIGN OF THE ARGON LASER

As a result of the discoveries and the kind of developmental efforts just described, the argon-ion lasers used today for medical applications can produce 1 to 20 W of power in continuous-wave operation,[11] principally at the 488- and 514.5-nm blue-green visible wavelengths. A typical argon laser tube is made of beryllium oxide, which is hardier than fused quartz and has better thermal conductivity. There are Brewster windows on each end to allow lasing of only one polarity and external mirrors to facilitate mirror changes and adjustments. The metal disk arrangement just described and a solenoid or other magnetic source together create an axial magnetic field for the central portion of the laser cavity. An oxide-coated cathode at one end of the tube emits the arc discharge and a molybdenum or stainless steel anode is at the opposite end. A water jacket surrounding the tube may be used to provide cooling in addition to the radiative cooling that occurs in the metal disks. The discharge tube must also have some sort of gas return line along the tube length, because, since electrons are too light to maintain an even pressure at the other end of the tube, positive ions tend to collect at the cathode and disrupt the pressure equilibrium during DC operation. Axis holes in the metal cooling disks should allow access to the gas bypass. A complete laser system must also include power sources: protective devices such as interlocks and ballast resistors; the starting circuit; a gas reservoir to replenish the gas, which tends to leak out slowly; gutters, which remove gas impurities; and gauges and meters to regulate and measure the gas pressure, current, and energy output. Higher-powered argon-ion lasers have mirrors that reflect many wavelengths, and the user selects the particular wavelength desired using an optical filter or prism.[7,12,13]

Medical argon lasers usually operate at only a few watts of power and emit all the light produced at wavelengths of 488 to 514.5 nm; singling out one wavelength is generally unnecessary. As a medical tool, argon-ion laser radiation can be coupled into an optical fiber attached to a lightweight handpiece that often can be removed and exchanged for a handpiece with different focusing optics to create different spot sizes. A mechanical shutter can be used to control the exposure time during treatment; in this way, varying pulsed effects as well as continuous-wave irradiation can be achieved.

A growing variety of laser accessories are being developed and tested for use in specific medical applications; these include special probes and systems for use in dermatology, angioplasty, gynecology, and ophthalmologic microsurgery.[14–18]

PHYSICS AND BIOPHYSICS

The light amplification produced by the stimulated emission of radiation in the argon-ion laser is accomplished by sending a large amount of electric energy through pressurized argon gas, whose electrons absorb this energy and move to ionic levels. An electron voltage of 15.75 eV is necessary to ionize a neutral atom. A second electron collision must occur to further excite the ion to energy levels at least 19.68 eV above the argon-ion ground state. Thus, this two-step excitation process requires a relatively large amount of energy, with current densities of up to 10 amps/mm^2. Laser emission occurs when electrons drop from 4p to 4s energy levels (including one 4p' to 3d transition), because the 4s level is the upper level for a vacuum-UV transition to the ion ground state and this very high energy transition of about 72 nm has a much shorter lifetime than the 4p-to-4s transition.[7] This means more electrons remain at the upper ion levels than at the lower ion levels (which are nearly empty), resulting in population inversion. Continued energy input causes the excited ions to emit the same energy instead of just absorbing it. This amplification process is maintained and directed by sending the energy back and forth through the lasing medium with the mirrors at each end of the laser cavity, though a certain amount of energy is lost through the mirrors. Laser action occurs as long as gain conditions exceed the losses, but output efficiencies are often only a few hundredths to a tenth of a percent.[13,19]

The line width of the ionic transitions are essentially entirely due to Doppler broadening, with broadening here being a measure of nonuniformity in the energy emission. Individual atoms—especially in a hot gas—move about at random speeds and directions, in or against the direction of the laser radiation, so that the frequency response of an atom becomes shifted. Different atoms may move at different velocities and contribute to different parts of the emission spectrum in a particular instant, causing a nonhomogeneous broadening. However, because of the finiteness of emission, natural broadening is homogeneous, in that any atom at any instant is capable of contributing to all frequencies. Collision broadening, a homogeneous broadening due to the physical interaction of the excited atoms, and natural broadening together make up what is called a *lorentzian-function emitted spectrum*. The natural linewidth of the two strongest wavelengths emitted by argon lasers, 488 and 514.5 nm, is about 100 MHz. Due to collisions, the lorentzian width is about

600 MHz. The Doppler width, however, is about 5 GHz, so one can essentially disregard the other broadening effects. When a Doppler-broadened laser eventually reaches gain saturation—operation near the lasing threshold—if the homogeneous linewidth is greater than the spacing between modes of emission, as in the argon laser, the several possible lasing modes compete for ions and not all of them actually lase.[20] Approximately 45% of the output is at 488 nm, 37% is at 514.5 nm, and a tiny 6% is at either 496.5 or 476.5 nm. The remaining output consists of three or four wavelengths between 454.5 and 528.7 nm, from violet to blue to green.[7]

These wavelengths are effective or medical use because hemoglobin and other chromophores can absorb them well. Furthermore, the water in tissue often acts as a black body and rapidly absorbs laser energy. The intense, coherent energy of a laser can vaporize or necrotize tissue wherever a great deal of photon or electron absorption has occurred. Tissue adjacent to the target sites may undergo thermal damage due to scattering and diffusion of the applied energy, but this may or may not be desired, depending on the area and purpose of the medical procedure. Choosing a laser and developing the proper dosimetry for a particular procedure depend on an understanding of these interactions.[21,22]

Clinical Uses of the Argon Laser

Shortly after the argon laser was discovered in 1964, the first medical application of lasers was described. Zwang, at the Palo Alto Medical Clinic, used it to treat diseases of retinal vessels, and Lash and Maser, plastic surgeons who were also practicing in Palo Alto, began to use it to treat cutaneous vascular lesions. Beginning in the 1960s and continuing to the present time, Leon Goldman, then a dermatologist in Cincinnati, began to investigate the use of lasers in the treatment of cutaneous disease. In the 1970s and 1980s plastic surgeons Bard Cosman, Joel Noe, and David Apfelberg all contributed to the further use of the argon laser in the treatment of port-wine stains.

The two most important chromophores in the skin that absorb argon laser light are oxyhemoglobin and melanin. Although the emission spectrum of the argon laser does not coincide with the absorption peaks of the oxyhemoglobin (418, 542, and 577 nm) spectrum or melanin's absorption spectrum, there is sufficient absorption of argon laser light by oxyhemoglobin and melanin for selective tissue damage in the target to occur. This process results in the thrombosis and obliteration of vessels or the destruction of pigmented structures. In addition, however, because the argon laser light is delivered in a continuous wave, heat diffuses from these chromophores to surrounding tissue and causes nonspecific thermal damage. This characteristic of all the continuous-wave lasers discussed in this chapter is responsible for the major drawback of these lasers—scarring, textural changes, and pigmentary alteration.

Argon laser light may theoretically penetrate 1 mm into the skin. The actual depth of penetration, however, is determined by the degree of competition for light absorption between melanin and hemoglobin. The melanin in the epidermis of a dark-skinned person absorbs the argon laser light, decreasing its transmission to the dermal blood vessels. Conversely, there is less melanin to absorb the argon light in a light-skinned person, so more of it reaches the dermal blood vessels in port-wine stains, which extend to a depth of at least 1 mm. Because both melanin and hemoglobin absorb the light emitted from the argon laser, it can be used to treat multiple types of cutaneous vascular lesions as well as superficial pigmented lesions.

PORT-WINE STAINS

The exact incidence of port-wine stains is unknown, but they are conjectured to occur in approximately 0.3% of live births.[23,24] Most lesions are located on the face, followed by the trunk, the neck, and the lower and upper extremities.[24] Early in life, the lesions are light pink and flat, but after puberty, the lesions darken, becoming deep red or purple. Multiple small surface irregularities known as *blebs* develop in 50% to 60% of patients with facial port-wine stains after 30 years of age and may protrude 2 to 3 mm above the surface of the skin. Functional impairment may result if these blebs form around the nose or eyes. In addition, these blebs may bleed spontaneously and can be easily traumatized, leading to significant bleeding, secondary infection, or the development of pyogenic granulomas.[25] Besides these medical reasons for treatment, the psychological benefits are obvious.[26] Before the development of the argon laser, patients with port-wine stains had to choose between wearing cosmetics; undergoing excision and grafting, radiation therapy, or cryosurgery;[27] and camouflaging them with tattoos.[28] However, none of these therapeutic modalities offered patients a good cosmetic result and several of them caused significant scarring.

Port-wine stains are composed of an increased number of ectatic vessels (20–150 mm in diameter), which are located in the superficial vascular plexus of the papillary dermis, well within the range of the penetration depth of the argon laser. When appropriate energy fluences are used, the argon laser produces coagulation necrosis of vessels, with subsequent obliteration and clinical blanching. The histologic changes occurring after argon laser treatment consist of a nonspecific fibrosis in the upper dermis with some loss of the superficial vascular elements.[29,30] The collagen damage extends beyond the middermis. Unlike burn scars, the appendageal structures are usually preserved.[31] Tan and colleagues[32] carried out a study in which they irradiated port-wine stains with the argon laser (fluence, 150 J/cm²). At 7 days, histologic analysis showed that the epidermis had necrosed, the dermal collagen was destroyed, and hair follicles and sebaceous lobules had degenerated. The necrosis was more marked in the upper dermis, and the damage in the blood vessel walls correlated with that of the surrounding dermis. Fibrin was seen in the lumina of the vessels. One month after laser exposure, the papillary dermal collagen, blood vessels, and necrotic appendages in the reticular dermis were found to have been replaced by scar tissue. No dilated blood vessels were seen. The few visible blood vessels had small lumina without thrombi.

Histochemical analysis has also been used to evaluate the tissue damage induced by the argon laser, and it is thought that this is a more accurate way of assessing the results of treatment than histologic study alone. Histochemical evaluation is done by staining tissue with nitro blue tetrazolium chloride. Reduction of this redox dye by nicotinamide adenine dinucleotide diaphorase (NADH-diaphorase) leads to the formation of an intense blue precipitate on frozen tissue sections. The activity of NADH-diaphorase ceases immediately upon cell death. When port-wine stains were exposed to the argon laser with fluences of 19 to 114 J/cm^2 (pulse duration, 0.2–0.3 sec), an arc-shaped epidermal and dermal necrosis was seen that was clearly demarcated from surrounding normal tissue.[33] The depth of thermal injury ranged from 0.28 to 0.45 mm and correlated with the exposure time rather than with the fluence. The vast majority of port-wine vessels were found to be affected.

Technique

Multiple techniques for treating port-wine stains using the argon laser have been devised. The continuous technique is the most common and is described in detail in the following section. The procedures are carried out with the patient under local anesthesia, using lidocaine without epinephrine. Before attempting to treat the entire port-wine stain, however, a test area should be treated first.

Test Area

1. The test area should be 1 to 2 cm in diameter and within the port-wine stain but in the least conspicuous area. Before the administration of local anesthesia, the area is outlined with a felt-tipped marker.
2. The following parameters are used: spot size, 1 mm; power, 0.8 W. The handpiece is held perpendicular to the skin at approximately 2 cm from the skin, depending on the focal length of the handpiece.
3. The test area is treated with continuous back-and-forth passes or enlarging concentric circles, starting in the center. The handpiece should be moved at a speed that produces an opalescent color, known as the *minimal blanching response*. This whitish color is due to the thermal coagulation of tissue protein. It is important to avoid overlapping areas.
4. The laser can be used in either a continuous-wave or shuttered mode with a pulse duration of 0.05 to 10.0 seconds. Although

novices may prefer to use the shuttered beam, more experienced practitioners may prefer to use the continuous beam, because it is faster and less fatiguing.

5. The response of the test area is assessed 4 months after treatment, by comparing the untreated port-wine stain and normal skin (Fig. 5-1). The criteria for judging the test area response are: the degree of lightening; the degree of textural improvement; any adverse textural changes—atrophic or hypertrophic scarring; and the presence or absence of hypopigmentation or hyperpigmentation.

6. If a hypertrophic scar develops within the test area, there are several options. Either another test site can be treated using a lower power or the test area can be reevaluated in another 4 months. Alternatively, a test can be done using the pulsed dye or another laser. Corticosteroids can be injected between the lesions to help reduce the hypertrophic scar.

Large Area

1. Local anesthesia is administered and a 1-mm spot size and a 0.8-W power (or higher if appropriate) are used.
2. The handpiece is held perpendicular to the skin and moved across the skin slowly to produce a minimal blanching response.
3. Nodular areas of the port-wine stain can be treated with 1.6 to 2.0 W of power.
4. Patients are instructed that the skin will turn from white to a dusky grayish purple within several hours. Postoperative edema may develop and last 1 to 2 days.

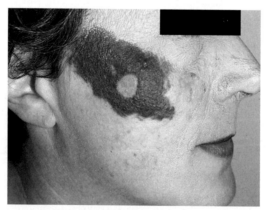

Fig. 5-1. Test spot within a purple, cobblestone-surface port-wine stain on the cheek of a woman. The port-wine stain color within the test spot has completely disappeared, leaving a flat, slightly erythematous surface at the same level as that of the normal surrounding skin. The erythema will fade with time. The port-wine stain surrounding the purple area has subsequently been treated. The extensive port-wine stain on the forehead and cheeks is covered with cosmetics. See Fig. 5-1 in color section. (Courtesy Joel M. Noe, MD.)

5. Postoperative crusting is routine and is treated with a topical an-
    tibiotic ointment.

Two other less commonly used methods that have been used are
the "stripe," or "zebra stripe," technique and the "polka-dot" method.
Apfelberg and associates[34] introduced the "striping" technique, in
which alternating rows of epidermis are treated at each session. It
was hoped that by leaving alternating rows of undamaged epidermis
the argon laser–induced scarring would be reduced. However, the
consensus regarding this technique is that it has no advantage over
the routine method and patients are reported to be unhappy with
the bizarre-looking stripes.

Apfelberg and associates[35] later published their observations in a
series of 51 patients with port-wine stains treated with the "polka-
dot" or "pointillistic" method, a method originally described by John
Dixon. In this technique, the argon laser is used to create multiple 1-
to 2-mm dots of blanching separated by 1 to 2 mm of undamaged
epidermis. In this series, scar-prone areas such as the nasolabial fold,
upper and lower lip, nose, and chin were treated, and hypertrophic
scarring occurred in only 6% of the patients.

Clinical Results of Port-Wine Stain Treatment with the Argon Laser

Apfelberg and co-workers[36] observed good to excellent results in approximately 70% of their adult patients with port-wine stains who
were treated with the argon laser. Similar results have been obtained
by other investigators[37] (Figs. 5-2 and 5-3).

The most common complications of argon laser treatment are scarring (Fig. 5-4) (hypertrophic and atrophic) and permanent hypopigmentation (Fig. 5-5), with the reported incidence of hypertrophic
scarring ranging from 9% to 26%.[24,38–40] The upper lip and chin are

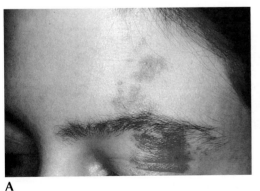 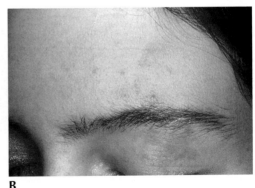

A   **B**

Fig. 5-2.   (A) Red port-wine stain on the eyelid and forehead before treatment with the argon laser.
(B) Fading of port-wine stain several months after treatment with the argon laser. There is no textural
change. See Fig. 5-2 in color section.

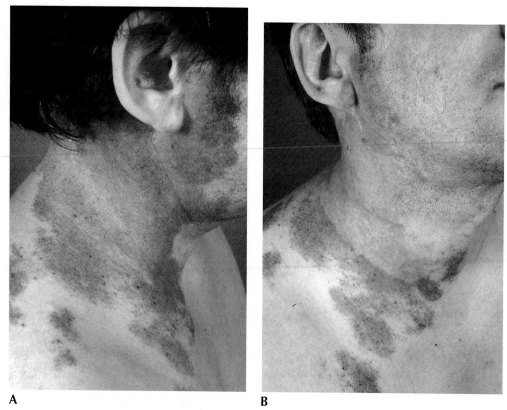

A   **B**

Fig. 5-3.   (A) Port-wine stain on the neck and side of the face before treatment with the argon laser. (B) Results of treatment. There is significant fading with no textural changes. See Fig. 5-3 in color section.

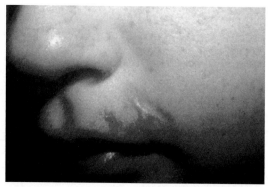

Fig. 5-4.   Argon laser–induced scar on the upper lip of a child. This is one of several sites more at risk for laser-induced thermal scarring.

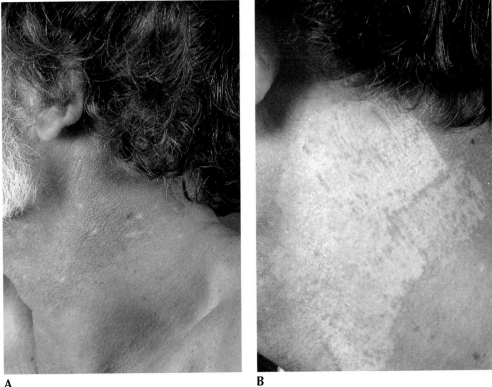

A   **B**

Fig. 5-5.   (A) Poikiloderma of Civatte on the left side of the neck of a fair-skinned man, with considerable photodamage. (B) Striking hypopigmentation at the sites treated with the argon laser. See Fig. 5-5 in color section.

the most prone to hypertrophic scarring. Gilchrest and colleagues[41] were the first to identify epidermal atrophy as another complication of argon laser treatment. When investigators report the incidence of scarring, however, they are usually referring to hypertrophic scarring. Most patients with port-wine stains have some degree of textural change in the skin after argon laser treatment, a finding not discussed in many reports.

In an attempt to maximize the risk-benefit ratio in patients with port-wine stains undergoing argon laser treatment, guidelines regarding patient selection and treatment have been proposed.

Test Area

All patients with port-wine stains who are being considered for argon laser therapy should have a test spot treated first. Cosman[42] believed the test spot is the single best means of determining whether a patient is likely to respond to treatment and whether scarring is likely to occur. The test area is not, however, a perfect predictor of patient satisfaction with the final outcome, in that patients tend to be less satisfied with the final result of treatment than with the result of the test site. One of the reasons for this is that patients tend to compare the initial test site with the remaining port-wine stain but then compare the treated port-wine stain with adjacent normal skin.[43] The test site should not be evaluated until 4 and possibly even 5 months later, because further improvement may occur during the fifth month.

Age of Patient

Noe and colleagues[44] have shown that patients over 37 years old are more likely to have a desirable result than those less than 37 years old.

Color

Port-wine stains in infants are flat pink and smooth, but as the child ages, the color darkens to red, then purple, and the texture of the skin surface becomes irregular. The darker the color of the port-wine stain (i.e., purple), the better the result from argon laser treatment. Thus, age and color are related; older patients usually have darker lesions.[44]

Histology

The histology of the port-wine stain is also a predictor of the results from treatment.[45] Features noted on biopsy specimens that are indicative of a desirable result include a vascular area (percentage of dermal area composed of vessels) of more than 5%, a mean vessel area (the average space per vessel) exceeding 2500 μm^2, and a percent fullness of the vessels of more than 15%. The percent fullness (percentage of vessels containing luminal erythrocytes) has been noted to be the best histologic predictor of response. This makes sense, because it is the most direct measurement of the amount of hemoglobin available to absorb argon light.[44]

Location of Port-Wine Stain

Port-wine stains on the face and neck usually lighten after treatment in 70% to 75% of patients, but there are no adequate data regarding lesions on the extremities. As stated earlier, hypertrophic scars are more likely to occur on the upper lips and chin than at other sites.[46,47]

Skin Type

Patients with fair skin respond better to argon laser treatment because of the inherent lack of pigment that allows the laser light to be transmitted with less interference.

HEMANGIOMAS

Hemangiomas are vascular abnormalities that appear a few days to several weeks after birth. They start off as a localized area of pallor, followed by the development of one or more red papules that coalesce to form single or multiple lesions on the body, usually on the head. Hemangiomas undergo a rapid growth phase for approximately the next 9 months, followed by a period of 2 to 3 years during which the hemangioma is static. Eighty percent of hemangiomas involute spontaneously by the time the children are 5 to 7 years old. If a hemangioma does not start to involute by 7 years of age, it is probably not going to do so. When a hemangioma begins to involute, a white area is usually noted within the lesion.

There are three types of hemangiomas: (1) capillary or superficial hemangiomas (65% of hemangiomas), which are composed of small, superficial vascular channels; (2) cavernous or deep hemangiomas (15% of hemangiomas), which are composed of deeper, larger vascular spaces; and (3) capillary-cavernous, or superficial and deep mixed, hemangiomas (20% of hemangiomas), which have features of both. Superficial hemangiomas usually involute with no scar or minimal atrophy. Deep hemangiomas do not usually involute completely, and patients are left with folds of atrophic telangiectatic skin with subcutaneous fibrofatty tissue replacing the involuted areas.[1]

In the past, physicians advocated that most childhood hemangiomas be observed and not treated, because they spontaneously involute. Treatment was only recommended if (1) the lesion was extensive; (2) repeated ulcerations, bleeding, or infections occurred; or (3) the lesion obstructed a vital organ (eye, nose, mouth, anus, or penis). Treatments have included excisional surgery, compression therapy,[48] irradiation, cryosurgery, the systemic or intralesional administration of corticosteroids,[49] and, most recently, systemic interferon therapy.

Recently, however, some clinicians have begun to reconsider the usefulness of early definitive treatment and now tend to advocate it. Grabb and associates[45] reported on a group of 20 patients with hemangiomas followed for 14 years. The hemangiomas involuted in only five of the patients during this time. Some did not involute until the patient was 18 years old. This showed that a hemangioma can have a significant psychological impact on a child for a longer time than was appreciated in the past. The awareness of the psychological effects of hemangiomas on these children and their parents may be somewhat responsible for this change in attitude toward treatment. Advances in laser technology, making possible the treatment of hemangiomas with an attendant low risk of scarring, have also played a role. In 1981 Apfelberg and associates[50] published their findings in three children with hemangiomas who underwent argon laser treatment. After treatment, growth was arrested and premature resolution occurred. At this time, however, these investigators did not recommend that the argon laser be considered a routine treatment for hemangiomas. In 1983, Hobby[51] reported that arrested growth and premature regression were observed in six patients with hemangiomas treated with the argon laser. Hobby recommended early intervention, because treatment results were better for patients with very small lesions. Achauer and VanderKam[52] also found that smaller lesions respond better to treatment than large bulky lesions do. In another series, Achauer and VanderKam[53] treated 10 infants with ulcerated hemangiomas of the anogenital region who had been treated unsuccessfully with conservative therapy. After treatment, all hemangiomas healed rapidly (within 1 to 5 weeks) and involution was accelerated. Although some scarring and textural changes did occur, the authors noted that both occurred after the spontaneous involution of an ulcerated hemangioma. These authors recommended that the argon laser be used in such infants with hemangiomas to promote wound healing, thus minimizing the scarring that prolonged ulceration causes. Hobby[54] has advocated that argon laser treatment be considered in patients with strawberry hemangiomas who have:

1. A growing hemangioma that is predominantly capillary or superficial. The results are better in younger patients with smaller lesions.
2. A lesion with a superficial component that is not growing but is causing functional problems, such as amblyopia, airway obstruction, or hygienic dysfunction.
3. A lesion that is subject to chronic trauma with resultant ulceration and bleeding.
4. A lesion causing a pathologic level of parental anxiety.
5. A lesion in a 6-year-old patient that has shown no signs of further resolution for at least 1 year.
6. A hemangioma that still has a vascular component and is scheduled to be removed using a conventional surgical procedure. Treatment with the argon laser helps to devascularize the lesion and make the surgical procedure easier.

More recently the pulse dye laser has been added to the armamentarium of treatments for hemangiomas (see Chap. 6). This laser can safely and effectively treat superficial hemangiomas in both the proliferative and involution phases. It can also be used in the treatment of thin and thick hemangiomas, as long as the lesion is not primarily deep or cavernous, and in most instances is the laser-of-choice for this purpose. However, multiple treatments with the pulsed dye laser are usually necessary, in contradistinction to the argon laser, which can produce a maximum therapeutic response in one or two treatments. On the plus side, however, scarring and pigmentary loss are less common in patients who undergo treatment with the pulsed dye laser.

TELANGIECTASES

The argon laser can effectively treat telangiectases of the face, trunk, and upper limbs, but results of treatment on the lower extremities have been disappointing.[55] There are two techniques that are used to treat telangiectases: the continuous-wave method and the shuttered method. Regardless of the method used, the laser beam is used to trace out the abnormal vessel, which in effect "heat seals" it. The beam diameter is chosen to match that of the dilated vessel. Immediately after treatment the vessels have an opalescent gray appearance. The clinical outcome cannot be fully evaluated for at least 6 weeks, however, because the larger vessels may recanalize during that time. If a patient does not show improvement after the first treatment, the power output may be increased at the next treatment. Telangiectases of the face and neck respond well to treatment with the argon laser.[56] Although scarring is rare, a slight depression or atrophic scar within the skin that follows the course of the ectatic vessel may be seen. Lower-extremity vessels with a diameter of 0.3 mm or less can be treated with continuous-wave lasers. The best results are obtained for vessels that are 0.1 mm in diameter. The most common side effect is linear hyperpigmentation, which can be minimized by only treating vessels with a diameter of 0.2 mm or less using the lowest power output possible and a spot size no larger than the vessel's diameter. Elevating the leg, applying ice compresses, and having the patient wear compression stockings postoperatively may also help minimize the occurrence of this troublesome complication.

In summary, the argon laser is very useful and effective in the ablation of small- to large-diameter ectatic vessels. The results are equal to, and sometimes better than, those produced by any of the visible light continuous-wave and quasi–continuous-wave lasers.

OTHER TELANGIECTATIC DISORDERS

The Red Nose

The term *red nose* refers to a diffuse erythema of the nose, with or without telangiectasis. It is often caused by acne rosacea and accompanied by inflammatory papules and pustules. Another frequent cause in light-skinned people is chronic actinic damage. Excessive use of corticosteroid creams may also produce excessive telangiectases of the nose.[57] A diffuse erythema or telangiectasis of the nasal dorsum may occur after rhinoplasty, a condition termed the *postrhinoplasty red nose syndrome*.[58,59] Other cases of red nose include radiation treatment, infection, trauma, and the carcinoid syndrome. Before the advent of laser treatment, treatment options included electrosurgery with an epilating needle, electrolysis, and cryosurgery, but none of these methods was very efficacious in reducing the generalized redness of the nose. Several authors have reported on the successful treatment of the red nose with the argon laser.[59,60] Dicken[60] has shown that low-energy fluences are very effective in treating the condition, with a very low incidence of hypopigmentation and scarring. If the vessels are large enough, they can be traced individually with the laser beam. If the vessels are too narrow to be traced individually, the entire area is treated using a 1.0-mm spot size.

Spider Nevi

The treatment of spider nevi (nevi aranei) with the argon laser yields consistently good results[55,56] (Fig. 5-6). The 0.5- or 1.0-mm spot size is used to coagulate the central feeder vessel, and the surrounding vessels can then be traced using a spot size equal to their diameter.

Telangiectasis Associated with Collagen Vascular Disease

Cosmetically troublesome telangiectases are common in patients with lupus erythematosus, dermatomyositis, or scleroderma. Zachariae and associates[61] reported on the outcome from treatment with the argon laser in two patients with juvenile dermatomyositis, five with chronic discoid lupus erythematosus, and one with the Rothmund-Thomson syndrome, all of whom had the telangiectases associated with these diseases. Marked improvement with no activation of the underlying disease was observed in all.

Other Vascular Lesions

The argon laser is very effective for the treatment of other vascular lesions. Dermatologic lesions that have a vascular component also respond to argon laser treatment (Table 5-1; Figs. 5-7 to 5-9).

Angiokeratomas

Angiokeratomas start as pink to red compressible papules that are 1 to 3 mm in diameter, then darken and develop a keratotic, warty surface. Microscopically they contain ectatic vessels in the papillary dermis. These dilated vessels form large lacunae that may be entirely trapped by the epidermis. Flores and associates[62] have shown that argon laser treatment can cure angiokeratoma of Fordyce, and Pasyk and colleagues[63] successfully treated two patients with angiokeratoma circumscriptum using the argon laser. Occella and co-work-

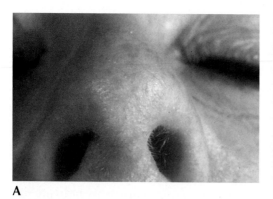 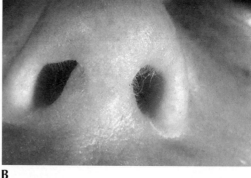

A   **B**

Fig. 5-6.   (A) Spider ectasia on a patient's nose before treatment with the argon laser. (B) Complete disappearance of lesion after therapy. See Fig. 5-6 in color section.

Table 5-1. Other vascular lesions treated with the argon laser

Vascular lesions	Lesions with a vascular component
Angiokeratoma	Angiolymphoid hyperplasia
Cherry angiomas	Adenoma sebaceum
Venous lakes	Granuloma faciale
Pyogenic granuloma	Kaposi's sarcoma

ers[64] successfully treated two patients affected by angiokeratoma circumscriptum and angiokeratoma of Fordyce. Each angiokeratoma is irradiated until whitening or flattening occurs. The adjacent normal skin is not treated. Resolution and complete healing usually take 4 to 6 weeks to occur.

Cherry Angiomas

Cherry angiomas respond completely to therapy with the argon laser, regardless of the body location. No scarring has been seen on

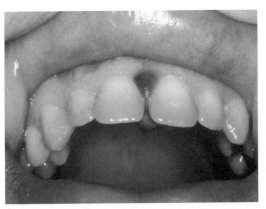

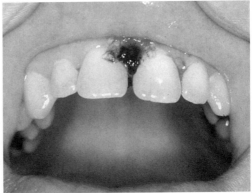

A

B

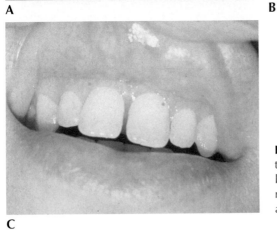

C

Fig. 5-7. (A) Epidemic Kaposi's sarcoma on the gingivae before treatment with the argon laser. (B) Appearance immediately after treatment. (C) Complete disappearance of the lesion after therapy.

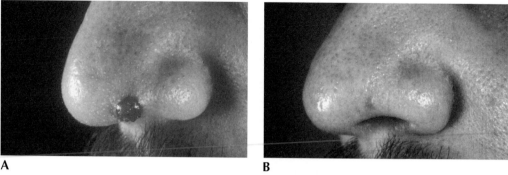

A   B

Fig. 5-8.   (A) Kaposi's sarcoma on the left side of a patient's nose before treatment. (B) Almost complete disappearance of the lesion after therapy. See Fig. 5-8 in color section.

the trunk or extremities after treatment.[55,65] The lesions are treated in the same manner as angiokeratomas.

Venous Malformations

Venous lakes are dark blue, soft, compressible blebs that are found on the lips, ears, and face. Histologically they consist of dilated veins or venules lined by a single layer of endothelial cells. The argon laser has proved to be a valuable tool in their treatment. The subepidermal location of venous lakes allows for optimal penetration of the laser beam. Neumann and Knobler[66] published their findings in a se-

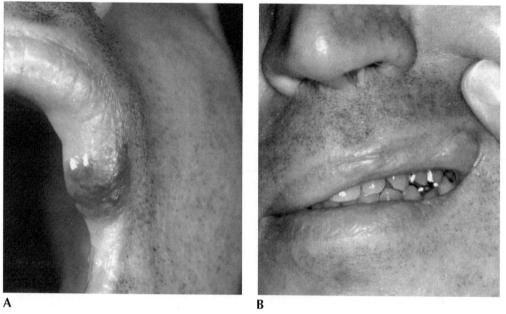

A   B

Fig. 5-9.   (A) Large venous lake on lips before therapy with the argon laser. (B) Complete disappearance of the lesion after therapy. See Fig. 5-9 in color section.

ries of 51 patients with venous lakes treated with the argon laser. An excellent cosmetic result was observed in 90% of the patients, with 5% showing scarring. Patients usually need to be anesthetized during treatment. Many practitioners recommend that the lesion be compressed with a diascope to reduce its size. The lesion may then be treated through the glass slide. The overlying skin on the lip turns white during treatment, signifying epidermal thermal coagulation. If the venous lake is less than 5 mm in diameter, usually only one treatment is necessary. Larger venous malformations may require two or three treatments performed at monthly intervals (Fig. 5-10). Venous malformations of mucosal surfaces respond more rapidly and with less scarring to argon laser treatment than those on glabrous skin do.

Angiolymphoid Hyperplasia

Angiolymphoid hyperplasia is a rare benign condition involving the development of single or multiple plum-colored nodules or plaques. Histologically the nodules contain proliferating capillary vessels with a dense mixed-cell infiltrate. Successful treatment of this clinical entity with the argon laser has been reported, although recurrences are often seen[67] (Fig. 5-11).

Adenoma Sebaceum

Adenoma sebaceum is a facial angiofibroma, and these lesions are pathognomonic for tuberous sclerosis. Previous ways of treating the condition have included curettage, liquid nitrogen cryosurgery,[68] electrocautery, and dermabrasion.[69] However, the cosmetic results of these therapies were not satisfactory and regrowth was common. The vascular component of some angiofibromas, if prominent, makes them amenable to removal with the argon laser (Fig. 5-12). Their successful removal using the argon laser, without subsequent scarring or regrowth, has been reported by Arndt[70] and Pasyk and Argenta.[71]

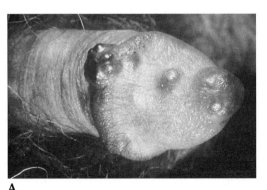
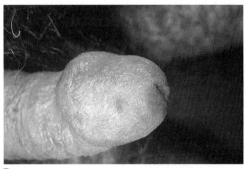

A   B

Fig. 5-10.   (A) Vascular malformation on the glans penis before treatment with the argon laser using 1.0-W power with a 1-mm spot size. (B) Complete disappearance of the lesions 6 months after therapy. See Fig. 5-10 in color section.

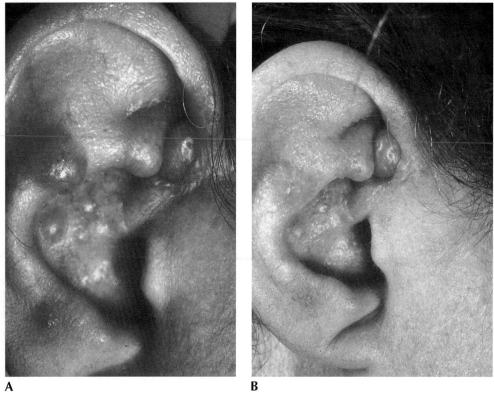

A   **B**

Fig. 5-11.   (A) Blue nodules of angiolymphoid hyperplasia on the ear before treatment with the argon laser. (B) Almost complete disappearance of lesions after argon laser therapy. There is no textural change.

Because patients usually have numerous facial angiofibromas, it is sometimes best to treat them while under general anesthesia.

PIGMENTED LESIONS

Epidermal Pigmented Lesions

The argon laser has been used successfully to treat superficial pigmented lesions such as lentigines, the pigmented macules occurring in the Peutz-Jeghers syndrome, seborrheic keratoses, postinflammatory hyperpigmentation, and junctional nevi.[71–74] The melanin in these lesions absorbs the argon blue-green light, producing thermal damage. Café au lait spots and Becker's nevi are usually not treated with the argon laser because the results are not consistent. Pigmented lesions are usually anesthetized before treatment with the argon laser, and a 1-mm spot size and 0.4 to 0.8 W of power are used. The lesion is irradiated with a focused or slightly defocused laser beam until it is slightly opalescent. Postoperative care includes a topically administered antibiotic ointment and a nonadherent dressing. The outcome of treatment may be assessed at 1 month.

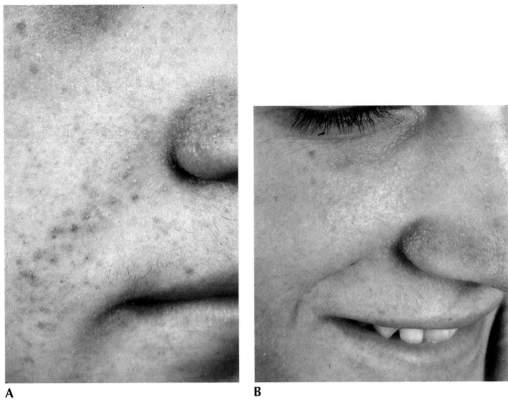

A   **B**

Fig. 5-12.   (A) Papules typical of adenoma sebaceum associated with tuberous sclerosis before argon laser therapy. (B) Complete subsidence of lesions 6 months later. See Fig. 5-12 in color section.

Lentigo Maligna

Arndt[75,76] successfully treated a patient with facial lentigo maligna with the argon laser, but 4 years later a new pigmented lesion, shown by biopsy findings to be lentigo maligna, appeared at the margin of the treated area. It is not known whether this represented a recurrence or was outside the original treated area. In any event, the argon laser is not the treatment of choice for lentigo maligna, because the atypical melanocytes in these lesions extend into the hair follicle, possibly placing them beyond the 1-mm skin-depth penetration of the argon laser light. This method of treatment should be considered only if surgical excision is not feasible.

Dermal Pigmented Lesions

Dermal melanin selectively absorbs argon laser light, but nonselective thermal damage to surrounding connective tissue is an inevitable consequence. Although good results have been reported for the argon laser treatment of dermal pigmented lesions, such as nevus of Ota (Fig. 5-13), scarring and fibrosis are often unwanted results. The treatment of melanocytic nevi with the argon laser often yields excellent results, but textural changes or scarring may occur.

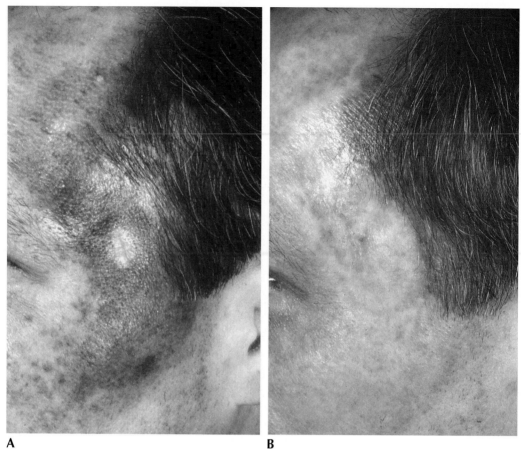

A   **B**

Fig. 5-13. (A) Nevus of Ota on the left side of a patient's face, showing a marked decrease in pigmentation at the site of an argon laser test site. (B) Appearance after treatment of the entire lesion. There was a striking decrease in pigmentation associated with slight hypopigmentation and atrophy. See Fig. 5-13 in color section.

The argon laser has also been used to remove decorative and traumatic tattoos. Although some of the tattoo pigments absorb the argon laser light, scarring usually occurs. The Q-switched ruby, Nd:YAG, and alexandrite lasers can disrupt tattoo pigment in a more specific and less traumatic fashion.

Continuous-Wave Dye Lasers

The continuous-wave dye laser, or tunable dye laser, which is most often pumped by an argon laser, can deliver a broad wavelength spectrum specific to the organic dye used. The dye proper is usually not changed; instead the wavelength emitted is altered to ±20 nm through the use of a prism. The rhodamine dye used in the dye laser designed for use in the treatment of cutaneous lesions is energized by an argon laser to produce an adjustable band of light energy with wavelengths of 488 to 638 nm (including the argon laser wavelengths of 488 and 514 nm). Although this energy is emitted as a continuous wave, it can be mechanically or electronically shuttered to be as short as 20 msec or it can be emitted as a continuous wave with an adjustable repetition rate. The beam is transmitted via fiberoptics to a variable spot size handpiece that permits the laser surgeon to select a beam size of 0.1 to 6 mm. The continuous-wave dye laser can be operated freehand or used in conjunction with a robotized scanning device.

This continuous-wave laser is usually tuned using rhodamine dye to deliver yellow light at a wavelength of 577 or 585 nm that coincides with one of the absorption peaks of oxyhemoglobin.[77] At this wavelength there is less absorption of the laser light by melanin and deeper penetration into the dermis. Theoretically these wavelengths should cause more selective damage to blood vessels, with less absorption by and potential damage to the melanin-containing epidermis. However, Cotterill[78] found that the continuous-wave dye laser (with a wavelength of 577 nm), with the beam emitted in microsecond or longer pulses, was effective in treating a variety of vascular lesions. The lesions included spider nevi, facial telangiectases, pyogenic granulomas, and port-wine stains. The reported incidence of scarring was less than 1%, and there was no keloidal scarring. Textural changes were not reported, and hypopigmentation was rare.

PORT-WINE STAINS

The continuous-wave dye laser, emitting 577- and 585-nm wavelengths, has been used in the treatment of port-wine stains to produce more specific thermal damage to ectatic vessels than that produced by the argon laser. Lanigan and associates[79] reported on the use of a continuous-wave dye laser (577 nm) in the treatment of 100 adults and children with port-wine stains. A good or excellent result was obtained in 63%; some improvement occurred in 17%. There was a 14% incidence of atrophic scarring and a 5% incidence of hypertrophic scarring. These results are similar to those achieved for the argon laser treatment of port-wine stains.[80–82] The argon and continuous-wave dye lasers achieve better results in older patients with raised, purple port-wine stains. In contrast, the pulsed dye laser produces the best results in younger patients with flat, pink lesions. In a randomized study of 20 patients with port-wine stains, Malm and colleagues[83] also showed that continuous-wave dye laser and argon laser treatments were equally beneficial. Even though the 577-nm wavelength of the continuous-wave dye laser is more specifically absorbed by hemoglobin than the wavelength of the argon laser, the results from continuous-wave dye laser treatment appear to be comparable to those from argon laser treatment, because selective vascular destruction is more dependent on the pulsewidth than the wavelength of the laser light.

In an attempt to improve the treatment of port-wine stains in both children and adults, Scheibner and Wheeland[84] devised a tracing technique using the continuous-wave dye laser (577 nm). Because port-wine stains are composed of a network of dilated individual capillaries (30–300 μm in diameter), if only the vessels and not the uninvolved skin are treated, injury to normal skin can be avoided. The technique they developed involves the use of binocular magnifiers (Carl Zeiss, West Germany) with ×8 magnification and a 190-mm focal length. Each blood vessel can then be traced individually using a 100-μm spot size at a rate of 0.5 cm/s using a continuous discharge at a wavelength of 577 nm. No anesthesia is necessary, and the laser surgeon must be very careful not to irradiate normal intervening skin. A small test area is done in advance to determine the lowest power setting that will cause the disappearance of the dilated blood vessels. A power setting greater than 0.8 W is never used. The test treatment is begun at a power of 0.08 W and then the power is increased slowly until the treated blood vessel disappears completely. If any graying, blanching, charring, or shriveling of the epidermis occurs, the power is too high. Although the power setting seems low compared with those used by other investigators, the irradiance is actually very high because of the narrow beam size. After a successful test treatment, 1- to 2-inch square (2.5- to 5-cm^2) areas can be treated in 1 hour. These areas are done in concentric circles radiating out from a central point. Treatment is usually done monthly until the entire port-wine stain has been treated. Areas that require more treatment should be redone 6 to 12 months after completion of the first round of treatments.

Eighty-two adults with port-wine stains of the head and neck were treated using this method.[84] Excellent results were obtained in 44% and good results in 43%. Each patient required an average of 1.7 treatment sessions. In a pediatric population, the results were not as good.[85] Of 92 children (ages, 2–15 years) treated with the same technique, 38% had excellent results, 25% had good results, and 33% had only fair results. No hypertrophic scarring or textural or pigmentary changes occurred in either the pediatric or adult group. This technique requires a great deal of expertise, however, and is so tedious that few have ever mastered it.

Robotized scanning devices have been adapted for use with the continuous-wave dye laser in an attempt to convert the continuous beam into a shuttered beam. By using a shuttered beam, treatment with this laser can theoretically adhere more closely to the principles of selective photothermolysis, thereby preventing many of the adverse effects (i.e., hypertrophic and atrophic scarring and pigmentary alterations) associated with continuous-wave dye laser treatment. Dover and associates[86] compared the effects of the flashlamp-pumped pulsed dye laser and a continuous-wave dye laser equipped with a Hexascan (both at 585 nm) on test sites within 29 pink or purple, raised or flat, port-wine stains in patients at least 3 months of age. The pulsed dye laser was used to treat one test area with a 5-mm spot size and a fluence of 6.0 to 7.5 J/cm^2, and a continuous-wave dye laser equipped with a Hexascan was used to treat a second test area with a 3-mm spot size and the appropriate threshold fluence for each patient. Patients were evaluated for 6 weeks after treatment. It was found that, although both lasers produced statistically significant lightening after one treatment, the pulsed dye laser produced a greater degree of lightening. In addition, it produced less pigmentary alteration. Neither laser caused atrophic or hypertrophic scarring. Overall, despite the addition of the Hexascan to the continuous-wave dye laser system, the pulsed dye laser still proved to be slightly superior. However, this scanning device does appear to decrease the risk of scarring while maintaining the beneficial effects of the continuous-wave dye laser.[87]

FACIAL TELANGIECTASES

The continuous-wave dye laser may be used to treat facial telangiectases. Orenstein and Nelson[88] treated 21 patients freehand with the continuous-wave dye laser (577 nm) using a 100-μm focused beam with a power of 0.7 to 1.0 W and a pulse duration of 0.05 to 0.10 second. All of the patients treated had an excellent response, usually within one to two treatment sessions. There was no hypertrophic scarring or pigmentary or textural changes noted in any patients. Ross and co-workers[89] compared the flashlamp-pumped pulsed dye laser (585 nm) to the continuous-wave dye laser (585 nm) with a robotized handpiece in the treatment of facial telangiectases. The continuous-wave dye laser was used at a fluence of 20 and 27 J/cm^2 with a 13-mm hexagonal treatment area. The flashlamp-pumped pulsed dye laser was used at a fluence of 6.0 and 6.5 to 6.75 J/cm^2 with a 5-mm spot size and a pulse duration of 460 μsec. The flashlamp-pulsed dye laser was found to be faster to use, although the continuous-wave dye laser was faster to use utilizing the robotized handpiece than the freehand technique was. Six weeks after treatment, both the investigators and the patients judged the pulsed dye laser to be more efficacious in treating facial telangiectases. Despite this fact, almost 50% of the patients preferred treatment with the continuous-wave dye laser with the Hexascan because it did not produce the significant purpura the pulsed dye laser produced. The results might have differed if the pulsed dye laser had been used with the 2- or 3-mm spot size, in which case less prominent purpura would have been induced.

The size of the vessels involved is also important. Although the flashlamp-pumped pulsed dye laser is excellent for obliterating smaller telangiectatic vessels (100 μm in diameter) and vessels within port-wine stains (30–300 μm in diameter), many cutaneous laser surgeons believe it is not as effective for treating larger telangiectatic vessels. Studies comparing the pulsed dye, continuous-wave dye, and copper vapor lasers in the treatment of these larger vessels are needed.

KTP and Krypton Lasers

The KTP laser is a frequency-doubled Nd:YAG laser that produces only green light at a wavelength of 532 nm. The Nd:YAG wavelength of 1064 nm is frequency-doubled with a KTP crystal (potassium titanyl phosphate) to produce the 532-nm output. This laser produces a train of pulses at a frequency of 25,000 Hz with a pulse duration of about 200 nsec. The Nd:YAG laser rod is continuously pumped with a krypton arc lamp and is Q-switched. Fiberoptics direct the green light from the source to the output, and a maximum output of 12 W can be achieved. Because the 532-nm wavelength of the KTP laser closely corresponds to one of hemoglobin's absorption peaks (542 nm), this laser can be used to treat cutaneous vascular lesions. Although a great deal of research using this laser has been done in the field of otolaryngology, its use by cutaneous laser surgeons has been limited.

Apfelberg and colleagues[90] published their findings from a side-by-side comparison of the treatment of various vascular lesions using the argon and KTP/532 lasers. Both lasers were found to produce equivalent clinical results in the treatment of port-wine stains, capillary-cavernous hemangiomas, and decorative tattoos. The outcome of treatment in most of the patients was fair to good, but an excellent result was achieved in only a few patients. Posttreatment biopsy specimens from patients treated with the argon and KTP/532 lasers showed identical histologic changes: obliteration of vessels in the upper 1 mm of the dermis, dermal fibrosis, and normal reepithelialization. This indicates that further evaluation of the KTP laser in the treatment of cutaneous vascular lesions is warranted. This laser is a reliable source of high-energy green light, plus its energy output is higher and the laser is less likely to need service than some other lasers producing light in the same region of the spectrum.

The krypton laser has a gas medium that emits yellow light at 568 nm and two bands of green light at 521 and 530 nm. The green light can be filtered out, leaving just yellow wavelengths for the treatment of vascular lesions. This continuous-wave laser is used in a fashion identical to that described for the other lasers in this chapter, including those used with robotic scanners, and it is reasonable to expect the clinical results from the treatment of vascular or pigmented lesions with the krypton laser to be no different from those produced by other lasers emitting light in the yellow or green region of the spectrum. Because of the benign composition of its gas medium, however, an advantage of this laser is that the potential exposure to solvents and organic dyes inherent in the use of both types of dye lasers is avoided.

Copper Vapor Laser

The heavy-metal vapor lasers, introduced in 1966 as industrial lasers, were developed by Walker and colleagues.[91] The two metals used in heavy-metal vapor lasers are copper and gold. Copper emits light at 578.2 nm (yellow light) and 510.5 nm (green light). Gold emits energy at 628 nm. The laser cavity consists of a neon gas–filled ceramic tube that contains copper or gold pellets at specific locations near each end. To produce the metal vapor, a high-voltage, pulsed electronic circuit excites a gas discharge, which generates heat, causing the vaporization of copper. Laser light is then produced by the interaction of the electrons from the gas discharge with the atoms of the vaporized metal. Industrial applications of the copper vapor laser include the detection of fingerprints and separation of isotopes of uranium and plutonium; it is also used as a substitute for strobes in high-speed flash photography.[92] In 1980 the copper vapor laser came available for use in medicine, and it, and more recently, a copper bromide laser have been adapted for cutaneous use.[93] Cutaneous laser surgeons have been using these copper lasers to treat vascular lesions with the yellow or green light, or both, and pigmented lesions with the green light.

The two wavelengths produced by the copper vapor laser can be emitted either separately or together. The yellow (578-nm) light is identical to the wavelength produced by the pulsed dye and continuous-wave dye lasers. A filter is used to change from the yellow to the green option. The copper vapor laser is a pulsed laser that emits a train of very short pulses with a duration of 20 nsec and at an interval between pulses of 67 to 125 μsec. The laser emits a train of 10,000 to 15,000 pulses per second (10–15 kHz). Because the number of pulses produced per second is so high, the human eye cannot "perceive" each pulse individually. The light is also "perceived" by the tissue as a continuous beam. The laser light is delivered to the skin surface via a 10-mm-diameter quartz optical fiber. The spot size of the beam ranges from 100 to 800 μm, but the most commonly used spot size is 150 μm.

The copper vapor laser differs from the flashlamp-pumped pulsed dye laser in terms of the pulse duration, pulse energy levels, and the spot size, with a subsequent difference in its effect on tissue. The copper vapor laser is a high-repetition–rate pulsed laser with a pulse duration (20 nsec) far less than the thermal relaxation time of most typical facial telangiectatic vessels (20–100 msec). Thus, a single pulse from the copper vapor laser does not have enough energy to coagulate a blood vessel.[94] However, the additive effect of multiple pulses from this laser can cause many telangiectatic vessels in the skin to coagulate in a fashion no different from the coagulation induced by the 578-nm light from a continuous-wave dye laser.

Light at 578 nm coincides with a peak in the absorption spectrum of oxyhemoglobin, and thus is relatively well absorbed by hemoglobin in ectatic blood vessels. However, melanin in the skin does not absorb yellow light well. Thus, the yellow light emitted by the copper vapor laser is somewhat selectively absorbed by vascular ectatic tissue, with less accompanying damage to the overlying epidermis. This is in contrast to the argon laser, which emits a blue-green light that is better absorbed by oxyhemoglobin but also is better absorbed by melanin as well.[94]

PORT-WINE STAINS

The optimal laser to use in the treatment of port-wine stains should emit light that is absorbed by the capillaries in the lesion to a dermal depth of 1.2 nm but that does not affect melanin in the epidermis.[95] The copper vapor laser meets some of these requirements, in that it emits the right wavelength of light—578 nm, which corresponds to one of the absorption peaks of oxyhemoglobin. However, melanin absorbs maximally from 300 to 500 nm with a steady decrease beyond 500 nm. Thus, the energy emitted by the copper vapor laser is mostly absorbed by the blood vessels of the port-wine stain and not by melanin in the epidermis (Fig. 5-14).

Not only must the energy emitted by the laser be of the appropriate wavelength, it must also be delivered briefly enough (the pulsewidth) so that the heat generated passes from the red blood cells to the vessel wall, because it is necessary to damage the vessel wall to ensure long-term improvement, but the thermal damage does not extend much beyond the vessel wall. Neumann and associates[96] have developed these theoretical considerations in the context of the copper vapor laser and a robotized scanner and performed a comparative study in 12 patients with mature port-wine stains treated once each with the copper vapor laser (yellow wavelength, 578 nm) and argon laser. The immediate histologic effects of copper vapor laser and argon laser treatment at fluences ranging from 8.0 to 32 J/cm^2 (pulsewidth, 50–200 msec) were assessed using a histochemical method, in which frozen tissue sections were stained with nitroblue tetrazolium chloride. As noted earlier, this causes viable cells to be stained blue and thermally damaged cells to be unstained, thereby permitting the accurate differentiation of viable and nonviable tissue. At 8, 10, and 12 J/cm^2 (corresponding pulsewidths of 50, 62, and 74 msec), argon laser–induced injury was confined to epidermal cell layers and damage to the dermis was none to minimal. Energy densities of 15 J/cm^2 or greater produced a sharply demarcated area of necrosis involving all epidermal and dermal structures. In contrast, when the copper vapor laser was used at the same energy densities (8, 10, and 12 J/cm^2), the epidermis remained viable, with thermal damage in the papillary and reticular dermis restricted to the blood vessel wall and perivascular cuff of collagen. The surrounding dermal structures were not affected. At a fluence of 15 J/cm^2 (pulsewidth, 94 msec), besides the vascular injury, the epidermal basal cell layer was also damaged. When fluences of 17 to 20 J/cm^2 (pulsewidth, 120–200 msec) were used, a diffuse necrosis was produced similar to that produced by the argon laser. Thus, if the exposure duration is long compared with the time it takes for the heat to diffuse to surrounding structures, the damage caused by the copper vapor laser will be nonspecific, no matter how selective the absorption of the laser light. In fact, under some circumstances, it appears that the copper vapor laser used with a robotized scanning device may produce selective photothermolysis. In summary, this study demonstrated that the thermal damage produced by the copper vapor laser was confined to the vessel wall and the cuff of collagen and the epidermis was not affected. However, at identical fluences, the argon laser caused thermal damage to the epidermis because of its absorption of the laser light. Nevertheless, the copper vapor laser was found to produce only moderate blanching when used at vessel-selective fluences.[96]

Few clinical studies have been performed assessing the merits of the copper vapor laser in the treatment of port-wine stains. Dinehart and colleagues[97] believe that the copper vapor laser is best suited for the treatment of dark purple port-wine stains, using the freehand technique for smaller lesions and a robotized scanning device for larger lesions. However, they believe that the pulsed dye laser is still the treatment of choice for pink or red port-wine stains in the pediatric population. They may initiate the treatment of dark purple port-wine stains with the copper vapor laser and finish with the pulsed dye laser. Because the effectiveness of treatment with the copper vapor laser is very operator dependent, however, it can be difficult to treat a large port-wine stain uniformly. To solve this problem, the copper vapor laser can be equipped with a robotized scanning device.

Sheehan-Dare and Cotterill[98] used both a copper vapor laser (at 578 nm) and argon laser to make test areas in 31 patients with port-wine stains. Both lasers were used with a Hexascan delivery system and the sites treated with minimally blanching fluences. They found that the copper vapor laser produced better fading and the light was more absorbed within the lesions.

Dinehart and co-workers[97] use an average power setting of 250 to 350 mW in the chopped or shuttered mode to treat a port-wine stain.

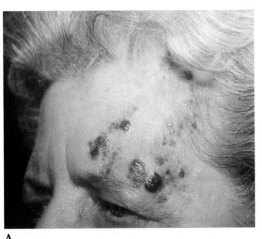 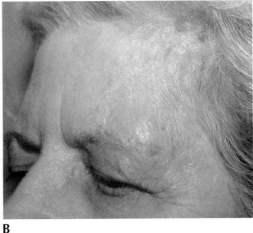

A   **B**

Fig. 5-14.   (A) Papular and nodular, purple port-wine stain on the left forehead of a woman before treatment with the copper vapor laser. (B) Good to excellent result when assessed several months later. See Fig. 5-14 in color section. (Courtesy of Milton Waner, MD.)

For optimal results, they recommend the use of magnifying loupes ($\times 3.5$–$\times 6$). Although small lesions may be treated freehand, a robotized scanning device is useful for the treatment of large port-wine stains. This device ensures that a uniform dose is delivered to the entire lesion. Scabbing occurs, but the skin heals within 2 weeks of treatment. Postoperative wound care consists of application of topical antibiotic ointments or synthetic dressings.

FACIAL TELANGIECTASES

The copper vapor laser has been shown to be safe and effective in the treatment of facial telangiectases (Fig. 5-15). Key and Waner[99] treated 20 patients with facial telangiectases using the 578-nm wavelength of the copper vapor laser and the following parameters: spot size, 150 mm; focal length, 1 cm from the distal tip of the handpiece; and power, 300 to 650 mW. All telangiectatic vessels were traced individually by the physician using the freehand method. Eighteen of the 20 patients experienced satisfactory clearing of their telangiectasia. Although fine punctate scabbing developed in half of the patients, this resolved in 10 to 12 days. Postinflammatory hyperpigmentation developed in 15% of patients and resolved in less than 2 months in response to the topical application of bleaching agents. A small depressed scar developed in only one patient. The only patients who did not show a good response were those who had telangiectatic acne rosacea. Waner and Dinehart[100] have shown that the copper vapor laser and the pulsed dye laser are equally effective in treating facial

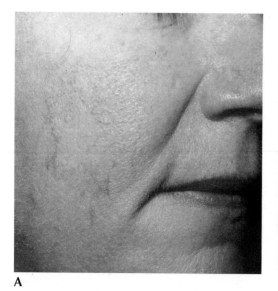
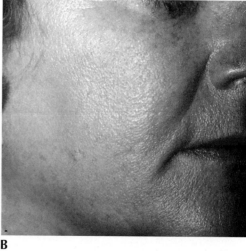

A   B

Fig. 5-15.   (A) Telangiectasia on the right cheek of a woman before copper vapor laser treatment. (B) Complete disappearance of lesions postoperatively. See Fig. 5-15 in color section. (Courtesy of Milton Waner, MD.)

telangiectases, but found in their study that patients better tolerated treatment with the copper vapor laser than treatment with the pulsed dye laser (a 5-mm spot size was used), and this was due to two reasons. First, immediately after treatment with the copper vapor laser, barely perceptible, thin, crusted, white lines develop, similar to those produced by the argon and continuous-wave dye laser. This is in sharp contrast to the appearance of the skin after treatment with the pulsed dye laser, in that treatment with the pulsed dye laser using the 5-mm spot size causes purpuric spots to form that are difficult to camouflage and persist for 10 to 12 days, though use of the 2-mm spot size now available on the pulsed dye laser results in less severe postoperative purpura. Second, patients treated with the copper vapor laser were found to experience less pain, swelling, and postinflammatory hyperpigmentation than those treated with the pulsed dye laser. However, although these authors favor the copper vapor laser for the treatment of discrete facial telangiectases, they believe the pulsed dye laser is more effective for treating telangiectatic rosacea and poikiloderma of Civatte.

When treating telangiectasia on the face with the copper vapor laser, a power setting of 450 to 650 mW is used in the gated mode, which chops the light into 200-msec exposure intervals every 400 msec. Anesthesia is usually not required, although some patients cannot tolerate the pins-and-needles sensation experienced during treatment. These patients can be pretreated with a topical or local anesthetic. The use of magnification ($\times 3.5$–$\times 6$) is usually necessary. The vessel should be traced with the laser until it "disappears." Postoperative wound care should include the topical application of an antibiotic ointment and avoidance of the sun. The fine punctate scabbing that occurs resolves within 10 to 14 days.

Telangiectatic Leg Veins of the Lower Extremities

There have been no published studies evaluating the treatment of spider veins with the copper vapor laser, though anecdotal evidence indicates that the small matlike vessels of the lower extremities may sometimes be successfully treated with the copper vapor laser.

Pigmented Lesions

The green light (511-nm) option of the copper vapor laser is used to treat pigmented lesions because melanin absorbs green light better than yellow light. The copper vapor laser is excellent for removing lentigines and ephelides. However, the outcomes from the treatment of café au lait spots with the copper vapor laser are not consistent, in that some lesions recur with time. Some suggest that melasma can be successfully treated with the copper vapor laser, although there are no published data to support this.

The 511-nm beam is delivered in either the chopped or gated mode. A 150-μm spot size is used freehand with power settings of 160 to 250 mW. Immediately after treatment the lesion should be slightly darker or gray. A crust forms in 3 to 4 days, which falls off in two weeks.

POSTSCLEROTHERAPY HYPERPIGMENTATION

Hyperpigmentation of the skin is a common side effect of sclerotherapy for the removal of varicose and spider veins of the lower extremities. It typically appears within 6 weeks of treatment and usually resolves without treatment over the next 6 months. The hyperpigmentation fades in most patients within 2 years, but occasionally, it persists for as long as 5 years after sclerotherapy. Histologic evaluation of this pigment has shown it to be hemosiderin in the superficial dermis.

Thibault and Wlodarczyk[101] used the copper vapor laser to treat 16 white women with postsclerotherapy pigmentation of at least 6 months' duration. In view of the absorption spectrum of hemosiderin (greater absorption of light at 511 nm than at 578 nm), the green light (511-nm) option was utilized and the laser was used in the continuous mode with a 400-μm spot size. The intensity and depth of pigmentation were evaluated, and on the basis of the findings, a power of 225 to 350 mW was selected. After one treatment session, 69% of the patients showed significant lightening of their hyperpigmentation but 25% felt that there was only slight improvement. None of the patients felt the hyperpigmentation had totally resolved.

COMPLICATIONS

Transient hyperpigmentation develops in 10% of patients who undergo treatment with the copper vapor laser for the removal of facial telangiectases.[99] Pickering and colleagues[102] reported a 3.5% incidence of scarring for patients with port-wine stains treated with the copper vapor laser, but only a small fraction of the treated area was affected in these patients. Waner and associates[100] have not noted any cases of scar formation. Hypopigmentation is another infrequent complication of copper vapor laser treatment.

SUMMARY

The copper vapor laser and copper bromide laser are versatile lasers, because they both emit a 578-nm (yellow) and a 511-nm (green) light, and the two may be used alone or in combination. Vascular lesions can be treated with the 578-nm wavelength and pigmented lesions with the 511-nm wavelength. Although the copper vapor laser does not treat vascular and pigmented lesions by selective photothermolysis (except in limited instances), it is a valuable tool for the treatment of certain clinical entities.

Robotic Optical Scanners and Automated Handpieces

Before the development of the flashlamp-pumped pulsed dye laser, the argon laser was the treatment of choice for many port-wine stains. However, a major drawback to the argon and other continuous-wave or quasi–continuous-wave lasers is that they can produce hypertrophic scarring and textural changes of the skin that may be caused by nonspecific thermal damage. The reported incidence of atrophic and hypertrophic changes is 6%, with an even higher incidence in children and in patients with port-wine stains in certain anatomic areas, such as the lip and neck.[72,103] Scarring has also been responsible for limiting the use of continuous-wave lasers on the trunk and extremities.

In an attempt to decrease the incidence of hypertrophic scarring and textural changes, new treatment techniques have been explored. One such modification involves altering the physical environment. Gilchrest and co-workers[41] tried to limit scarring by cooling the skin before and after treatment. However, although there was a decrease in the incidence of epidermal atrophy in patients on whom this technique was used, the incidence of hypertrophic scarring was unchanged. Several other authors have also not been able to demonstrate any advantage to cooling the skin in the prevention of hypertrophic scarring.[104,105] Another variation in treatment technique was to use a geometric variation in the pattern of the treatment area. Two patterns, dots and zebra stripes, were developed. The dot method was originally suggested by John Dixon[46] and consists of the formation of multiple 1- to 2-mm dots of blanching, produced by minimal power, with the dots placed 1 to 2 mm apart. The interspaces are then filled in at 12-week intervals. This method has been shown to lead to a reduction in the incidence of hypertrophic scarring, even in high-risk areas such as the upper and lower lip, nose, and nasolabial fold. Unfortunately, the method requires great skill on the part of the operator. The technique is also slow and tedious, and there is great variation in results.[35] The zebra-stripe method pioneered by Apfelberg and associates[106] consists in forming alternating rows or stripes, placed in the minimal skin tension lines of the face. The untreated stripes are treated later. The stripe technique is faster than the dot technique but is less precise. In addition, because the stripe method involves movement of the entire arm, it is especially difficult to master and reproduce the same results. Many patients have also been dissatisfied with the stripe technique, because they are often left with permanent bizarre stripes on their face.

Any method that involves manual movement of the handpiece has the potential to lead to complications. This is because it is difficult to maintain a constant speed across the entire lesion, with the result that a consistent energy fluence is often not delivered to each area. In an attempt to provide rapid, reproducible, and homogeneous laser treatments, robotic scanning devices and automated handpieces have been designed.[107-109] These devices are connected to the laser source via a fiberoptic cable and involve the use of an automated program, which places pulses of laser light in a precise, nonadjacent pattern, thereby ensuring that uniform laser energy is delivered to the entire lesion. This nonadjacent pattern limits undesired thermal injury to the surrounding dermis.

Currently, there are three types of robotic scanners—the Scanall, Multiscan, and Autolase—and three types of automated handpieces—the Hexascan, Smartscan, and CC-Scan.[109] Many of these devices are compatible with the argon, argon-dye, copper vapor, krypton, and continuous-wave frequency-doubled Nd:YAG laser.

The most commonly used of these devices has been the Hexascan.[110] The handpiece contains a power meter and a focusing device, and uniform 1-mm spot sizes are produced. A shutter provides pulse durations ranging from 30 to 990 msec. The 1-mm spot size forms a hexagonal irradiation pattern, and hexagons of various diameters can be produced: 3, 5, 9, 11, and 13 mm. The spots are placed 2 mm apart at 50-msec intervals to minimize nonspecific thermal injury. A 13-mm hexagon comprising 127 pulses can be created in 20 seconds.

The Autolase scanner has been available since 1991. The scanner is compatible with all high-repetition–rate pulsed laser (copper vapor and KTP) and continuous-wave laser (argon and continuous-wave dye). However, currently such a scanner is only available for the copper vapor laser. The Autolase exposure time can be adjusted in 5-msec increments from 20 msec to a maximum of 250 msec. Three hexagonal pattern sizes are available: 4, 7, and 10 mm.

A new KTP laser system, termed the *Orion system,* was recently released, which includes a scanning option called the *Smartscan.* The Orion can deliver 1- to 500-msec pulsewidths and 1 to 50 pulses/sec of 532-nm or 1064-nm radiation. The scanning device allows pulsewidths of between 1 and 50 msec.

Initially, the Hexascan was used with the argon laser to treat port-wine stains. Mordon and colleagues,[108] who developed this device, compared the effectiveness of the conventional point-by-point technique with that of the Hexascan in the treatment of port-wine stains. Their study population was large, consisting of over 100 patients treated with one of the two techniques. They found the results in patients treated using the Hexascan to be superior to those in patients treated using the conventional point-by-point technique. The incidence of scarring associated with Hexascan use was only 1%, compared with the 7% associated with use of the point-by-point technique.

McDaniel[111] has used the argon laser–pumped, tunable dye laser (yellow wavelength at 585 nm) with the Hexascan to treat vascular lesions, including port-wine stains, in infants as young as 3 weeks of age and observed proliferating hemangiomas that protruded up to 3 mm to abate after treatment. McDaniel has found side effects to be rare. Hypertrophic scarring has not been seen, although transient textural changes have occurred, and hypopigmentation and hyper-pigmentation are also rare. Other disorders that have been treated with this laser include telangiectases of the face, spider angiomas, cherry angiomas, poikiloderma of Civatte, venous lakes, and pyogenic granulomas. More studies using the Hexascan and 585-nm laser light to treat vascular lesions are necessary to define its role in the treatment of vascular lesions.

Dover and colleagues[86] compared the effects of the flashlamp-pumped pulsed dye laser and a continuous-wave dye laser used with a Hexascan (both at 585 nm) on test sites within port-wine stains in 29 patients. Both lasers were found to produce slight lightening after one treatment, but the pulsed dye laser produced slightly greater lightening and less hypopigmentation and hyperpigmentation.

The Hexascan has also been used in conjunction with the argon laser (514-nm green light) in the treatment of benign pigmented

Table 5-2. Hexascan treatment parameters

I. Vascular Lesions
    585 nm (yellow).
    Pulse length, 30–100 msec (pulsewidth for the selected fluence is controlled by a microprocessor).
    Use of maximum energy output produces the shortest pulse time with best clinical results.
    Treat every 6–12 weeks.
    A. Small-diameter vessels—port-wine stains, telangiectases, spider nevi:
        1. Treat with fluence of 18, 20, 22, or 24 J/cm².
        2. For infants; patients with lesions of neck or chest, severe actinic damage or scarring, or lesions on bony prominences; or darkly pigmented patients, start with 18–20 J/cm².
        3. For adults with lesions on the face or patients with trunk or hypertrophic lesions, start with 20–22 J/cm².
    B. Large-diameter vessels—port-wine stains, telangiectases, hemangiomas of less than 2 mm: Treat with fluence of 22–24 J/cm².
    C. Hemangiomas (2–3 mm or greater):
        1. Treat with fluence of 22, 24, or 26 J/cm².
        2. Can retreat in 2 weeks if lesion is rapidly proliferating.
II. Melanocytic Lesions
    514 nm (green).
    Pulse length, 30–50 msec.
    Treat every 4–6 weeks.
    A. Face: Treat with fluence of 10–12 J/cm².
    B. Trunk and extremities:
        1. Treat with 10, 12, or 14 J/cm².
        2. In darkly pigmented patients, start with 8–10 J/cm²; perform test treatment.

---

lesions. Although the shortest Hexascan pulse length is longer than that required for the selective photothermolysis of blood vessels and melanosomes, good results can still be obtained. Solar lentigines lighten significantly or disappear after one or two treatments, with maximal fading usually occurring within 3 to 4 weeks. The ideal fluence for treatment has been found to be 10 to 12 J/cm², but darkly pigmented people should be treated with lower fluences of 8 to 10 J/cm² (Table 5-2). It may be appropriate to treat a test area before the treatment of a large lesion. Other superficial pigmented lesions that respond well to treatment with the argon laser using the Hexascan are café au lait spots, ephelides, nevus spilus, and Becker's nevus, though the results from the treatment of melasma have been mixed.

Dermal pigmented lesions, such as nevus of Ota and congenital nevi, do not respond well to treatment with the argon laser (514-nm green light) delivered by Hexascan, because dermal penetration is not possible. Few side effects have been seen in the treatment of superficial pigmented lesions. Transient hypopigmentation, persistent hyperpigmentation, and epidermal atrophy are rare.

References

1. Gordon JP, Zeiger HJ, Townes CH. Molecular microwave oscillator and new hyperfine structure in the microwave spectrum of NH³. Phys Rev 1954;95:282–284.
2. Maiman TH. Stimulated optical radiation in ruby. Nature 1960;187:493–494.
3. Javan A, Bennett WR Jr, Herriott DR. Population inversion and continuous optical maser oscillation in a gas discharge containing a He-Ne mixture. Phys Rev Lett 1961;6:106.
4. Lengyel BA. Evolution of lasers and masers. Am J Physics 1966;34:903–913.
5. Bridges WB. Laser oscillation in singly ionized argon in the visible spectrum. Appl Phys Lett 1964;4:128–130.
6. Convert G, Armande M, Martinot-Lagarde P. Effet laser dans des melanges mercure-gaz rares. Compt Rend 1964;258:3259–3260.
7. Paananen RA. Progress in ionised-argon lasers. IEEE Spectrum 1966;3:88–99.
8. Bennett WB Jr, Knutson JW Jr, Mercer GN, Detch JL. Super-radiance, excitation mechanisms, and quasi-CW oscillation in the visible Ar+ laser. Appl Phys Lett 1964;4:180–182.
9. Gordon EI, Labuda EF, Bridges WB. Continuous visible laser action in singly ionized argon, krypton, and xenon. Appl Phys Lett 1964;4:178–180.
10. Labuda EF, Gordon EI, Miller RC. Continuous-duty argon ion lasers. IEEE J Quan Elec 1965;QE-1:273–279.
11. Bellina JH, Bandiermonte G. Principles and practice of gynecologic laser surgery. New York, London: Plenum, 1984:23–24.
12. Wilson J, Hawkes JFB. Lasers: principles and applications. New York: Prentice Hall, 1987:68.
13. Coherent SuperGraphite™ Series Ion Lasers Product Info and Specifications. Coherent, 1978.

14. Goldman L, Taylor WA. Development of a laser intravascular fiber optic probe for the treatment of superficial telangiectasia of the lower extremity in man. SPIE Novel Optical Fiber Techn Med Appl 1984;494: 76–78.

15. Russo V, Sottini S, Margheri G, Crea F. A novel corolla-irradiating fiber optic probe for laser angioplasty. SPIE Optical Fibers Med 1988;906: 301–304.

16. Russo V. Requirements of an up to date fibre optics delivery system for laser medicine. SPIE Adv Laser Medicine 1989;113–117.

17. Razum NJ, Keller GS, Bradley JG et al. Quartz contact probe for use with argon and Nd:YAG lasers. SPIE Optical Fibers Med 1990;1201: 313–317.

18. Wolinski W, Kazmirowski A, Kesid J et al. Argon-dye laser photocoagulator for the microsurgery of the interior structures of the eye. SPIE Lasers Med 1990;1353:172–176.

19. Carruth JAS, McKenzie AL. Medical lasers: science and clinical practice. Bristol, Boston: Adam Hilger, 1986:8–12.

20. Carruth JAS, McKenzie AL. Medical lasers: science and clinical practice. Bristol, Boston: Adam Hilger, 1986:13–19.

21. Anderson RR, Parrish JA. The optics of human skin. J Invest Dermatol 1981;77:13–19.

22. Anderson RR, Parrish JA. Selective photothermolysis: precise microsurgery by selective absorption of pulsed radiation. Science 1983;220: 524–527.

23. Jacobs HA, Walton RG. The incidence of birthmarks in the neonate. Pediatrics 1976;58:218–222.

24. Karvonen SL, Vaajalakti P, Mareuk M et al. Birthmarks in 4346 Finnish newborns. Acta Derm Venereol (Stockh) 1992;72:55–57.

25. Hobby LW. Treatment of port-wine stains and other cutaneous lesions. Contemp Surg 1981;18:22–45.

26. Geronemus RG, Ashinoff R. The medical necessity of evaluation and treatment of port-wine stains. J Dermatol Surg Oncol 1991;17:76–79.

27. Hidano A, Ogihara Y. Cryotherapy with solid carbon dioxide in the treatment of nevus flammeus. J Dermatol Surg Oncol 1977;3:213–216.

28. Conway H, Montry RE. Permanent camouflage of capillary hemangioma of the face by intradermal injection of insoluble pigments (tattooing): indications for surgery. NY State J Med 1965;65:876–885.

29. Finley JL, Barsley SH, Geer DE et al. Healing of port-wine stains after argon laser therapy. Arch Dermatol 1982;117:486–489.

30. Finley JL, Arndt KA, Noe JM, Rosen S. Argon laser–port-wine stain interaction: inadequate effects. Arch Dermatol 1984;120:613–619.

31. Solomon H, Goldman L, Henderson B et al. Histopathology of the laser treatment of port-wine lesions. J Invest Dermatol 1968;50:141–146.

32. Tan O, Carney M, Margolis R et al. Histologic responses of port-wine stains treated by argon, carbon dioxide and tunable dye lasers. Arch Dermatol 1986;122:1016–1022.

33. Neumann RA, Knobler RM, Leonhartsberger H et al. Histochemical evaluation of the coagulation depth after argon laser impact on a port-wine stain. Lasers Surg Med 1991;11:606–615.

34. Apfelberg DB, Kosek J, Maser MR, Lash H. Histology of port-wine stains following argon laser treatment. Br J Plast Surg 1979;32:232.

35. Apfelberg DB, Smith T, Maser M et al. Dot or pointillistic method for

improvement of results in hypertrophic scarring in the argon laser treatment of port-wine hemangiomas. Lasers Surg Med 1987;6:552–558.

36. Apfelberg DB, Maser MR, Lash H. Argon laser treatment of cutaneous vascular abnormalities: progress report. Ann Plast Surg 1978;1:14–18.
37. Goldman L, Dreffer R. Laser treatment of extensive mixed cavernous and port-wine stains. Arch Dermatol 1977;113:504.
38. Apfelberg DB, Kosek J, Maser MR, Lash H. Histology of port-wine stains following argon laser treatment. Br J Plast Surg 1979;32:232.
39. Apfelberg DB, Maser MR, Lash H, Rivers J. The argon laser for cutaneous lesions. JAMA 1981;245:2073.
40. Cosman B. Experience in the argon laser therapy of port-wine stains. Contemp Surg 1981;18:21.
41. Gilchrest BA, Rosen SH, Noe JM. Chilling port-wine stains improves the response to argon laser therapy. Plast Reconstr Surg 1982;67:278.
42. Cosman B. Clinical experience in the laser therapy of port-wine stains. Lasers Surg Med 1980;1:133–152.
43. Kalick SM, Goldwyn RM, Noe JM. Social issues and body image concerns of port-wine stain patients undergoing laser therapy. Lasers Surg Med 1981;1:205.
44. Noe JM, Barsky SH, Geer DE. Port-wine stains and the response to argon laser therapy: successful treatment and the predictive role of color, age and biopsy. Plast Reconstr Surg 1980;65:130.
45. Grabb WC, Dingman RO, O'Neal RM et al. Facial hamartomas in children: neurofibroma lymphangioma, and hemangiomas. Plast Reconstr Surg 1980;66:509.
46. Dixon JA, Huether S, Rotering R. Hypertrophic scarring in argon laser treatment of port-wine stains. Plast Reconstr Surg 1984;73:771–777.
47. Brauner G, Schliftman A, Cosman B. Evaluation of argon laser surgery in children under 13 years of age. Plast Reconstr Surg 1991;81:37–43.
48. Miller SH, Smith RL, Schochat SJ. Compression treatment of hemangiomas. Plast Reconstr Surg 1976;58:573–579.
49. Brown SH, Neerhant RC, Fonkalsrud EW. Prednisone therapy in the management of large hemangiomas in infants and children. Surgery 1971;71:168.
50. Apfelberg DB, Greene RA, Maser MR et al. Results of argon laser exposure of capillary hemangiomas of infancy: preliminary report. Plast Reconstr Surg 1981;67:188.
51. Hobby LW. Further evaluation of the potential of the argon laser in the treatment of strawberry hemangiomas. Plast Reconstr Surg 1983;71:481.
52. Achauer BM, VanderKam VM. Argon laser treatment of strawberry hemangiomas in infancy. West J Med 1985;143:628.
53. Achauer BM, VanderKam VM. Ulcerated anogenital hemangioma of infancy. Plast Reconstr Surg 1991;87:861–866.
54. Hobby L. Discussion of article by Achauer BN, VanderKam VM. Strawberry hemangioma of infancy. Early definitive treatment with the argon laser. Plast Reconstr Surg 1991;88:486–491.
55. Arndt KA. Argon laser therapy of small cutaneous vascular lesions. Arch Dermatol 1982;118:220–224.
56. Apfelberg DB, Maser MR, Lash HL. Treatment of nevus araneus by means of an argon laser. J Dermatol Surg Oncol 1978;4:172–174.
57. Kligman AM, Frosch PJ. Steroid addiction. Int J Dermatol 1979;18:23–31.

58. Safian J. A new anatomical concept of post-operative complications in aesthetic rhinoplasty. Plast Reconstr Surg 1973;51:162.

59. Noe JM, Finley J, Rosen S, Arndt KA. Post-rhinoplasty "red nose": Differential diagnosis and treatment by laser. Plast Reconstr Surg 1981; 67:661–664.

60. Dicken CH. Argon laser treatment of the red nose. J Dermatol Surg Oncol 1990;16:33–36.

61. Zachariae H, Bjerring P, Crmaers M. Argon laser treatment of cutaneous vascular lesion in connective tissue diseases. Acta Derm Venereol (Stockh) 1988;68:179–182.

62. Flores JT, Apfelberg DB, Maser MR et al. Angiokeratoma of Fordyce: successful treatment with the argon laser. Plast Reconstr Surg 1984;74: 835.

63. Pasyk KA, Argenta LC, Schelbert EB. Angiokeratoma circumscriptum: successful treatment with the argon laser. Ann Plast Surg 1988;20: 183–190.

64. Occella C, Bleidl D, Rampini P et al. Argon laser treatment of cutaneous multiple angiokeratomas. Dermatol Surg 1995;21:170–172.

65. Apfelberg DB, Maser MR, Lash H, Flores J. Expanded role of the argon laser in plastic surgery. J Dermatol Surg Oncol 1983;9:145–151.

66. Neumann RA, Knobler RM. Venous lakes of the lips—treatment experience with the argon laser and 18 months follow-up. Clin Exp Dermatol 1990;15:115–118.

67. Metze D, Neumann R, Chott A. Angiolymphoid hyperplasia. Histologic study and successful therapy with the argon laser. Hautarzt 1991;42: 101–106.

68. DaSilva OA, DaSilva PA, Verde SF, Martins O. Treatment of adenoma sebaceum by cryosurgery. Report of a case. J Dermatol Surg Oncol 1980;6:586.

69. Earhart RN, Nuss DD, Martin RJ et al. Dermabrasion for adenoma sebaceum. J Dermatol Surg 1976;2:412.

70. Arndt KA. Adenoma sebaceum: successful treatment with the argon laser. Plast Reconstr Surg 1982;70:91–93.

71. Pasyk KA, Argenta LC. Argon laser surgery of skin lesions in tuberous sclerosis. Ann Plast Surg 1988;20:426–433.

72. Arndt KA, Noe JM, Rosen S. Cutaneous laser therapy—principle and methods. Chichester: Wiley, 1983:165–186.

73. Wheeland RG. Lasers in skin disease. New York: Thieme, 1988:7–51.

74. McBurney EL. Dermatologic laser surgery. Otolaryngol Clin North Am 1990;23:77–97.

75. Arndt KA. Argon laser treatment of lentigo maligna. J Am Acad Dermatol 1984;10:953–957.

76. Arndt KA. New pigmented macule appearing four years after argon laser treatment of lentigo maligna. J Am Acad Dermatol 1986;14:1092.

77. Greenwald J, Rosen S, Anderson RR et al. Comparative histological studies of the tunable dye (at 577 nm) laser and argon laser: the specific vascular effects of the dye laser. J Invest Dermatol 1981;77:305–310.

78. Cotterill JA. Preliminary results following treatment of vascular lesions of the skin using a continuous wave dye laser which emits at 577 nm. Clin Exp Dermatol 1986;11:628–635.

79. Lanigan SW, Carwright P, Cotterill JA. Continuous wave dye laser therapy of port-wine stains. Br J Dermatol 1989;121:343–352.

80. Cosman B. Experience in the argon laser therapy of port-wine stains. Plast Reconstr Surg 1980;65:119–129.

81. Apfelberg DB, Maser MR, Lash H. Experience in the argon laser therapy of port-wine stains. Ann Plast Surg 1977;1:14–18.

82. Goldman L, Dreffer R, Rockwell JR Jr, Perry E. Treatment of port-wine stains by the argon laser. J Dermatol Surg 1976;2:385–388.

83. Malm M, Rigler R, Jurell G. Continuous wave (CW) dye laser vs. CW argon laser treatment of port-wine stain (PWS). Scand J Plast Reconstr Surg 1988;22:241–244.

84. Scheibner A, Wheeland R. Argon-pumped tunable dye laser therapy for facial port-wine stain hemangiomas in adults—a new technique using small spot-size and minimal power. J Dermatol Surg Oncol 1989; 15:277–282.

85. Scheibner A, Wheeland R. Use of the argon-pumped tunable dye laser for port-wine stains in children. J Dermatol Surg Oncol 1991;17:735–739.

86. Dover JS, Geronemus R, Stern RS et al. Dye laser treatment of port wine stains: comparison of the continuous wave dye laser with a robotized scanning device and the pulsed dye laser. J Am Acad Dermatol 1995;32:237–240.

87. McDaniel DH. Cutaneous vascular disorders: advances in laser treatment. Cutis 1990;45:339–360.

88. Orenstein A, Nelson JS. Treatment of facial vascular lesions with a 100-micron spot 577-nm pulsed continuous wave dye laser. Ann Plast Surg 1989;23:310.

89. Ross M, Watcher MA, Goodman MM. Comparison of the flashlamp pulsed dye laser with the argon tunable dye laser with robotized handpiece for facial telangiectasia. Lasers Surg Med 1993;13:374–379.

90. Apfelberg DB, Bailin P, Rosenberg H. Preliminary investigation of KTP/532 laser light in the treatment of hemangiomas and tattoos. Lasers Surg Med 1986;6:38–42.

91. Walter WT, Solimene N, Piltch M, Gould G. Efficient pulsed gas discharge lasers. IEEE J Quantum Electronics 1966;4:474–479.

92. Hecht J. Copper and gold vapor lasers. In: The laser guidebook. New York: McGraw-Hill, 1992:197–210.

93. Goldman L, Taylor APT, Putnam T. New developments with the heavy metal vapor lasers for the dermatologist. J Dermatol Surg Oncol 1987;13:163–165.

94. Tan O, Stafford T, Murray S, Kurban A. Histologic comparison of the pulsed dye laser and copper vapour laser effects on pig skin. Lasers Surg Med 1990;10:551–558.

95. Tan OT, Murray S, Kurban AK. Action spectrum of vascular specific injury in pulsed irradiation. J Invest Dermatol 1989;92:868–871.

96. Neumann RA, Knobler RM, Leonhartsberger H, Gebhart W. Comparative histochemistry of port-wine stains after copper vapor laser (578 nm) and argon laser treatment. J Invest Dermatol 1992;99:160–167.

97. Dinehart SM, Waner M, Flock S. The copper vapor laser for treatment of cutaneous vascular and pigmented lesions. J Dermatol Surg Oncol 1993;19:370–375.

98. Sheehan-Dare RA, Cotterill JA. Copper vapour laser treatment of port wine stains: clinical evaluation and comparison with conventional argon laser therapy. Br J Dermatol 1993;128:546–549.

99. Key JM, Waner M. Selective destruction of facial telangiectasia using a

copper vapor laser. Arch Otolaryngol Head Neck Surg 1992;118: 509–513.

100. Waner M, Dinehart SM. A comparison of the copper vapor and flash-lamp pulsed dye lasers in the treatment of facial telangiectasia. J Dermatol Surg Oncol 1993;19:992–998.

101. Thibault P, Wlodarczyk J. Postsclerotherapy hyperpigmentation. The role of serum ferritin levels and the effectiveness of treatment with the copper vapor laser. J Dermatol Surg Oncol 1992;18:47–52.

102. Pickering J, Walker E, Butler P, Halewyn C. Copper vapor laser treatment of port-wine stains and other vascular malformations. Br J Plast Surg 1990;43:273–282.

103. Dover JS, Arndt KA, Geronemus RG, Olbricht SM, Noe JM, Stern RS. Illustrated cutaneous laser surgery: a practitioner's guide. Norwalk, CT: Appleton & Lange, 1990:73–106.

104. Welch AJ, Motamedim M, Gonzales A. Evaluation of cooling techniques for the protection of the epidermis during Nd:YAG laser radiation of the skin. In: Joffe SN, ed. Neodymium-YAG laser in medicine and surgery. New York: Elsevier, 1983:196–204.

105. Yanai A, Fukuda O, Soyano S et al. Argon laser therapy of port wine stains: effects and limitations. Plast Reconstr Surg 1985;75:520–527.

106. Apfelberg D, Flores JT, Maser M, Lash H. Analysis of complications of argon laser treatment for port wine hemangiomas with reference to stripe treatment. Lasers Surg Med 1983;2:357–372.

107. Rotteleur G, Mordon S, Buys B et al. Robotized scanning laser handpiece for the treatment of port wine stains and other angiodysplasias. Lasers Surg Med 1988;8:283–287.

108. Mordon SR, Rotteleur G, Buys B, Brunetaud JM. Comparative study of the "point-by-point technique" and the "scanning technique" for laser treatment of port wine stain. Lasers Surg Med 1989;9:398–404.

109. Chambers IR, Clark D, Bainbridge C. Automation of laser treatment of port wine stains. Phys Med Biol 1990;7:1025–1028.

110. McDaniel DH, Mordon S. Hexascan. A new robotized scanning laser handpiece. Cutis 1990;45:300–305.

111. McDaniel DH. Clinical usefulness of the Hexascan: treatment of cutaneous vascular and melanocytic disorders. J Dermatol Surg Oncol 1993;19:312–319.

6 ——— The Flashlamp-Pumped Pulsed Dye Laser for Cutaneous Vascular Lesions

Jerome M. Garden

Advances in the field of laser therapy for cutaneous diseases have evolved rapidly for the past several years. This progress has been especially apparent in the treatment of benign cutaneous blood vessel diseases. The development of the dye laser, used in a pulsed mode, has allowed therapists to treat these lesions in patients of all ages and in all anatomic sites. In particular, this laser has increased our ability to effectively treat port-wine stains (PWSs) and other vascular abnormalities, with an attendant decrease in the risk of undesirable side effects.

Basic Concepts

To understand the reasons for the therapeutic advancements, it is important to look at several basic laser parameters. All lasers emit specific wavelengths, depending on the type of lasing medium in the optical cavity. Many different wavelengths potentially can be used as a source of lesional irradiation. The main lesional chromophore in cutaneous blood vessel processes, such as PWSs, hemangiomas, spider angiomas, and telangiectasia, is hemoglobin, with oxyhemoglobin assumed to be the major hemoglobin species present. Oxyhemoglobin is an excellent target for laser emission, because it is located intravascularly in a high concentration. It has major absorption peaks at 418, 542, and 577 nm.[1,2] Although the strongest peak is at 418 nm, making the 418-nm wavelength the one most readily absorbed, the laser emission wavelength chosen for therapy coincides with the 577-nm peak.

There are two reasons for using the weaker 577-nm wavelength. First, the major competing chromophore in the skin is melanin, which absorbs very well in the ultraviolet range and has a diminishing absorption capacity throughout the visible range. Therefore the absorption of melanin at 418 nm is significantly greater than its absorption at 542 nm or 577 nm, with the latter wavelength being the least absorbed and thus the desirable one to be used in this setting. The other reason is the penetration depth of laser emission. For the nonionizing, visible range of wavelengths, the longer the wavelength the deeper the tissue penetration. Therefore the 577-nm wavelength has the advantage of both coinciding with an oxyhemoglobin absorption band, at which the melanin absorption is decreased, and of penetrating deeper into tissue.[3] Recent evidence has indicated that even longer wavelengths are still selectively absorbed by oxyhemoglobin, thereby producing vascular damage, but penetrate deeper than the 577-nm wavelength.[4–6]

The tissue response to laser emission is not only wavelength dependent but also time dependent. Because the effect of most cutaneous medical lasers is achieved mainly through photothermal conversion, a longer tissue exposure time results in a greater thermal response. Mathematical tissue modeling has been used to predict the optimal laser time emissions that will effect the selective destruction of cutaneous blood vessels.[2] An index used to assist in these computations is the thermal relaxation time, which is the time it takes a heated container, such as the cutaneous blood vessel, to lose half of its maximum heat. Depending on the size of the blood vessel, the predetermined emission wavelength, the optimum pulse duration (i.e., the time the laser remains on) can be estimated using these formulas. The goal of these calculations is to determine the amount of time needed to heat and denature the vasculature without damaging the surrounding tissue.[1]

Selective heating of the targeted blood vessels can best be accomplished through the containment of high temperatures in the vessels, followed by the slow diffusion of cooler temperatures to the perivascular area. If the pulse duration produces vascular destruction but is not on long enough to allow the diffusion of undesirably high temperatures to the surrounding tissue, tissue sparing occurs. Clinical studies were conducted to evaluate the normal skin response, followed by others that assessed the PWS response. Analysis of the 350-nsec to 20-μsec pulse duration, at 577 nm, revealed that this produced vessel-selective, laser-induced damage,[7–9] but these pulse durations were unable to produce PWS lightening.[10] Although thermal damage was confined to the target vessels with no apparent perivascular change, the vessels were subsequently able to repair sufficiently that no permanent clinical change occurred.

When pulse durations were extended to the 20- to 500-μsec range, at a wavelength of 577 nm, vessel-selective damage resulted in lesional lightening. Histologic evaluation revealed the presence of an intervascular coagulum and not the extravasation of red blood cells seen in lesions treated at the shorter pulse durations.[8,11] The longer pulse durations, especially those greater than 200 μsec, were found to be increasingly more likely to produce lesional lightening, yet the perivascular changes remained unremarkable, with only a few areas of scattered focal epidermal spongiosis. The epidermal changes occurred most commonly adjacent to areas of superficial blood vessels, which may represent direct thermal diffusion to the epidermis. On the basis of these findings it appears that the intravascular photothermal conversion must last long enough to cause permanent endo-thelial damage but not so long as to allow high temperatures to dif-fuse into the perivascular area.

Besides the appropriate wavelength and pulse duration for op-timizing the selective destruction of cutaneous blood vessels, the amount of energy delivered to the tissue (fluence) is another impor-tant laser parameter.[12] On the basis of mathematical projections at 577 nm and modeled for cutaneous blood vessels, energy fluences can be estimated that can elevate the core vessel temperature to 70°C, thereby producing the desired permanent endothelial denatura-tion.[1] When initially studied in normal skin, the fluences necessary to produce purpura and vessel damage were found to be remarkably similar to the estimated values. Indeed, when much higher energy densities were tested in normal skin, there was significant perivascu-lar damage along with collagen denaturation. These data helped clinicians develop a therapeutic energy range for PWSs.

The fluence needed to produce purpura in normal skin at a wave-length of 577 nm and pulse duration of 360 μsec was found to be 3.5 to 4.25 J/cm², depending on the skin temperature[13,14] and color.[15] Both factors were found to influence the laser-tissue interaction. From the standpoint of temperature, the colder the tissue, the more fluence is needed to produce purpura, either because of vessel con-striction and the resulting decrease in the target size, or the need to heat the tissue over a greater range. With regard to skin color, higher fluences are needed for increasingly darker skin types, because of the presence of epidermal melanin, which acts as a shield or barrier to the incoming photons. The PWS, with its dilated vessels, requires more energy to produce lesional lightening. Temperature and color play a role in the lesional response similar to the one they play in normal skin.[16]

Another laser parameter that has been analyzed is the spot size, which is the area of tissue impacted by the laser beam during each pulse. Animal studies have shown that the laser-induced tissue effects are inconsistent when a circular spot size of less than 3 mm in diame-ter is used.[17] It is believed that optical effects, probably secondary to dermal scattering, are important factors in determining the clinical outcome that occurs with a changing spot size. Recent clinical work in which a 2-mm spot size was used in the treatment of solitary tel-angiectatic vessels demonstrated the necessity of using higher flu-ences than those used with 3-mm or greater spot sizes.

The selective thermal destruction of blood vessels with sparing of surrounding tissue that occurs when optimal laser and tissue para-meters are used has been termed *selective photothermolysis*.[18] It accom-plishes the incorporation of laser light into the general tissue area, thereby producing selective photothermal damage, without the need for structure-specific laser focusing. It is this approach which has been responsible for achieving more desirable clinical outcomes.

While the theoretical concepts of selective photothermolysis were being developed, it was necessary to have a laser capable of producing the desired optimal laser parameters. The flashlamp-pumped, pulsed dye laser was chosen because of its inherent flexibility. An emission in the 577-nm range was achieved by selecting the appropriate organic dye as the lasing medium and tuning the wavelength to the desired one using a filter. In recent modifications, different organic dyes are mixed at set concentrations, thereby producing the desired wavelength emission and eliminating the need for a filter. The pulsed-dye laser also has the advantage of being able to excite the dye for long enough to achieve a pulse duration in the 400- to 500-μsec range, with sufficient energy to produce spot sizes at 3 mm and above. Other lasers available for the treatment of cutaneous lesions either do not emit the desired wavelengths (argon, CO_2, Nd:YAG, ruby, and KTP laser) or are unable to produce pulse durations in the desired range (argon, CO_2, Nd:YAG, ruby, KTP, copper vapor, krypton, and argon laser–pumped tunable dye laser). Although many of these lasers can be effective in the treatment of cutaneous blood vessel lesions, they are less tissue selective, which has limited their use. In addition, more technical expertise is required on the part of the user and, most importantly, the risk of associated side effects is greater.[19,20]

Clinical Effectiveness

There are many types of cutaneous blood vessel lesions that can be successfully treated with the flashlamp-pumped, pulsed dye laser, including PWSs, capillary hemangiomas, telangiectases, spider and senile angiomas, permanent erythema resulting from rosacea or trauma, angioma serpiginosum, angiofibromas, venous ectasia, and minor varicosities. It appears that any small-caliber vessel, superficial tissue process is amenable to pulsed dye laser therapy.[21-23] However, the most data and experience have been acquired in the treatment of patients with PWSs.

PORT-WINE STAINS

The emitted energy is the laser parameter that is varied in the treatment of PWSs. Ongoing studies are evaluating longer wavelengths of up to 600 nm and pulsed durations at 1.5 msec to determine whether they produce better results. Currently a wavelength of 585 nm and pulse duration of 400 to 500 μsec are used. The fluences found to be therapeutic range from 3.5 J/cm^2, which is used in the pediatric population, to 9.0 J/cm^2, which is used in adults with thick, dark purple PWSs. The spot size generally used is either 5 to 10 mm, but the efficacy of a 10-mm spot size is currently being investigated. Originally test sites were placed over the PWSs using fluences 1½ to 2 times those needed to produce threshold purpura. This was defined as the least amount of energy necessary to cause normal, nonlesional skin to become purpuric within a set amount of time after laser exposure.

However, as experience accumulated threshold testing was found to be unnecessary and test site fluences are now chosen on the basis of the patient's age, the anatomic area, and the thickness and color of the lesion.

When the laser light impacts the tissue, two events occur. The patient experiences discomfort, described by many as a hot pinprick sensation or the sensation of an elastic band snapping against the skin, and the tissue becomes purpuric. The sensation is generally well tolerated by adult patients, except in more sensitive places, such as the upper lip or periorbital areas. The perceived sensation may be greater when larger spot sizes are used. Topically administered or injected local anesthesia is helpful.[24,25] Although local anesthetic agents may help adolescent or pediatric patients tolerate the procedure, other agents also may be necessary. Nitrous oxide may be beneficial in older children, and infants may be helped by chloral hydrate or other orally administered mild sedatives. However, many children need greater sedation, involving the use of intramuscularly or intravascularly administered anesthetic agents used for outpatient procedures. Popular anesthetics for young infants include propofol and ketamine. When treating nonperioral areas, halothane can be administered with ease for relatively short cases, without the need for intubation.[26]

The purpura that occurs after exposure to the laser light appears immediately or within a few minutes and gradually darkens over the following 24 hours. Histologically, the purpura represents the formation of an intravascular coagulum.[11] Within 24 hours a leukocytoclastic vasculitis also develops in treated vessels. Resorption of the vessel occurs over 4 weeks. The vessels are replaced by normal-diameter vessels within a few months of treatment.[27] Clinically, the purpura remains for an average of 7 to 14 days.[28] During this time, a topical antibiotic ointment is used in pediatric patients. Adult patients, however, may place a cosmetic coverup over the treated area, if desired, immediately after therapy. Occasionally some epidermal scaling or crusting forms in patients treated with higher energies. In the adult patient, this is treated with a topical antibiotic ointment. A dermatitis occasionally develops after multiple treatments, which responds well to treatment with mild topical corticosteroids.

Test sites are first placed over the PWS to determine the clinical efficacy and optimal energy dosage. Multiple sites are generally placed using various energies. Because the PWS is nonhomogeneous, different energies may be needed to achieve the same clinical effect throughout the lesion. The goal is to use the least amount of energy to achieve the most acceptable outcome. However, as already noted, there is a finite therapeutic window, in that too little energy does not produce enough lightening and too much energy may cause undesired pigmentary and texture changes, with the potential of scarring.

Although the PWS darkening that occurs after treatment resolves in 7 to 14 days, it may last slightly longer in patients in whom the 7-mm spot size and higher fluences are used. Lesional lightening may take 2 to 3 months.[21-23,28] In fact, after the darkening resolves, the lesion may appear redder for several weeks and unchanged for an additional 4 to 6 weeks before lightening appears. It is almost always necessary to retreat a lesional area to promote lightening. These retreatment sessions are scheduled every 2 to 3 months until maximum lightening is achieved. It is not uncommon for patients to undergo many treatment sessions. Lesional lightening may be achieved even after 20 treatment sessions.[29] However, the percentage of lightening that occurs in response to each treatment continues to decrease, and eventually it becomes appropriate to stop therapy.

Results can range from total clearing to very little perceptible change. It is assumed that a more superficial vessel with a smaller caliber will clear easier than a larger vessel situated deep in the dermis. Because PWSs are composed of vessels of various calibers with differing depths of involvement, inconsistent lightening occurs, both among patients and in the same patient.

Studies have revealed that 36% to 44% of the adult patients with PWSs experience 75% or more lightening and approximately 75% of patients experience at least 50% lightening after a total of four treatments.[30,31] These results were based on a limited number of retreatments, however. It is likely that continued lightening would have occurred with more retreatment sessions (Fig. 6-1). Those adult patients who do not show substantial lightening after repeated treatments fortunately account for less than 10% of the total number of patients treated. Some of these patients have nodular and thickened PWSs, which do not respond well to this laser treatment. These types of PWSs may respond better to treatment with continuous-wave or quasi–continuous-wave lasers, such as the argon, copper vapor, Nd:YAG, or krypton lasers, which incorporate a greater degree of the nonselective thermal energy necessary to decrease both the soft-tissue and vascular components.[19]

Of interest are the patients with PWSs who do not respond well to laser treatment even though they have lesions clinically identical to those in other patients who do show an acceptable degree of lightening. Apparently the clinical appearance of the lesion cannot necessarily be used as the basis for predicting the therapeutic outcome. PWSs in different anatomic sites also respond differently to this laser treatment, as is seen for treatment with other types of lasers. PWSs on the central cheek and upper lip are more resistant to therapy, as are lesions on the lower extremities and the distal aspects of the upper extremities. On the other hand, PWSs in the periorbital and lateral facial areas, as well as those on the neck, chest, and upper arm, generally respond the best to this laser treatment.[32,33]

Of greater significance than the degree of lesional lightening in adult patients with PWSs has been the paucity of adverse effects. Changes such as permanent hypopigmentation or hyperpigmentation or skin texture atrophy or depression occur in less than 10% of the patients in less than 2% of the lesion.[30] A recent retrospective study of 297 patients with PWSs treated by the pulsed dye laser

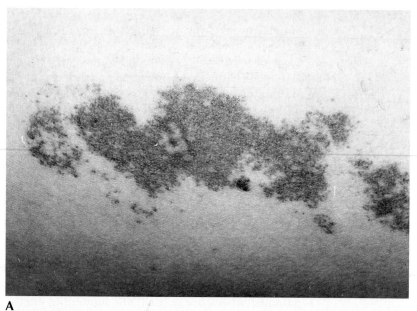

A

B

Fig. 6-1. (A) Port-wine stain on left thigh of 25-year-old woman. (B) Site after nine treatments with the flashlamp-pumped, pulsed dye laser. See Fig. 6-1 in color section.

showed an incidence of atrophic scarring of approximately 1% and no hypertrophic scarring.[34] Many of the cases of pigmentary changes or skin depression, or both, are transient, with almost complete normalization occurring over time. Most importantly, skin induration and scarring have only rarely occurred. There are only a few anecdotal reports of small areas of lesions becoming indurated or scarred, which is a small number considering the tens of thousands of treatment sessions that have been performed using this laser.[35]

The clinical outcome of treatment with the flashlamp-pumped, pulsed dye laser in the pediatric population with PWS also has been remarkable.[23,36–40] It appears to be more effective in achieving lesional lightening in children than in adults, however. The PWS lightening reported to occur in these pediatric patients ranges from 100% clearing in all treated patients,[36] to greater than 95% clearing in 18% with the rest showing 65% to 70% response,[38] to 42% of patients showing more than 75% clearing and 84% of patients more than 50% clearing,[39] to 87% of patients showing at least 50% lightening.[40] The age ranges of patients and number of treatment sessions (from two to more than six) differed for these series, however, thus making direct comparison difficult. Nevertheless, these data do show that the response is definitely greater in the young pediatric population.

The small caliber of the vessels in the PWSs of pediatric patients, compared with the caliber of the vessels in adults, may be a factor. PWSs typically appear pink to red in childhood and gradually darken and thicken in adulthood as the result of progressive widening of the vessels. Unfortunately, there are infants who have deeply colored PWSs which may lighten with greater difficulty.[37] It is still often necessary, however, to perform test site placement procedures and repeated procedures to the same area in the pediatric population. Regardless of whether the patient is a child or adult, after therapy is completed, there is always the potential of a residual lesion, which does not continue to sufficiently respond to warrant further procedures, to darken with time. Indeed, this already has occurred in several patients. One would expect this to happen as the result of the vessels dilating with age. It is hoped that these treated lesions do not revert back to their original appearance, because many of the vessels in the lesion with therapy are now a normal caliber. However, should the underlying cause of PWS be a defect in the innervation of PWS vessels, the incidence of recurrence may prove to be greater than expected.

The fluences necessary for the treatment of pediatric patients with PWSs are less than those needed in adults, with a smaller therapeutic window. However, fluences as low as 3.5 J/cm² have been used successfully in some pediatric PWSs in certain anatomic areas, such as the neck and chest, employing the 10-mm spot size. The risk of textural changes is greater in the pediatric population. Even fluences above 6.5 J/cm² have a tendency to produce these cutaneous changes in younger patients. It is therefore appropriate to treat young patients using lower fluences and more treatment sessions, rather than the reverse, to reduce the risk of these side effects.

Overlapping of the individual circular pulses is recommended in an effort to prevent a honeycomb pattern of clearing. This not only improves the appearance of the PWS as it clears but it also reduces the total number of treatments needed. Overlapping should be limited to approximately 10% to 15% of the spot size.[41] This is especially true for pediatric patients with PWSs, because there may be an increased risk of scarring if too much overlap occurs. Although treatment with the pulsed dye laser is far less painful than treatment with continuous-wave lasers, as mentioned earlier, each pulse does produce discomfort and, as the number of pulses increases, the pain associated with the treatment increases. Thus, pain may become the limiting factor of treatment if appropriate, anesthetic intervention, such as that described earlier, is not used.

The greatest risk to the patient and to the treating staff is eye damage. Because of good absorption of 585-nm light by the pigmented and vascular portions of the retina, there is a great potential for significant retinal damage to occur if the appropriate protective eyewear is not worn. Goggles made from didymium, which has a narrow band of absorption high in the 500-nm visible spectrum, are ideal for eye protection, at the same time allowing the operator to see. Patients can wear these protective goggles, they can wear opaque goggles, or their eyes can be covered with gauze. If periorbital treatment is being performed, the patient can wear nonplastic eye shields.

TELANGIECTASIS

Cutaneous vascular lesions, other than PWSs, also respond well to the flashlamp-pumped pulsed dye laser. Face, neck, and trunk telangiectases can generally be treated using a 3- or 2-mm spot size. These include telangiectases that form as the result of almost any cause, including actinic damage, rosacea, connective tissue disease, hepatic dysfunction, or trauma.[42-44] The darkening of the treated area resolves faster than that associated with PWSs, lasting 5 to 10 days. However, the posttherapy darkening is still of concern to many patients. Fortunately, the smaller 2-mm spot size causes the posttherapy bruised appearance to be significantly diminished. The discomfort experienced during therapy is also less when the smaller spot size is used.

It is only occasionally necessary to perform test sites in patients with telangiectases, and when this is done, a fluence of 5.75 to 7.00 J/cm^2 is usually chosen. However, it appears that fluences higher than 7.0 J/cm^2 are necessary when using the 2-mm spot size. Lesional lightening may occur immediately after the posttherapy darkening resolves or up to 4 to 6 weeks later. Retreatment may be necessary, but this is less often necessary than it is for the treatment of PWSs. The final therapeutic outcome is usually excellent, with almost total eradication of the telangiectases and with only rare cases of skin texture changes or depression.

Vessels on the face respond best (Fig. 6-2). Although lower-extremity telangiectases do not respond as well,[45] very small caliber red vessels can be effectively treated. The fine-caliber, "star-burst"–type vessels, those less than 0.2 mm in diameter, which often develop as a consequence of sclerotherapy, may also respond well to pulsed dye laser therapy, performed in one or two treatment sessions. A com-

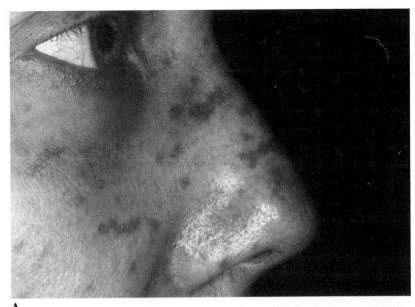

A

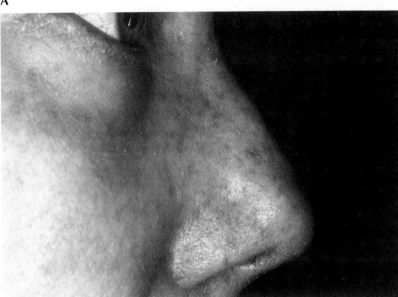

B

Fig. 6-2.   (A) Matted telangiectasia on right nose of 35-year-old woman. (B) Site after two treatments with the flashlamp-pumped, pulsed dye laser. See Fig. 6-2 in color section.

bined approach, in which other therapeutic modalities, such as sclerotherapy, are used on the larger-caliber vessels and the laser is used on the small-caliber vessels, which are more difficult to inject, has proved effective. Unfortunately, even in the treatment of these small-caliber vessels, postlaser hyperpigmentation may persist for months. Studies in which wavelengths of up to 600 nm and pulse durations of 1.5 msec were used for the treatment of up to 0.6-mm lower-extrem-

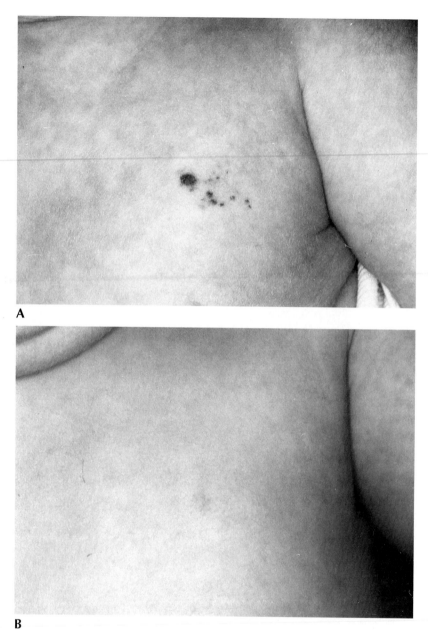

A

B

Fig. 6-3. (A) Capillary hemangioma, superficial and deep type, in a 2-month-old female infant. (B) Site after five treatments with the flashlamp-pumped, pulsed dye laser. There has been resolution of the superficial component only. See Fig. 6-3 in color section.

Table 6-1.   Criteria for use of laser therapy for hemangiomas

Potential for functional impairment

Risk of ulceration:

  Rapid enlargement

  Recurrent trauma

  Moist area

Cosmetic disfigurement:

  Highly visible lesion

  Extensive surface area

Source: Data from Garden JM, Bakus AD, Paller AS. Treatment of cutaneous hemangiomas by the flashlamp-pumped pulsed dye laser: prospective analysis. J Pediatr 1992;120:555–560.

ity vessels have shown promising results. Elliptical spot sizes delivered at fluences of 15 J/cm^2 or greater have been shown to be effective using pulsewidths of both 450 and 1.5 msec. Posttherapy hyperpigmentation, even using these different parameters, remains an undesirable sequela, however.

Capillary hemangiomas have shown a good response to flashlamp-pumped pulsed dye laser therapy.[46–49] However, only the superficial type appears to respond to laser therapy, whereas the deep cavernous type is unaffected (Fig. 6-3). The best outcome is achieved in the early phase of the clinical presentation, before or immediately at the onset of the proliferative stage. The flatter superficial lesions, those that are raised 3 mm or less off the skin surface, almost completely resolve with treatment. Low energy doses are delivered every few weeks until the lesion flattens and resolves. It is more difficult to interrupt active proliferation and achieve total resolution in lesions that are raised more than 3 mm above the skin surface. After completed therapy, textural changes consisting of atrophy and hypopigmentation develop in some areas. Criteria have been suggested to help the laser clinician decide whether it is appropriate to use the laser for the treatment of capillary or mixed hemangiomas (Table 6-1).[48]

OTHER BENIGN VASCULAR DISORDERS

Areas of permanent cutaneous erythema or diffuse telangiectasis, as occur in the settings of rosacea, postrhinoplasty red-nose, and poikiloderma of Civatte[50]; after trauma; or in scars, respond to the flashlamp-pumped pulsed dye laser. The therapeutic approach used is similar to the one used for PWSs, and involves the use of a 5-mm or greater spot size and treating, if necessary, a wide surface area. Outcomes have been very favorable, with a significant reduction in and elimination of the underlying permanently dilated vessels and the manifested erythema. Investigations evaluating the use of the 10-mm spot size using low fluences immediately below the purpura threshold have yielded encouraging results. It may be possible using this large spot size to treat telangiectases and permanent erythema but not induce significant purpura.

In addition, it has been observed that flashlamp-pumped pulsed dye treatment not only reduces the erythema of scars in many patients with hypertrophic scars secondary to prior treatment of their vascular lesions, but also reduces the size of the scar.[51] The precise mechanism responsible for this is unknown, but it has been suggested that a therapy-induced reduction in the lesional vessel volume results in a decrease in the total tissue volume. However, this most likely only partially explains its effectiveness, because nonvascular malformation–associated scars also have been noted to respond to pulsed dye laser treatment.[52] Therefore it is likely that this laser treatment has some effect on scar tissue other than just its effect on the vasculature. It is unknown whether laser therapy has any permanent positive effect on the fibroblasts.

Solitary vascular lesions such as venous lakes and spider or cherry angiomas also respond favorably to treatment with the flashlamp-pumped pulsed dye laser.[21–23] However, as with PWSs and hemangiomas, the thicker lesions do not respond as well. Enlarged pyogenic granulomas are especially difficult to treat, even if multiple, repetitive, high-energy pulses are delivered to the lesion, but can, at times, be very responsive.

NONVASCULAR LESIONS

Other cutaneous clinical processes that have been treated by the flashlamp-pumped pulsed dye laser include plaque-type psoriasis[53,54] and warts.[55] Both appear to respond but only in a limited manner. Psoriatic lesions do flatten, but generally incompletely, and can recur. Warts that are not located over the periungual or plantar surfaces and are flat may resolve readily with laser therapy. However, the initial failure rate and follow-up recurrence rate associated with the treatment of very keratotic lesions or those over the periungual or plantar surfaces are much greater than the rates associated with the treatment of less keratotic lesions and lesions in other areas. It is assumed that the laser interaction with the underlying vasculature plays a beneficial but uncertain role in the eradication of both diseases.

An interesting recent development has been the use of the pulsed dye laser for the treatment of stretchmarks. Larger spot sizes have been used in this setting, with some early successes in the treatment of both new and older lesions. Not all lesions respond, but those that do can show significant resolution.

Summary

The flashlamp-pumped pulsed dye laser may be the therapeutic instrument of choice for the treatment of most superficial cutaneous vascular lesions, especially in the pediatric population. Most types of cutaneous blood vessel diseases have been treated with and re-sponded favorably to pulsed dye laser therapy. However, the best response is seen for processes that are superficially located and have small-caliber vessel involvement; a favorable outcome may be achieved for other types of vascular lesions, but only with greater dif-ficulty. Limitations in the ability of the flashlamp-pumped pulsed dye laser to treat all lesions consistently well have fueled efforts to im-prove its design and use. Research into ways to optimize the wave-length, pulse duration, spot size, and energy for the treatment of specific lesions is ongoing.

References

1. Anderson RR, Parrish JA. Microvasculature can be selectively damaged using dye lasers: a basic theory and experimental evidence in human skin. Lasers Surg Med 1981;1:263–276.
2. Van Gemert MJC, Hulsbergen Henning JP. A model approach to laser coagulation of dermal vascular lesions. Arch Dermatol Res 1981;270: 429–439.
3. Anderson RR, Parrish JA. The optics of human skin. J Invest Dermatol 1981;77:13–19.
4. Tan OT, Murray S, Kurban AK. Action spectrum of vascular specific in-jury using pulsed irradiation. J Invest Dermatol 1989;92:868–871.
5. Tan OT, Morrison P, Kurban AK. 585 nm for the treatment of portwine stains. Plast Reconstr Surg 1990;86:1112–1117.
6. Goldman L, Kerr JH, Larkin M, Binder S. 600 nm flash pumped dye laser for fragile telangiectasia of the elderly. Lasers Surg Med 1993;13: 227–233.
7. Greenwald J, Rosen S, Anderson RR et al. Comparative histological stud-ies of the tunable dye laser and argon laser: the specific vascular effects of the dye laser. J Invest Dermatol 1981;77:305–310.
8. Garden JM, Tan OT, Kerschmann R et al. Effect of dye laser pulse dura-tion on selective cutaneous vascular injury. J Invest Dermatol 1986;87: 653–657.
9. Nakagawa H, Tan OT, Parrish JA. Ultrastructural changes after pulsed laser radiation. J Invest Dermatol 1985;84:396–400.
10. Hulsbergen Henning JP, van Gemert MJC, Lahaye CTW. Clinical and histological evaluation of portwine stain treatment with a microsecond-pulsed dye-laser at 577 nm. Laser Surg Med 1984;4:375–380.
11. Morelli JG, Tan OT, Garden J et al. Tunable dye laser (577 nm) treat-ment of portwine stains. Lasers Surg Med 1986;6:94–99.
12. Van Gemert MJC, Welch AJ, Amin AP. Is there an optimal laser treat-ment for portwine stains? Lasers Surg Med 1986;6:76–83.
13. Paul BS, Anderson RR, Jarve J, Parrish JA. The effect of temperature and other factors on selective microvascular damage caused by pulsed dye laser. J Invest Dermatol 1983;81:333–335.
14. Tan OT, Kerschmann R, Parrish JA. Effect of skin temperatures on selec-tive vascular injury caused by pulsed dye laser irradiation. J Invest Der-matol 1985;85:441–444.
15. Tan OT, Kerschmann R, Parrish JA. The effect of epidermal pigmenta-tion on selective vascular effects of pulsed laser. Lasers Surg Med 1985; 4:365–374.

16. Ashinoff R, Geronemus RG. Treatment of a portwine stain in a black patient with the pulsed dye laser. J Dermatol Surg Oncol 1992;18:147–148.
17. Tan OT, Motemedi M, Welch AJ, Kurban AK. Spotsize effects on guinea pig skin following pulsed irradiation. J Invest Dermatol 1988;90:877–881.
18. Anderson RR, Parrish JA. Selective photothermolysis: precise microsurgery by selective absorption of pulsed radiation. Science 1983;220:524–527.
19. Tan OT, Stafford TJ, Murray S, Kurban AK. Histologic comparison of the pulsed dye laser and copper vapor laser effects on pig skin. Lasers Surg Med 1990;10:551–558.
20. Dover JS, Geronemus R, Stern RS et al. Dye laser treatment of port-wine stains: comparison of the continuous-wave dye laser with a robotized scanning device and the pulsed dye laser. J Am Acad Dermatol 1995;32:237–240.
21. Garden JM, Geronemus RG. Dermatologic laser surgery. J Dermatol Surg Oncol 1990;16:156–168.
22. Garden JM, Bakus AD. Clinical efficacy of the pulsed dye laser in the treatment of vascular lesions. J Dermatol Surg Oncol 1993;19:321–326.
23. Geronemus RG. Pulsed dye laser treatment of vascular lesions in children. J Dermatol Surg Oncol 1993;19:303–310.
24. Kennard CD, Whitaker DC. Iontophoresis of lidocaine for anesthesia during pulsed dye laser treatment of portwine stains. J Dermatol Surg Oncol 1992;18:287–294.
25. Tan OT, Stafford TJ. EMLA for laser treatment of portwine stains in children. Lasers Surg Med 1992;12:543–548.
26. Rabinowitz L, Esterly N. Anesthesia and/or sedation for pulsed dye laser therapy: special symposium. Pediatr Dermatol 1992;9:132–153.
27. Tan OT, Whitaker D, Garden JM, Murphy G. Pulsed dye laser (577 nm) treatment of portwine stains: ultrastructural evidence of neovascularization and mast cell degranulation in healed lesions. J Invest Dermatol 1988;90:395–398.
28. Garden JM, Tan OT, Parrish JA. The pulsed dye laser: its use at 577 nm wavelength. J Dermatol Surg Oncol 1987;13:134–138.
29. Kauvar AB, Geronemus RG. Repetitive pulsed dye laser treatments improve persistent port-wine stains. Dermatol Surg 1995;21:515–521.
30. Garden JM, Polla LL, Tan OT. The treatment of portwine stains by the pulsed dye laser: analysis of pulse duration and long-term therapy. Arch Dermatol 1988;124:889–896.
31. Glassberg E, Lask GP, Tan EML, Uitto J. The flashlamp-pumped 577 nm pulsed tunable dye laser: clinical efficacy and in vitro studies. J Dermatol Surg Oncol 1988;14:1200–1208.
32. Holy A, Geronemus RG. Treatment of periorbital portwine stains with the flashlamp-pumped pulsed dye laser. Arch Ophthalmol 1992;110:793–797.
33. Renfro L, Geronemus R. Anatomical differences of portwine stains in response to treatment with the pulsed dye laser. Arch Dermatol 1993;128:182–188.
34. Levine VJ, Geronemus RG. Adverse effects associated with the 577- and 585-nanometer pulsed dye laser in the treatment of cutaneous vascular lesions: a study of 500 patients. J Am Acad Dermatol 1995;32:613–617.
35. Swinehart JM. Hypertrophic scarring resulting from the flashlamp-pumped pulsed dye laser surgery. J Am Acad Dermatol 1991;25:845–846.

36. Tan OT, Sherwood K, Gilchrest BA. Treatment of children with portwine stains using the flashlamp-pumped tunable dye laser. N Engl J Med 1989;320:416–421.
37. Garden JM, Burton CS, Geronemus R. Dye laser treatment of children with portwine stains. N Engl J Med 1989;321:901–902.
38. Goldman MP, Fitzpatrick RE, Ruiz-Esparaza J. Treatment of portwine stains (capillary malformation) with the flashlamp-pumped pulsed dye laser. J Pediatr 1993;122:71–77.
39. Ashinoff R, Geronemus RG. Flashlamp-pumped pulsed dye laser for portwine stains in infancy: earlier versus later treatment. J Am Acad Dermatol 1991;24:467–472.
40. Reyes BA, Geronemus R. Treatment of portwine stains during childhood with the flashlamp-pumped pulsed dye laser. J Am Acad Dermatol 1990;23:1142–1148.
41. Dinehart SM, Flock S, Waner M. Beam profile of the flashlamp-pumped pulsed dye laser: support for overlap of exposure spots. Lasers Surg Med 1994;15:277–280.
42. Polla LL, Tan OT, Garden JM, Parrish JA. Tunable pulsed dye laser for the treatment of benign cutaneous vascular ectasia. Dermatologica 1987;174:11–17.
43. Gonzalez E, Gange RW, Momtaz KT. Treatment of telangiectases and other benign vascular lesions with the 577 nm pulsed dye laser. J Am Acad Dermatol 1992;27:220–226.
44. Lowe NJ, Behr KL, Fitzpatrick R, Goldman M, Ruiz-Esparza J. Flashlamp pumped dye laser for rosacea-associated telangiectasia and erythema. J Dermatol Surg Oncol 1991;17:522–525.
45. Goldman MP, Fitzpatrick RE. Pulsed dye laser treatment of leg telangiectasis with or without simultaneous sclerotherapy. J Dermatol Surg Oncol 1990;16:338–344.
46. Glassberg E, Lask G, Rabinowitz LG, Tunnessen WW. Capillary hemangiomas: case study of a novel laser treatment and a review of therapeutics options. J Dermatol Surg Oncol 1989;15:1214–1223.
47. Ashinoff R, Geronemus RG. Capillary hemangiomas and treatment with the flashlamp pumped dye laser. Arch Dermatol 1991;127:202–205.
48. Garden JM, Bakus AD, Paller AS. Treatment of cutaneous hemangiomas by the flashlamp-pumped pulsed dye laser: prospective analysis. J Pediatr 1992;120:555–560.
49. Morelli JG, Tan OT, West WL. Treatment of ulcerated hemangiomas with the pulsed tunable dye laser. Am J Dis Child 1991;145:1062–1064.
50. Geronemus RG. Poikiloderma of Civatte. Arch Dermatol 1990;126:547–548.
51. Alster TS, Kurban AK, Grove GL et al. Alteration of argon laser-induced scars by the pulsed dye laser. Lasers Surg Med 1993;13:368–373.
52. Alster TS, Williams CM. Treatment of keloid sternotomy scars with 585 nm flashlamp-pumped pulsed dye laser. Lancet 1995;345:1198–1200.
53. Hacker SM, Rasmussen JE. The effect of flashlamp-pulsed dye laser on psoriasis. Arch Dermatol 1992;128:853–855.
54. Ros AM, Garden JM, Bakus AD, Hedblad MA. Psoriasis response to the pulsed dye laser. Lasers Surg Med 1996;19:331–335.
55. Tan OT, Hurwitz RM, Stafford TJ. Pulsed dye laser treatment of recalcitrant verrucae: a preliminary report. Lasers Surg Med 1993;13:127–137.

7 ____ The Nd:YAG Laser in Cutaneous Surgery

Michael Landthaler
Ulrich Hohenleutner

In contrast to argon, dye, Q-switched ruby, and CO_2 lasers, which are used routinely for the treatment of skin lesions, the Nd:YAG laser is used much less commonly for cutaneous surgery. Because its 1060-nm radiation can be easily directed by flexible light guides, the Nd-YAG laser is mainly used for endoscopic surgical procedures, such as urologic and gastroenteric procedures.

Biophysical Considerations

The Nd:YAG laser is a solid-state laser containing a crystal rod of yttrium-aluminum-garnet (YAG) doped with 1% to 3% of neodymium ions. The Nd:YAG rod is placed within the laser cavity, where powerful xenon arc lamps excite the Nd ions, providing emission in the invisible near-infrared region at 1064 nm. Nd:YAG lasers produce continuous wave (cw) or pulsed (Q-switched) radiation.[1,2] The output of the Q-switched Nd:YAG laser is controlled by a fast electrooptical switch (quality switch [Q-switch]), which releases the energy stored in the cavity in one intense, single pulse with a duration in the nanosecond range.[1]

Another type of laser is the frequency-doubled Nd:YAG laser, which produces a wavelength of 532 nm. High-power Nd:YAG lasers can be doubled in frequency by placing a potassium-titanyl-phosphate crystal inside the laser cavity and focusing the beam into the crystal. By passing the beam through the crystal, the invisible near-infrared, 1064-nm–wavelength light is transformed into green visible light at a wavelength of 532 nm. Power up to 20 W is possible, and the light can be transmitted through conventional fiberoptic delivery systems. The tissue effect of this green light is similar to that of the argon laser.[1]

Usually the cw Nd:YAG laser energy is delivered to the skin by flexible fiberoptics. The distal end of the fiber is coupled to a focusing handpiece. Recently, solid sapphire crystal probes fixed to the end of the fiber have expanded the versatility of the Nd:YAG laser.

In memoriam of Dr. D. Haina, who died suddenly in March 1989.

Since their introduction in 1985, they have become increasingly popular in various fields of surgery. The output powers necessary for contact surgery are much lower than those needed for noncontact modalities, and incision, vaporization, as well as coagulation are possible with the proper output settings. The time it takes to make an incision in thick skin depends on the diameter of the scalpel tip and the power setting. The incision time is shorter and less radiation tissue damage occurs when thinner scalpels and higher power settings are used.[3] According to Gallucci and associates,[4] Nd:YAG contact laser therapy is associated with a significant reduction in postoperative morbidity among patients with tumors operated on after having received radiotherapy for head and neck cancer. Reportedly the potential for tumor cell seeding is also significantly less than that associated with the use of traditional scalpels.[5]

The cw Nd:YAG lasers currently used in therapy typically have an output power of up to 80 to 100 W. Because the 1060-nm wavelength is less scattered in human skin than the shorter, visible wavelengths and poorly absorbed by hemoglobin, melanin, and water, it penetrates deeply into the skin. The average pathlength in skin, defined as the depth of the tissue layer that reduces the incident energy to 1/e (36.8%), is 0.75 mm. A reduction to 10% occurs in a 3.5-mm-thick skin layer. The values for the argon laser are 0.5 for 36.8% reduction and 1.5 mm for 10% reduction (Figs. 7-1 and 7-2).[6]

The Nd:YAG laser is therefore suitable for deep coagulation of the skin. However, the depth of coagulation cannot be increased infi-

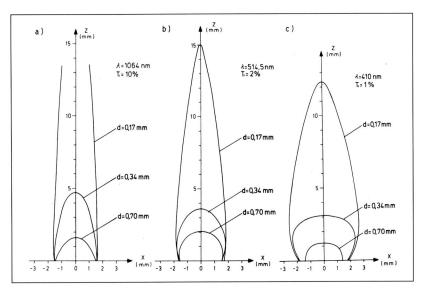

Fig. 7-1. Light distribution inside the skin for different wavelengths. Short wavelengths are more scattered inside the skin, resulting in a broader distribution compared with the radiation of the Nd:YAG laser. (Reproduced with permission from Haina D, Landthaler M, Braun-Falco O, Waidelich W. Optische Eigenschaften menschlicher Haut. In: Waidelich W, ed. Laser 83. Optoelektronik in der Medizin. Berlin, Heidelberg, New York, Tokyo: Springer, 1984.)

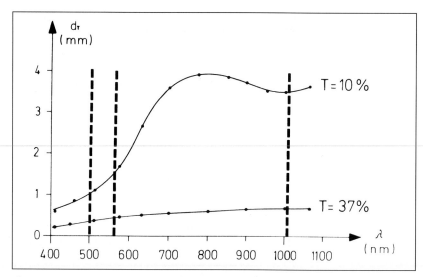

Fig. 7-2. Average penetration depth and 10% depth (T) in relation to wavelength. Increase in transmission occurs with increasing wavelength. (Reproduced with permission from Haina D, Landthaler M, Braun-Falco O, Waidelich W. Optische Eigenschaften menschlicher Haut. In: Waidelich W, ed. Laser 83. Optoelektronik in der Medizin. Berlin, Heidelberg, New York, Tokyo: Springer, 1984.)

nitely by simply increasing the laser power, because the skin surface will carbonize and vaporize beyond a certain power density. Carbonization of tissue can be prevented by cooling the surface during irradiation. A simple cooling technique is to rinse the skin surface during irradiation with cold tap water or ice-cold Ringer's solution. Because the radiation is only poorly absorbed in water, another approach is to irradiate through transparent ice cubes. Using this technique, thermal skin damage can be prevented in a skin layer as deep as 1 mm.[7,8] An additional advantage of this ice-cube technique is that it can compress the tissue to be treated and thereby increase the effective depth of laser therapy (e.g., in exophytic hemangiomas).

The coagulation depth of the Nd:YAG laser can also be increased by expanding the beam diameter (Table 7-1).[9] In our experience, a maximum coagulation depth of about 5 to 6 mm can be achieved in human skin by cooling the skin surface during irradiation.

To assess the coagulation and vaporization depth, in vivo trials with Nd:YAG laser irradiation were carried out in miniature pigs. The total depth of the defect was determined by measuring the depth of vaporization plus the depth of coagulation (Fig. 7-3). Within the delivered power range, the total depth of the defect was linearly correlated with the laser power and exposure time. It was found that, as the result of heat diffusion, the coagulation zones in skin were significantly broader than the beam diameter used, especially when longer exposure times were used.[10]

Table 7-1. Effect of different lasers and irradiation parameters on maximum coagulation depth in human skin

Irradiation parameters	Maximum coagulation depth (mm)		
	Nd:YAG	Argon	CO_2
	5.5	0.5	0.3
0.2 sec/1-mm beam diameter	0.45	0.35	<0.1
10 sec/1-mm beam diameter	1.7	1.2	0.6
10 sec/2-mm beam diameter	2.3	1.7	0.9
10 sec/2-mm beam diameter	5.5	3.5	—

Source: From Haina D, Landthaler M, Braun-Falco O, Waidelich W. Comparison of the maximum coagulation depth in human skin for different types of medical lasers. Lasers Surg Med 1987;7:355–362. Copyright © 1987 John Wiley & Sons, Inc. Reprinted by permission of Wiley-Liss, Inc., a subsidiary of John Wiley & Sons, Inc.

In contrast to other lasers, the Nd:YAG laser is unsuitable for the selective coagulation of vascular tissue, because the coagulation it produces in skin is completely nonspecific and independent of the hemoglobin content. However, by selecting optimal parameters of irradiation (i.e., short exposure times and relatively low laser output power, as well as cooling the skin surface during irradiation), unwanted thermal damage to the epidermis and dermis can be reduced to a certain extent.[11]

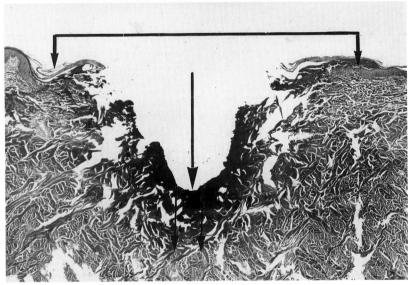

Fig. 7-3. Effect of Nd:YAG laser irradiation on miniature pig skin in vivo. (*Single arrow* = depth of vaporization, total depth of defect; *Lowest arrows* = depth of coagulation; *Bracketed arrows* = epidermal damage.) (H&E; ×45).

A thermal camera was used to measure temperatures in vitro during Nd:YAG laser irradiation of skin specimens of different thickness (1.7, 3.6, and 5.6 mm). The skin surface was radiated with a 1.8-mm spot size and 40-W laser power, and the skin temperature was measured at its border with the subcutaneous fat. It was found that irradiation of a 1.7-mm-thick sample of cheek skin for 4 seconds resulted in a temperature rise at the dermosubcutaneous junction to more than 60°C, whereas an exposure time of 22 seconds was required to raise the temperature to 60°C in a 5.6-mm-thick skin sample from the back.[12] These findings show that the irradiation parameters for Nd:YAG laser treatment have to be determined on the basis of the skin thickness of the different body regions, in order to prevent unwanted deep thermal damage in subcutaneous tissues.

Clinical Applications

VASCULAR LESIONS

Port-Wine Stains with Nodular Surface

Although the argon and particularly the flashlamp-pumped pulsed dye laser are the treatments of choice for port-wine stains (PWSs),[13-15] in our experience these lasers cannot produce optimal results in the treatment of nodular PWSs. Whereas most of the ectatic vessels are generally in the upper dermis in the macular PWSs seen in younger patients, the dilated vessels in violaceous or purple lesions and lesions with a nodular surface are deep in the dermis and even down in the subcutaneous fat.[16] Using the usual irradiation parameters, the argon laser or flashlamp-pumped pulsed dye laser can only coagulate vessels to a maximum depth of about 1 to 2 mm.[17,18] The Nd:YAG laser can easily achieve a greater depth of coagulation, and this laser has proved to be effective in the treatment of these nodular lesions.[19]

Treatment Technique

Treatment can usually be performed on an outpatient basis with the patient under local anesthesia. Single laser pulses with a spot size of about 2 mm and an exposure time of 0.3 to 1.0 second are applied. The laser power used varies between 20 and 40 W, resulting in an irradiance of 800 to 1600 W/cm² and a fluence of 400 to 1600 J/cm². The single pulses are set 2 mm apart to avoid confluent coagulation. During therapy, the skin surface is continuously rinsed with cold tap water by means of an injection syringe. As mentioned earlier, another way to cool the skin surface is to lase through transparent ice cubes, which also has the effect of producing deeper coagulation, because the exophytic nodules can easily be compressed by the ice cubes.[7,8]

A somewhat different technique was described by Apfelberg and Smith,[20] who treated patients with a spot size of 1 to 2 mm separated by 1 to 2 mm of untreated skin using a power density of 3584 W/cm² and a fluence of 3.9 J/cm². They did not cool the skin surface during irradiation.

Clinical Results

Immediately after Nd:YAG laser irradiation, the treated areas show a white-gray discoloration. Within 2 to 4 days a crust forms, and in regions such as the eyelids and the lips swelling may last for up to 5 days. Patients are instructed to clean the skin with water only and to dry it carefully to prevent trauma. The crust is shed within 2 to 4 weeks of therapy, and treatment can be repeated at 6 to 8 week intervals.

This technique can produce marked lightening of PWSs with a nodular surface and a reduction in macrocheilia (Fig. 7-4).

Most of our adult patients with nodular PWSs have been treated with a combination of Nd:YAG and argon laser therapy; the Nd:YAG laser is used to treat the nodular areas and the argon laser is used to treat the macular areas. This combined approach has the advantage of reducing the risk of scarring, because in our experience this risk is lower for argon laser treatment. Fifteen patients (12 male and 3 female, aged 24 to 65 years) were treated using this combination. Excellent results (i.e., total lightening) could never be obtained, but substantial lightening or flattening of the PWS was seen in all (Fig. 7-5). Scarring occurred in four patients. Overall this therapy produces a sufficient cosmetic result.

A similar procedure was described by Dixon and Gilbertson,[21] who treated 37 patients with dark nodular PWSs using the argon and Nd:YAG lasers. In four patients, residual nodules were treated by Nd:YAG laser coagulation using a glass slide to compress the nodule. Power settings varied from 20 to 40 W; the spot size was 2 mm and the exposure time was 0.2 second. Care was taken, as in our technique, to space exposure sites 2 mm apart to avoid the overlapping of treated areas.

Pathology

The morphological changes produced by Nd:YAG laser treatment are generally the same as those produced by argon laser therapy and consist of necrosis of the epidermis and dermis and destroyed vessels filled with coagulated erythrocytes (Fig. 7-6).[19] The lamina densa of the basement membrane is preserved after the Nd:YAG laser irradiation of vascular lesions (Fig. 7-7).[22] The epidermis begins to regenerate within a few days, and the acute inflammatory infiltrate is followed by a chronic inflammatory reaction, resulting in the resorption of necrotic tissue and formation of granulation tissue. Later, ectatic vessels are replaced by newly formed fibrous tissue and collagen matures. There are, however, three differences between the two laser treatments in terms of the morphologic changes they produce:

1. The depth of coagulation is enhanced with the Nd:YAG laser.
2. Coagulation of the dermal stroma is more pronounced after

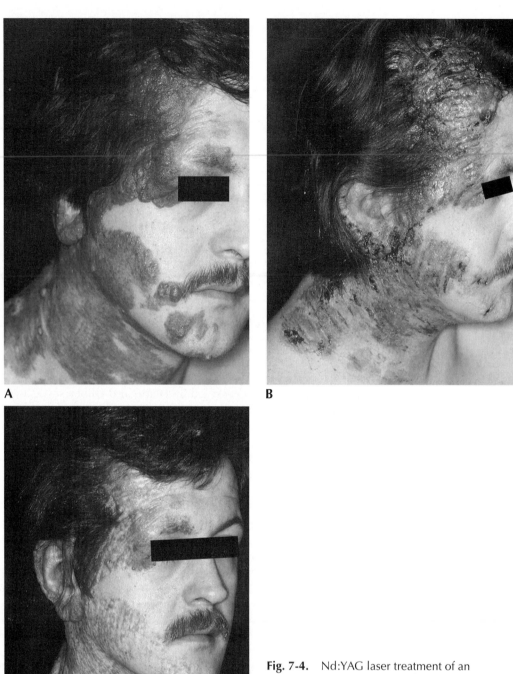

A

B

C

Fig. 7-4.   Nd:YAG laser treatment of an extensive port-wine stain with angiomatous nodules in a 28-year-old man. (A) Before treatment. (B) Crusting 7 days after treatment. (Spot size, 2 mm; exposure time, 0.5–1.0 second; output power, 30 W.) (C) Result of one treatment with patient under general anesthesia. See Fig. 7-4 in color section.

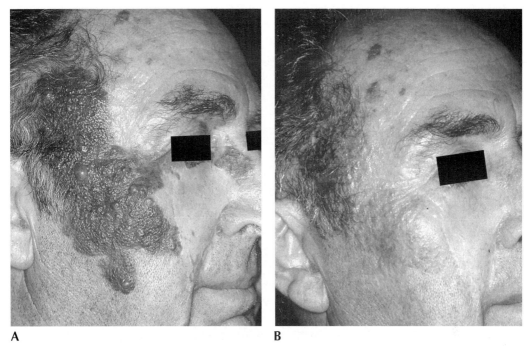

A   **B**

Fig. 7-5.   Combined Nd:YAG laser and argon laser treatment of a port-wine stain with a nodular surface in a 50-year-old man. (A) Before therapy. (B) Result of five treatments with patient under local anesthesia. (Nd:YAG laser irradiations: spot size, 2 mm; exposure time, 0.5 second; output power, 30 W. Argon laser irradiations: spot size, 2 mm; exposure time, 0.3 second; output power, 3 W.) See Fig. 7-5 in color section.

Nd:YAG laser treatment, resulting in a pronounced fibrosis. Because a certain amount of fibrosis of the dermis may be required to obtain good and stable treatment results in mature PWSs, this is not necessarily a disadvantage. On the other hand, the risk of scarring is greatly increased.

3. Epidermal and dermal tissue repair takes longer after Nd:YAG laser coagulation, in that it may take up to 4 to 6 weeks before a normal epidermis is restored and necrotic dermal tissue is completely resorbed and replaced by fibrous tissue. This can be explained by the deep thermal damage caused by Nd:YAG laser irradiation.

Macular Port-Wine Stains

Continuous-wave Nd:YAG laser irradiation is not indicated for the treatment of pink and red macular PWSs, but Lafitte and colleagues[23] have used a frequency-doubled Nd:YAG laser at 5-kHz repetition rate (quasi-cw), producing a wavelength of 532 nm, in combination with an automatic scanning device. They successfully treated 79 patients with PWSs using this approach, including 37 patients under 20 years of age. Compared with the results from argon laser therapy of PWSs, healing was more rapid in patients treated with the

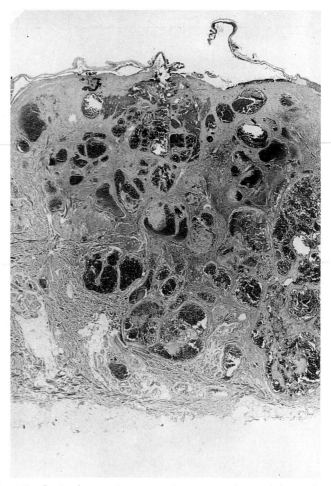

Fig. 7-6. Histologic changes in a port-wine stain with a nodular surface 2 hours after Nd:YAG laser irradiation. (H&E; ×20). Coagulation of dermis and ectatic vessels occurred to a depth of 3.5 mm. Vessels are filled with coagulated erythrocytes; the epidermis is coagulated and shows subepidermal blister formation.

frequency-doubled Nd:YAG laser, postoperative discomfort was reduced, and less edema and scarring occurred. In terms of lightening, the results obtained with the frequency-doubled Nd:YAG laser were superior to those obtained with the argon laser. However, frequency-doubled Nd:YAG laser treatment cannot compare with flashlamp-pumped pulsed dye laser treatment, which is the golden standard of macular PWS treatment.

Hemangiomas

Superficial hemangiomas of the skin and mucous membranes are suitable for Nd:YAG laser therapy. Oral hemangiomas are treated with single laser pulses of 1 to 2 mm in diameter, with untreated tis-

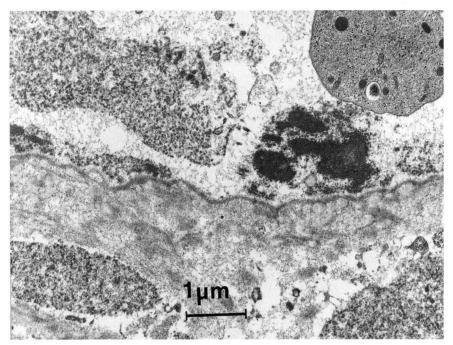

Fig. 7-7.   Electron micrograph of basement membrane 24 hours after Nd:YAG laser irradiation of a port-wine stain. (Spot size, 2 mm; pulse duration, 0.5 second; output power, 25 W.) (×15,000). The lamina densa of the basement membrane is preserved.

sue in between to avoid confluent coagulation. A laser power of up to 40 W with an exposure time of up to 1.0 second can be used. The exposure time should be long enough, however, to produce obvious shrinking of the angioma. In some patients, it is useful to compress the angioma with a glass slide or an ice cube during irradiation, which has the dual effect of enhancing the coagulation depth and promoting immediate shrinking of the lesion. The same method can be used for the treatment of lymphangiomas of the tongue.

Good to excellent results were obtained in 12 of 15 of our patients treated using these techniques (Fig. 7-8), and complications such as bleeding or infection were not observed. These results compare with the experiences of other authors. Dixon and colleagues[24] reported on four patients with cavernous hemangiomas of the oral mucosa treated with the Nd:YAG laser, which led to marked improvement of the lesion. Even when cure was not possible, the treatment alleviated the symptoms related to the volume of the angioma and also controlled the tendency to bleed. Apfelberg and Smith[20] cleared 13 capillary-cavernous hemangiomas using the Nd:YAG laser. Rosenfeld and Sherman[25] treated 38 patients with vascular lesions, including capillary and cavernous hemangiomas, PWSs, spider nevi, and multiple telangiectases. Good or excellent results were obtained in 16 of the 24 patients with hemangiomas. The acute side effects were limited to pain and some swelling; long-term complications consisted of

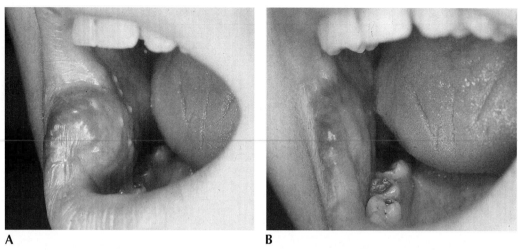

A   **B**

Fig. 7-8.   Cavernous oral hemangioma in a 20-year-old woman. (A) Before treatment. (B) Result of two treatments with patient under local anesthesia. (Spot size, 2 mm; pulse duration, 0.5–1.0 second; output power, 30 W.)

hypertrophic scarring, occurring in two patients, and hyperpigmentation, occurring in one. In a comparative study of six patients, David and associates[26] found the Nd:YAG laser to be more effective than the argon laser in the treatment of skin hemangiomas. Powell and co-workers[27] reported on the Nd:YAG laser excision of a giant gingival pyogenic granuloma of pregnancy, with excellent results.

Werner and colleagues[28] treated 31 patients (aged 3 months to 61 years) who had thick cutaneous and mucosal hemangiomas in the head and neck region, using Nd:YAG laser coagulation and surface cooling with transparent ice cubes or ice-cold Ringer's solution. Complete regression of the hemangioma was observed in 27 of the patients.

According to Apfelberg,[29] the Nd:YAG laser can be used successfully in either a contact or noncontact mode as a valuable and integral part of hemangioma therapy. In a series of six patients (aged 2 months to 53 years) with very difficult to treat vascular birthmarks, Nd:YAG laser treatment was used in combination with other modalities, such as intralesional steroids, arteriography with superselective embolization, tissue expansion, medical leeches, and the correction of coagulation deficiencies.

Another suitable indication for Nd:YAG laser application are fast-growing and complicated childhood hemangiomas (Table 7-2) (Fig. 7-9).[30–33] At our institution, such infants are placed under general anesthesia and treated on an outpatient basis. During irradiation the skin surface is rinsed with tap water to reduce epidermal damage. Overlapping of pulses is avoided, and radiation is applied until shrinkage of the hemangioma is observed clinically. The following irradiation parameters are used: power, up to 30 W; spot size, 2 mm; exposure time, up to 1 second; power density, up to 955 W/cm²; energy fluences, up to 955 J/cm².[33]

Table 7-2. Nd:YAG laser therapy of childhood hemangiomas

Study	Year	Number of patients	Results
Achauer and Vander Kam[30]	1989	55	72% excellent/good
Apfelberg et al[31]	1989	17 (Nd:YAG +steroids)	Marked shrinkage of lesions in 15 patients
Landthaler et al[33]	1995	4	Excellent/good in 3 patients
Grantzow et al[32]	1995	132	After one single treatment, regression in 77%; progression in 4%

Although a success rate of up to 70% has been reported for all studies evaluating the effectiveness of the Nd:YAG laser in the treatment of childhood hemangiomas, the decision to perform Nd:YAG laser treatment is a difficult one, because complications such as scarring are frequent and treatment has to be performed with the patient under general anesthesia. For these reasons, Nd:YAG laser therapy of childhood hemangiomas is associated with more risks than other laser treatments and should therefore only be performed in specialized and experienced units.[33]

A new approach to the therapy of thick subcutaneous hemangiomas is interstitial coagulation using a fiberoptic laser wand.[7,34–36] This involves the placement of a bare fiber inside the hemangioma using an injection syringe and applying the laser energy directly into the tissue, while the fiber is slowly withdrawn and the surrounding

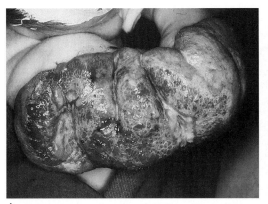 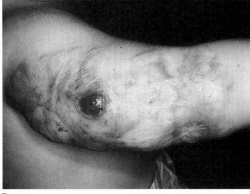

A   **B**

Fig. 7-9.   Extensive ulcerated and bleeding, mixed hemangioma in a 4-month-old female infant. (A) Before treatment. (B) Regression after four Nd:YAG laser treatments. See Fig. 7-9 in color section. (Reproduced with permission from Landthaler M, Hohenleutner U, Abd El-Raheem T. Laser therapy of childhood haemangiomas. Br J Dermatol 1995;133:275–281.)

tissue cooled by ice-cold Ringer's solution or ice cubes. The placement of the fiber and the coagulation of the hemangiomas can be controlled manually or guided by ultrasound imaging.[35,36]

Alani and Warren[34] reported their observations in 13 patients undergoing such treatment using a Nd:YAG laser power of 10 to 25 W. All lesions were reduced in size, without complications such as infections, hematomas, or injury to vital structures.

Werner and colleagues[35] used a different approach in their patients, irradiating using a laser power of 4 to 8 W for up to 40 seconds. In their technique, the laser fiber is moved as soon as an increase in sonographic density is noted at the tip of the light guide. Treatment is complete when an increase in sonographic density has occurred in all areas of the hemangioma. Such irradiation has to be performed carefully, however, so that sensitive neighboring structures such as the orbitae, the nasal skeleton, and the facial nerve are not irradiated. Extensive postoperative swelling often occurs and may last for up to 3 weeks. It takes up to 3 months for involution to occur. In 23 patients with hemangiomas larger than 3 cm in diameter, complete regression occurred in 14, without any cosmetic or functional impairment. Six hemangiomas were reduced incompletely but satisfactorily for the patient.

Other Vascular Lesions

Apart from PWSs with a nodular surface and thick hemangiomas, the Nd:YAG laser is rarely used for treatment of benign vascular lesions, but good results are possible in individual patients with such lesions. Shapsay and Olliver[37] used Nd:YAG laser pulses of 0.3 to 0.5 second in duration and a power of 20 to 25 W to treat patients with hereditary hemorrhagic telangiectasia (Osler-Weber-Rendu disease). The frequency and severity of hemorrhage was reduced, without significant complications.

Nonvascular Lesions

Human Papillomavirus Infections

Common warts and plantar warts as well as condylomata acuminata can be successfully coagulated by means of the Nd:YAG laser, using a relatively low laser power of up to 20 W and a spot size of 2 mm. The lesion should be irradiated until a complete whitish discoloration is seen, usually occurring after 0.5 to 1.0 second.

Using these parameters, the Nd:YAG laser is even suitable for the treatment of condylomata acuminata gigantea (Buschke-Löwenstein tumor).[38] Bowenoid papulosis can be treated by the Nd:YAG laser, and even extensive leukoplakia-like and verrucous lesions can be healed without causing mutilation of the external genitalia.[39,40]

Volz and associates[41] treated 20 men with the Nd:YAG laser for meatal and urethral condylomata acuminata and obtained a cure in

30% after one treatment; 40% of the patients needed up to five separate treatments before total cure occurred. According to Ferenczy,[42] the Nd:YAG laser has some specific applications in the treatment of large, relatively richly vascularized genital warts.

The lack of plume formation is an important advantage of the Nd:YAG laser over the CO_2 laser. Because the risk of bleeding is also lower, we prefer to use the Nd:YAG laser for the treatment of condylomata acuminata and other skin lesions in HIV-infected patients. However, in our experience the CO_2 laser is preferable to the Nd:YAG laser for the treatment of bowenoid papulosis and condylomata acuminata in non–HIV-infected patients, because of the more exact ablation possible, the reduced remaining coagulation zone, and the reduced postoperative pain, healing time, and risk of scarring.

A new approach to the Nd:YAG laser treatment of verrucae vulgares is laser hyperthermia (Regensburg's technique) (Table 7-3). Before Nd:YAG laser hyperthermia was used clinically, it was tested in vitro on samples of 5-mm-thick healthy skin excised as the safety margin of malignant melanomas. The skin was irradiated with a power output of 10 W, a single 20-second pulse, and a spot size of 8 mm. The surface temperature of the skin was raised from room temperature (23.1°C) to 40° to 41°C, as measured directly after irradiation by a contact thermocouple and thermometer (Fluke 51 Thermometer; John Fluke, USA). The temperature at the dermosubcutaneous border on the underside of the sample was 44° to 46°C. Thus, a temperature difference of 5°C between the surface and the deeper tissue was achieved by the Nd:YAG laser heating procedure. The temperature differences in vivo should be similar, but the absolute temperature rise may actually be lower because of the cooling effect of blood and lymph fluid.[43]

The aim of this hyperthermia technique is to raise the temperature of living skin, including the wart, from its normal level to about 45°C. Nd:YAG irradiation can easily accomplish this because of its ability to

Table 7-3. Regensburg's technique

REACHING THE ADEQUATE TEMPERATURE

No local anesthesia.

Apply Nd:YAG laser energy with a power of 10 W, a spot size of 8 mm, and a pulse time of 20 seconds.

Repeat this procedure until surface temperature of 40°C is reached.

MAINTAINING THE ADEQUATE TEMPERATURE

Continue to apply energy to keep a temperature of at least 40°C for a period of 30 seconds minimum.

CONTROLLING THE ADEQUATE TEMPERATURE

Measure the surface temperature by bringing the thermocouple in contact with the top of the treated lesion. (To measure the real temperature, heating has to be interrupted.)

Interrupt lasering for a moment when patient feels unbearable burning.

---

penetrate skin to a depth of up to 7 mm. The surface temperature of the skin must be measured during the heating procedure and should not exceed 40° to 42°C. According to our observations, the subsurface temperature of the skin reaches about 45°C when the surface temperature is raised to 40°C.

A primary study group comprised 39 patients with recalcitrant verrucae vulgares, which had been repeatedly and unsuccessfully treated before. Twenty-four of the patients complied well with treatment, following exactly the treatment regimen and the instructions. Seven followed the treatment procedure only irregularly, and eight did not continue with treatment. A good response was observed in 77% of patients who complied well with treatment, that is, the warts regressed completely after up to three treatment sessions performed at an interval of 2 weeks. However, sufficient keratolytic treatment must be done first, before the hyperthermia treatment.[44]

Epithelial Skin Tumors

The Nd:YAG laser can also be used in some patients for the treatment of skin tumors, as it is used for the treatment of tumors dealt with by other medical specialties, such as urology, neurosurgery, pulmonology, and gastroenterology. Basal cell carcinomas, squamous cell carcinomas, Bowen's disease, and other epithelial tumors are all indications for Nd:YAG laser therapy in selected patients.[45,46] However, because of the limited depth of coagulation, it should be used to treat only rather superficial and relatively small tumors. The tumor and a safety margin of 5 to 10 mm are covered with single laser pulses or are irradiated continuously until a complete whitish discoloration is observed. A laser power of up to 40 W, spot size of 2 mm, and exposure time of up to 3 seconds are employed. The tumor surface is rinsed with cool water during irradiation to prevent vaporization of tissue. Treatment can usually be performed with the patient under local anesthesia.

Edema and blistering occur initially, followed by the formation of a hemorrhagic crust. The time it takes for the wound to heal completely varies between 4 and 8 weeks. Complications such as bleeding or infection are rare. Hypertrophic scars are often observed after complete wound healing but regress in nearly all patients. Thus, the cosmetic result is mostly acceptable (Fig. 7-10).

We have treated 172 epithelial tumors in 50 patients; 85% were basal cell carcinomas, and 15% were squamous cell carcinomas, solar keratosis, or Bowen's disease.[47] Sixty percent of the tumors were located in the head and neck areas, 30% were on the trunk, and 10% were on the extremities. Minimum follow-up was 3 years, and 26 recurrences were observed, for a 3-year cure rate of 85%. It may be possible to improve the cure rate by extending safety margins and achieve a deeper coagulation by increasing the laser power and exposure time.[47]

Several reports about the use of the Nd:YAG laser for the treatment of epithelial skin tumors concern the treatment of squamous cell carcinoma of the external genitalia. Malloy and colleagues[48] re-

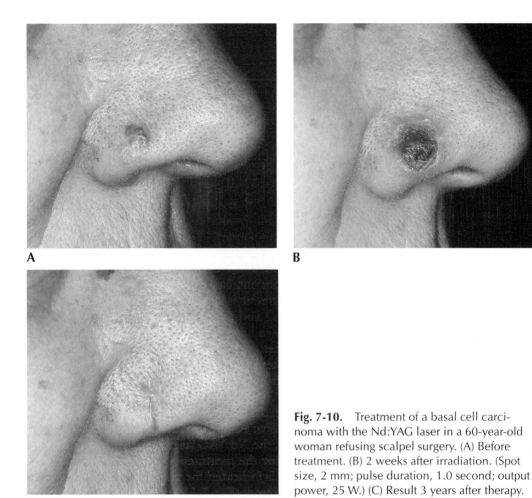

Fig. 7-10. Treatment of a basal cell carcinoma with the Nd:YAG laser in a 60-year-old woman refusing scalpel surgery. (A) Before treatment. (B) 2 weeks after irradiation. (Spot size, 2 mm; pulse duration, 1.0 second; output power, 25 W.) (C) Result 3 years after therapy.

ported on the Nd:YAG laser coagulation of tumors in situ (TIS) and T1 and T2 carcinomas. All their patients had refused the traditional therapy of partial penectomy. Circumcisions and deep biopsies were performed in all patients before laser coagulations. During the follow-up of 12 to 36 months, patients with TIS showed no evidence of recurrence. Six of the nine patients with T1 tumors remained tumor free. The tumor bulk was reduced in the patients with T2 tumors, but the tumors were not eradicated. Boon[49] reported on 16 patients with localized penile cancer (TIS, T1, and T2) treated with Nd:YAG laser coagulation. Eight of the 16 patients were exclusively treated with the Nd:YAG laser with a sapphire probe; the other eight were treated by scalpel excision followed by Nd:YAG laser irradiation. Thirteen patients were tumor free as of the time of the report, a recurrent tumor had developed in one patient on an untreated part of the glans penis after 14 months, one patient had shown TIS near the treatment area after 5 months, and an incomplete laser resection was followed by partial penectomy in one patient.

More recently, Malek[50] reported on a series of 30 men with biopsy-proven premalignant or malignant squamous cell lesions of the penis, who underwent treatment using CO_2, Nd:YAG, or frequency-doubled Nd:YAG lasers. Nd:YAG laser coagulation was used alone or in combination with CO_2 laser treatment for more histologically advanced lesions. Follow-up in 23 patients for up to 2 years showed that all but one (stage T3) remained free of penile cancer at the end of the 2 years.

These results show that the Nd:YAG laser may be useful for the management of epithelial tumors, but because of its limited coagulation capability, laser treatment should be confined to tumors that are less than 5 mm thick. The Nd:YAG laser expands the therapeutic possibilities of laser treatment for skin tumors, because it can destroy tissue by heat without direct contact, bleeding, or smoke formation. Wounds heal, even in skin previously damaged by radiotherapy or in scar tissue. Another advantage of Nd:YAG laser surgery is that it can be performed on an outpatient basis with the patient under local anesthesia. Only one treatment is necessary for most patients, and there is low risk of bleeding and infection. Furthermore, postoperative dressings are not required and precise positioning of the patient during the treatment is less crucial than it is during cold steel surgery. In addition, pacemakers do not cause problems and treatments can be repeated easily with no limit to the total dose, as there is with radiotherapy.

The disadvantages are the lack of histologic control, delayed wound healing, the expensive equipment, and the lack of long-term results. In our experience, the Nd:YAG laser has therefore not qualified as a routine method for the treatment of epithelial tumors, but Nd:YAG laser coagulation is indicated for tumors in old patients and in patients with multiple tumors (Fig. 7-11), tumors in damaged skin, or tumors in special locations such as the genital area and the oral mucosa. For example, even extensive verrucous oral leukoplakia in a

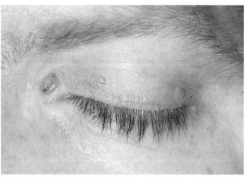 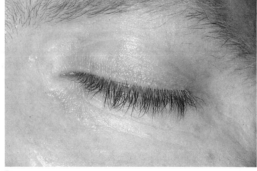

A   **B**

Fig. 7-11.   Basal cell carcinomas of the upper eyelid in a 27-year-old man with basal cell nevus syndrome. (A) Before therapy. (B) Result 1 year after one treatment. (Spot size, 2 mm; exposure time, 1.0 second; output power, 30 W.)

75-year-old woman was controlled by Nd:YAG laser treatments, performed on an outpatient basis with the patient under local anesthesia.[51] The same procedure was also used in a patient with extensive extramammary Paget's disease of the penis and scrotum.[52]

Kaposi's Sarcoma

In our experience, argon and Nd:YAG lasers have proved effective for the treatment of Kaposi's sarcoma in selected patients.[47] Treatment is performed with the patient under local anesthesia. Whereas the argon laser can only be used for the coagulation of superficial macular lesions, the Nd:YAG laser can be used for the treatment of small nodular lesions of the skin, oral mucosa, and the glans penis.[47,53,54] The cosmetic results may be lessened by the formation of hyperpigmented scars, however. Wishnow and Johnson[55] treated nodular lesions of the glans penis and lesions within the fossa navicularis with the Nd:YAG laser in a 42-year-old HIV-positive man. Removal of the two nodules during a single outpatient treatment restored the patient's ability to void normally.

It must be emphasized, however, that Nd:YAG laser therapy of Kaposi's sarcoma is only a palliative treatment. Although the removal of visible or functionally impairing lesions may improve the quality of life in some patients, tumor progression and the prognosis in these patients cannot be influenced. Advantages of the Nd:YAG laser in the treatment of lesions of Kaposi's sarcoma are its deep coagulating capability, the lack of bleeding, and the absence of plume production. The latter two are of particular importance, especially in HIV-positive patients with Kaposi's sarcoma.[47]

Melanin-Pigmented Lesions

Despite reports regarding Nd:YAG laser treatment of malignant melanomas of the skin,[56,57] the need for histologic control precludes the use of the Nd:YAG laser in the therapy of the primary tumor. Excisional surgery remains the treatment of choice. In our experience, the Nd:YAG laser may be helpful in some patients with multiple superficial cutaneous metastatic melanomas or other malignant tumors. Excellent results were obtained with the Nd:YAG laser in three patients with lentigo maligna. The lesions and a safety margin of 10 mm were completely irradiated with a spot size of 2 cm and an output power of 20 W. The irradiation time was long enough to result in complete necrosis, indicated clinically by immediate blister formation. No recurrences were discovered during the follow-up period of 2 to 3 years.[47]

It has been demonstrated recently that the frequency-doubled, Q-switched Nd:YAG laser is also suitable for the removal of cutaneous pigmented lesions, such as lentigines, café au lait macules, and nevus of Ota.[58–60] Linsmeier-Kilmer and associates[59] used this treatment in 49 patients, 37 with multiple lentigines, 7 with café au lait macules, and 5 with miscellaneous lesions, using a 532-nm wavelength, 2.0-mm spot size, 10-nsec pulsewidth. Treatment areas were divided into four quadrants, irradiated with fluences of 2, 3, 4, or 5 J/cm^2, and evaluated at intervals of 1 and 3 months after treatment. The response in patients with lentigines was related to the dose, with a pigment removal greater than 75% of the desired outcome. This was achieved in 60% of the lesions treated at higher energy fluences. Responses in the other lesions were variable, but fair to good improvement was noted in most patients. Spontaneously resolving, mild transient erythema, hyperpigmentation, or hypopigmentation were noted in some patients, but no scarring was observed.

Similar results were noted by Tse and associates[60] in patients with lentigines, café au lait macules, nevus of Ota, nevus spilus, or postinflammatory hyperpigmentations. A comparison of the Q-switched ruby laser with the Nd:YAG laser showed the former to cause more pain during treatment, but Nd:YAG laser treatment was associated with more postoperative discomfort. The ruby laser also seemed to produce a slightly better result.

Removal of Tattoos

Initially the CO_2 laser was the laser of choice for the removal of tattoos, but in recent years other lasers have been found to produce much better cosmetic results, replacing the CO_2 laser as the treatment of choice for tattoo removal. Therefore, the report of Kirschner,[61] who obtained results with a continuous-wave Nd:YAG laser comparable to those produced by the CO_2 laser, is now only of historical interest.

Brunner and associates[62] reported on the use of the pulsed, Q-switched Nd:YAG laser in the removal of 20 tattoos. Using a fluence of 3 to 5 J/cm^2, an asymmetrical pulse shape with a 50% energy output delivered in 18 nsec, and a spot size of 3 mm, they achieved excellent results in the removal of black ink tattoos. Immediately after irradiation the area was whitish and edematous, but these changes resolved within 10 minutes. They found that nearly complete removal could be obtained without scarring with up to three treatment sessions. The use of fluences exceeding 5 J/cm^2 resulted in scar formation. Pigment-containing macrophages are probably burst by the laser pulses, and the black pigment particles are then removed, but other colored pigments, such as red, green, and yellow, did not respond to this procedure.

Zelickson and co-workers[63] have recently examined the response of tattoo pigments treated with the Q-switched Nd:YAG (1064 and 532 nm), Q-switched ruby, and alexandrite lasers in vivo in hairless guinea pigs. Red-brown, dark brown, orange, and black pigments responded best to the Nd:YAG laser at 1064 nm, but red pigment responded best to the Q-switched Nd:YAG laser at 532 nm. Clinically, scarring was not observed after treatment with any of the lasers, but histologic and ultrastructural examinations revealed that epidermal and dermal damage was most evident after treatment with the Nd:YAG laser.

Kilmer and colleagues[64] published their findings from a prospective, blinded, controlled study that assessed the ability of the Q-switched Nd:YAG laser (1064 nm, 10 nsec, 5 Hz) to remove tattoos. Twenty-five patients with 39 blue-black or multicolored tattoos were randomly assigned to four quadrants, treated with 6, 8, 10, or 12 J/cm² at 3- to 4-week intervals in four treatment sessions. An excellent response (more than 75% ink removal) was seen in 77% of black tattoos, and more than 95% of the black ink cleared in 11 (28%) of 39 tattoos treated at fluences of 10 to 12 J/cm² in four treatment sessions. Colored pigments were not as effectively removed. The best results were noted in the patients treated with fluences of 10 and 12 J/cm². No significant side effects, including pigmentary changes or scarring, occurred. Histopathologic examinations showed that tattoo ink remained in clinically clean areas and confirmed the absence of fibrosis or granulomatous changes. These authors concluded that the Q-switched Nd:YAG laser (1064 nm) effectively treats black tattoos with an excellent cosmetic outcome, but other colors are only minimally responsive to treatment.

A study performed by Watts and co-workers[65] clearly demonstrated that the Q-switched Nd:YAG laser can also be used for removal of tattoo pigment in difficult areas such as the eyelids. These authors used this laser in 7 patients (14 eyelids) to remove permanent eyeliner tattoo. A reduction in pigmentation was achieved in all patients, although responses were variable. On average, five treatment sessions were necessary. Complications of treatment were limited to transient ocular bruising, but no cases of ectropion occurred after treatment, nor was any visible scarring induced.

OTHER APPLICATIONS

Contact Laser Scalpels

Since their introduction in 1985, artificial-sapphire contact probes (scalpels) have become increasingly popular for use with the Nd:YAG laser in various fields of surgery.[3] Although clinical experience with these contact laser scalpels is limited, early reports regarding their effectiveness have been published. Arai and Sato[66] have used contact laser scalpels with a distal probe diameter of 0.2 mm operating at 7 to 8 W to excise pigmented nevi, epidermal cysts, neurofibromas, ingrown toenails, and angiomas. Apfelberg and Smith[20] excised five large cavernous hemangiomas and two lymphangiomas using sapphire scalpels, and good results were obtained in six patients. The lesion was not resectable in the remaining patient. They found the contact laser scalpels to combine excellent cutting properties with the coagulative ability of the Nd:YAG laser, thus greatly extending the hemostatic, incisional, and vaporization capability of this laser.

Because of the benefits that accrue to the use of these scalpels in combination with continuous-wave Nd:YAG lasers, their future use seems secure.

Control of Connective Tissue Metabolism

In vitro experiments performed by Abergel and associates[67] using fibroblast cultures demonstrated suppression of collagen production at fluences of 1.1×10^3 J/cm^2. Keloid fibroblast cultures were found to be even more sensitive than control cells to the bioinhibition produced by the Nd:YAG laser. Irradiation with a fluence of 0.7×10^3 J/cm^2 was noted to reduce collagen production to the same (normal) level as that in control cultures. On the basis of the findings yielded by the tissue culture studies, clinical trials were initiated for the treatment of keloids with the Nd:YAG laser. With the patient under local anesthesia, the treatment area was irradiated by the Nd:YAG laser using a fluence of about 60 J/cm^2. The hypertrophic scars and keloids were treated with nonoverlapping areas until superficial blanching of the skin occurred. Treatments were repeated at 1- to 2-week intervals, and initial results consisted of flattening and softening of the lesion. These results represent a limited experience, however, and have not been reproduced. We have not found the treatment of hypertrophic scars with the Nd:YAG laser to be successful using either technique and therefore do not use it at all.

Tissue Welding

Another future application for the Nd:YAG laser may be tissue welding. In an experimental study, Abergel and colleagues[68,69] successfully closed skin wounds with the Nd:YAG laser, using a power of 1.0 W and a spot size of 0.02 cm^2, resulting in an irradiance of 50 W/cm^2. The procedure involved first the approximation of the wound edges with forceps, followed by closure of the wounds produced by continuous passage of the laser beam along the wound. The wounds welded by laser healed rapidly, and the tensile strength of the control and experimental wounds was similar at all times. Although the mechanism of laser welding is not clear, it seems likely that thermal energy causes protein denaturation, which causes the wound edges to be sealed. Because of its deep penetration and the resulting deep and homogeneous coagulation, the Nd:YAG laser seems especially suitable for tissue welding. Laser welding may have advantages over suturing, because it does not introduce foreign material into the wound and may provide improved cosmetic results. There are, as yet, however, no data regarding laser tissue welding in human subjects.

Summary

We have found that there are only limited indications for the continuous-wave Nd:YAG laser in cutaneous surgery but that it can comple-

Table 7-4. Continuous-wave comparison of Nd:YAG, argon, and CO_2 lasers

Variables	Nd:YAG	Argon	CO_2
Depth of coagulation	~5 mm	1 mm	—
Risk of bleeding	Low	Low	Moderate
Smoke/plume formation	None	None	High
Amount of time	Low	Low	High
Scarring	High	Low	Low
Wound healing	6–8 weeks	2 weeks	3–6 weeks

ment the other lasers used. At the Department of Dermatology at the University of Regensburg, less than 5% of patients undergoing laser procedures have been treated using the Nd:YAG laser.

Compared with the argon and CO_2 laser, the Nd:YAG laser has advantages as well as disadvantages (Table 7-4). Advantages include the relatively deep level of coagulation it achieves, as well as the low risk of bleeding and plume formation and, in most cases, the short treatment times associated with its use. Disadvantages are the higher risk of scarring and a delay in wound healing. The frequency-doubled Nd:YAG, Q-switched Nd:YAG, and frequency-doubled, Q-switched Nd:YAG lasers compete with the flashlamp-pumped pulsed dye, ruby, alexandrite, and pigmented lesion dye (Candela, Wayland, Massachusetts) lasers.

The future will show whether increasing experience, improved techniques, and further technical developments will extend the role of the Nd:YAG lasers in dermatology.

References

1. Nelson JS. Laser systems used in plastic surgery and dermatology. In: Achauer BM, Vander Kam V, Berns MW, eds. Lasers in plastic surgery and dermatology. Stuttgart, New York: Thieme, 1992:11–20.
2. Dover JS, Arndt KA, Geronemus RG et al. Illustrated cutaneous laser surgery. A practitioner's guide. Norwalk, CT: Appleton and Lange, 1990.
3. Hukki J, Krogerus L, Castren M, Schroder T. Effects of different contact laser scalpels on skin and subcutaneous fat. Lasers Surg Med 1988;8: 276–282.
4. Gallucci JG, Zeltsman D, Slotman GJ. Nd:YAG laser scalpel compared with conventional techniques in head and neck cancer surgery. Lasers Surg Med 1994;14:139–144.
5. Maker VK, Elseth KM, Radosevich JA. A reduced tumor cell transfer with contact neodymium-yttrium-aluminium garnet laser scalpels. Lasers Surg Med 1992;12:303–307.
6. Haina D, Landthaler M, Braun-Falco O, Waidelich W. Optische Eigenschaften menschlicher Haut. In: Waidelich W, eds. Laser 83. Optoelektronik in der Medizin. Berlin, Heidelberg, New York, Tokyo: Springer, 1984:187–197.
7. Berlien HP, Waldschmidt J, Müller G. Laser treatment of cutaneous and deep vessel anomalies. In: Waidelich W, Waidelich R, eds. Laser 87.

Optoelectronics in Medicine. Berlin, Heidelberg, New York, London, Paris, Tokyo: Springer, 1988:526–528.

8. Phillipp C, Shaltout J, Berlin HP. Die kontinuierliche Eiskühlung der Haut bei der Nd:YAG-Laserbehandlung von CVD [abstract]. Lasermedizin 1995;11:123.

9. Haina D, Landthaler M, Braun-Falco O, Waidelich W. Comparison of the maximum coagulation depth in human skin for different types of medical lasers. Lasers Surg Med 1987;7:355–362.

10. Landthaler M, Brunner R, Haina D et al. Der Neodym:YAG-Laser in der Dermatologie. Münch Med Wochenschr 1984;126:1108–1112.

11. Landthaler M, Haina D, Brunner R et al. Effects of argon, dye and Nd:YAG lasers on epidermis, dermis and venous vessels. Lasers Surg Med 1986;6:87–93.

12. Haina D, Landthaler M, Frank F et al. Zeitliche und räumliche Temperaturverteilung an Hautproben bei Nd:YAG Laserbestrahlung. In: Keiditsch E, Ascher PW, Frank F, eds. Verhandlungsbericht der Deutschen Gesellschaft für Lasermedizin. 2. Tagung. München, Zürich: Erdmann-Brenger, 1985:71–76.

13. Landthaler M, Haina D, Seipp W et al. Zur Behandlung von Naevi flammei mit dem Argonlaser. Hautarzt 1987;38:652–659.

14. Hohenleutner U, Abd-el Raheem T, Bäumler W et al. Nävi flammei im Kindes- und Jugendalter. Die Behandlung mit dem Blitzlampengepumpten Farbstofflaser. Hautarzt 1995;46:87–93.

15. Tan OT, Sherwood K, Gilchrest BA. Successful treatment of children with port wine stains using the flashlamp-pulsed tunable dye laser. N Engl J Med 1989;320:416–421.

16. Barsky SH, Rosen SH, Geer DE, Noe JM. The nature and evolution of port wine stains: a computer-assisted study. J Invest Dermatol 1980;74:154–157.

17. Landthaler M, Dorn M, Haina D et al. Morphologische Untersuchungen zur Behandlung von Naevi flammei mit dem Argonlaser. Hautarzt 1983;34:548–554.

18. Hohenleutner U, Hilbert M, Wlotzke U, Landthaler M. Epidermal damage and limited coagulation depth with the flashlamp-pumped pulsed dye laser: a histochemical study. J Invest Dermatol 1995;104:798–802.

19. Landthaler M, Haina D, Brunner R et al. Neodymium-YAG laser therapy of vascular lesions. J Am Acad Dermatol 1986;14:197–217.

20. Apfelberg DB, Smith T. Study of the benefits of the Nd:YAG laser in plastic surgery. In: Joffe SN, Oguro Y, eds. Advances in Nd:YAG laser surgery. Berlin, Heidelberg, New York, Paris, Tokyo: Springer, 1988:213–226.

21. Dixon JA, Gilbertson JJ. Argon and neodymium-YAG laser therapy of dark nodular port wine stains in older patients. Laser Surg Med 1986;6:5–11.

22. Klepzig K, Landthaler M, Haina D et al. Ultrastrukturelle Untersuchungen von Naevi flammei 24 Stunden nach Behandlung mit einem Argon- und Nd:YAG laser. In: Keiditsch E, Ascher PW, Frank F, eds. Verhandlungsbericht der Deutschen Gesellschaft für Lasermedizin, 2. Tagung. München, Zürich: Erdmann-Brenger, 1985:77–81.

23. Laffitte F, Mordon S, Chavoin JP et al. The frequency-doubled Nd:YAG laser with automatic scanning in the treatment of port wine stains: a preliminary report. Lasers Med Sci 1992;7:341–349.

24. Dixon JA, Davis RK, Gilbertson JJ. Laser photocoagulation of vascular malformations of the tongue. Laryngoscope 1986;96:537–541.

25. Rosenfeld H, Sherman R. Treatment of cutaneous and deep vascular lesions with the Nd:YAG laser. Lasers Surg Med 1986;6:20–23.

26. David LM, Dwyer RM, Goldmann RD. A comparison of Nd:YAG and argon lasers in treating hemangiomas of the skin [abstract]. Lasers Surg Med 1984;3:330.

27. Powell JL, Bailey CL, Coppland AT et al. Nd:YAG laser excision of a giant gingival pyogenic granuloma of pregnancy. Lasers Surg Med 1994; 14:178–183.

28. Werner JA, Lippert BM, Godbersen GS, Rudert H. Die Hämangiobehandlung mit dem Neodym:Yttrium-Aluminium-Granat-Laser (Nd: YAG-Laser). Laryngorhinootologie 1992;71:388–395.

29. Apfelberg DM. Management of difficult vascular birthmarks. In: Achauer BM, Vander Kam V, Berns MW, eds. Lasers in plastic surgery and dermatology. Stuttgart, New York: Thieme, 1992:61–69.

30. Achauer BM, Vander Kam V. Capillary hemangioma (strawberry mark) of infancy: comparison of argon and Nd:YAG laser treatment. J Plast Reconstr Surg 1989;84:60–69.

31. Apfelberg DB, Maser MR, White DN, Lash H. A preliminary study of the combined effect of neodymium:YAG laser photocoagulation and direct steroid instillation in the treatment of capillary cavernous hemangiomas of infancy. Ann Plast Surg 1989;22:94–104.

32. Grantzow R, Schmittenbecher PP, Schuster T. Frühbehandlung von Hämangiomen: lasertherapie. Monatsschr Kinderheilkd 1995;143:369–374.

33. Landthaler M, Hohenleutner U, Abd El-Raheem T. Laser therapy of childhood haemangiomas. Br J Dermatol 1995;133:275–281.

34. Alani HM, Warren RM. Percutaneous photocoagulation of deep vascular lesions using a fiberoptic laser wand. Ann Plast Surg 1992;29:143–148.

35. Werner JA, Lippert BM, Hoffmann P, Rudert H. Nd:YAG laser therapy of voluminous hemangiomas and vascular malformations. Adv Otorhinolaryngol 1995;49:75–80.

36. Hoffmann P, Offergeld CH, Hüttenbrink KB et al. Die perkutane und interstitielle Lasertherapie cavernöser Hämangiome [abstract]. Lasermedizin 1995;11:126.

37. Sharpsay SM, Oliver P. Treatment of hereditary hemorrhagic telangiectasia by Nd:YAG laser photocoagulation. Laryngoscope 1984;94:1554–1556.

38. Bahmer FA, Tang DE, Payeur-Kirsch M. Treatment of large condylomata of the penis with the neodymium-YAG laser. Acta Derm Venereol (Stockh) 1984;64:361–363.

39. Landthaler M, Baur S, Baltzer J, Haina D. Bowenoide Genitalpapeln. Behandlung mit dem Neodym-YAG Laser. Münch Med Wochenschr 1987;129:424–425.

40. Knoll LD, Segura JW, Benson RC, Goellner JR. Bowenoid papulosis of the penis: successful management with neodymium:YAG laser. J Urol 1988;139:1307–1309.

41. Volz LR, Carpiniello VL, Malloy TR. Laser treatment of urethral condyloma: a five-year experience. Urology 1994;43:81–83.

42. Ferenczy A. Laser treatment of genital human papillomavirus infections in the male patient. Obstet Gynecol Clin North Am 1991;18:525–535.

43. Pfau A, Abd El-Raheem T, Bäumler W et al. Nd:YAG laser hyperthermia in the treatment of recalcitrant verrucae vulgares (Regensburg's technique). Acta Derm Venereol (Stockh) 1994;74:212–214.

44. Pfau A, Abd El-Raheem T, Bäumler W et al. Treatment of recalcitrant

verrucae vulgares (Regensburg's technique)—preliminary results in 31 cases. J Dermatol Treat 1995;6:39–42.

45. Brunner R, Landthaler M, Haina D et al. Treatment of benign, semimalignant, and malignant skin tumors with the Nd:YAG laser. Lasers Surg Med 1985;5:105–110.

46. Bahmer F. The neodymium:YAG laser in dermatology. In: Steiner R, Kaufmann R, Landthaler M, Braun-Falco Q, eds. Lasers in dermatology. Berlin, Heidelberg, New York, London: Springer, 1991:73–84.

47. Landthaler M. Premalignant and malignant skin lesions. In: Achauer BW, Vander Kam V, Berns WM, eds. Lasers in plastic surgery and dermatology. Stuttgart, New York: Thieme, 1992:34–44.

48. Malloy TR, Wein AJ, Carpiniello VL. Carcinoma of penis treated with neodymium YAG laser. Urology 1988;31:26–29.

49. Boon TA. Sapphire probe laser surgery for localized carcinoma of the penis. Eur J Surg Oncol 1988;14:193–195.

50. Malek RS. Laser treatment of premalignant and malignant squamous cell lesions of the penis. Lasers Surg Med 1992;12:246–253.

51. Landthaler M, Brunner R, Haina D. Nd:YAG laser therapy of an oral verrucous leukoplakia. Dermatologica 1989;178:115–117.

52. Weese D, Murphy J, Zimmern PE. Nd:YAG laser treatment of extramammary Paget's disease of the penis and scrotum. J Urol (Paris) 1993;5:269–271.

53. Landthaler M, Fröschl M, Haina D, Braun-Falco O. Therapie des disseminierten Kaposi-Sarkoms (DKS). Münch Med Wochenschr 1989;131: 313–315.

54. Riederer A, Zietz C, Held M. Das HIV-assoziierte Kaposi-Sarkom im Kopf-Hals-Bereich: eine klinische, morphologische und therapeutische Übersicht. Laryngorhinootologie 1993;72:478–484.

55. Wishnow KI, Johnson DE. Effective outpatients' treatment of Kaposi's sarcoma of the urethral meatus using the neodymium:YAG laser. Lasers Surg Med 1988;8:428–432.

56. Wagner RI, Kozlov AP, Moskalik KG. Laser radiation therapy of skin melanoma. Strahlentherapie 1981;157:670–672.

57. Kozlov AP, Moskalik KG. Pulsed laser radiation therapy of skin tumors. Cancer 1980;46:2172–2178.

58. Goldberg DJ. Treatment of pigmented and vascular lesions of the skin with the Q-switched Nd:YAG laser [abstract]. Lasers Surg Med 1993;13 (suppl):55.

59. Linsmeier-Kilmer S, Wheeland RG, Goldberg DJ, Anderson R. Treatment of epidermal pigmented lesions with the frequency-doubled Q-switched Nd:YAG laser. Arch Dermatol 1994;130:1515–1519.

60. Tse Y, Levine CJ, Mcclain SA, Ashinoff R. The removal of cutaneous pigmented lesions with the Q-switched neodymium:yttrium-aluminium-garnet laser. J Dermatol Surg Oncol 1994;20:795–800.

61. Kirschner RA. Ablation of tattoos with the Nd:YAG laser. Laser Med Surg News 1986;5:21–25.

62. Brunner F, Hafner R, Giovanoli R et al. Entfernung von Tätowierungen mit dem Nd:YAG Laser. Hautarzt 1987;38:610–614.

63. Zelickson BD, Mehregan DA, Zarrin AA et al. Clinical, histologic and ultrastructural evaluation of tattoos treated with three laser systems. Lasers Surg Med 1994;15:364–372.

64. Kilmer SL, Lee MS, Grevelink M et al. The Q-switched Nd:YAG laser effectively treats tattoos. Arch Dermatol 1993;129:9711–9718.

65. Watts MT, Downes RN, Collin RO, Walker NPJ. The use of Q-switched Nd:YAG laser for removal of permanent eyeliner tattoo. Ophthal Plast Reconstr Surg 1992;8:292–294.
66. Arai K, Sato T. Clinical application of the Nd:YAG laser in dermatology and plastic surgery. In: Joffe SN, Oguro Y, eds. Advances in Nd:YAG laser surgery. Berlin, Heidelberg, New York, Paris, Tokyo: Springer, 1988:208–212.
67. Abergel RP, Mecker CA, Lam TS et al. Control of connective tissue metabolism by lasers: recent developments and future prospects. J Am Acad Dermatol 1984;11:1142–1150.
68. Abergel RP, Lyons RF, White RA et al. Skin closure by Nd:YAG laser welding. J Am Acad Dermatol 1986;14:810–814.
69. Abergel RP, Lyons RF, Dwyer R et al. Use of lasers for closure of cutaneous wounds: experience with Nd:YAG, argon, and CO_2 lasers. J Dermatol Surg Oncol 1986;12:1181–1185.

8 —— Selection of the Appropriate Laser for the Treatment of Cutaneous Vascular Lesions

Roy G. Geronemus
Jeffrey S. Dover

The beneficial effect of lasers on cutaneous disorders is best demonstrated in the treatment of vascular disorders. Both visible light (argon, continuous-wave dye, flashlamp-pumped pulsed dye, and copper vapor) and invisible light (CO_2 and Nd:YAG) lasers have been utilized in the treatment of cutaneous vascular disorders. Each of these lasers produces different wavelengths and pulsewidths and involves a different method of delivery, and the characteristics of each laser determine its effect on vascular tissue.

For the purposes of this discussion, the classification of vascular lesions, as described by Mulliken and Young,[1] is used. Hemangiomas are defined as vascular lesions that rapidly proliferate after birth and then enter a phase of spontaneous involution sometime by the end of the first year of life. All other vascular lesions are considered malformations, with the port-wine stain (PWS) representing a malformation of the capillary type. The classification of the other malformations is determined by the predominant vessel type—venous, arterial, arteriovenous, and lymphatic.

The diameter of cutaneous vessels may vary from 0.1 μm in a small telangiectasis to several millimeters in a venous malformation or cavernous hemangioma. In view of the wide disparity in the characteristics of vascular lesions of the skin and the differences in the characteristics of the various lasers, it is clear that no one laser can be used to treat all cutaneous vascular disorders. In some instances, it is often necessary to utilize more than one type of laser to treat a patient's vascular lesions. This discussion focuses on the rationale and criteria for the use of these various lasers in the treatment of different types of cutaneous vascular disorders. Each laser modality is described first, followed by a review of the major vascular anomalies and the laser preferred for the treatment of each.

Laser Modalities

FLASHLAMP-PUMPED PULSED DYE LASER

The flashlamp-pumped pulsed dye laser was developed to create specific vascular injury within dermal blood vessels 100 μm or less in diameter. The required parameters for specific vascular injury include a pulsewidth of less than 1 msec, a wavelength near an absorption peak of oxyhemoglobin (541 or 577 nm), and high peak energy densities of up to 10 J/cm². The short pulse duration and high peak power distinguish this laser from the other lasers available for the treatment of cutaneous vascular disorders. The pulsewidth, which is shorter than the thermal relaxation time of small vessels, selectively damages red blood cells as well as endothelial cells without causing thermal damage to surrounding collagen. This specific damage can be demonstrated histologically to a depth of 1.2 mm in treated PWSs. Agglutinated red blood cells, fibrin, and platelets are seen within the treated vessels without other dermal damage. One month after treatment, ectatic vessels are replaced with new normal-appearing vessels, with no fibrosis.[2]

The immediate effect on skin is the formation of a purpuric macule, which lasts 10 to 14 days. Crusting is uncommon after these treatments, so postoperative wound care is not routinely required. The need for anesthesia is minimal, but this depends on the age and pain tolerance of the patient. Young children may require sedation or anesthesia for the treatment of large lesions, but most adults can be treated quite extensively without the need for any local anesthesia. Although significant posttreatment darkening occurs often, it is of short-term cosmetic concern to the patient.

Argon Laser

Until the development of the flashlamp-pumped pulsed dye laser, the argon laser had been the treatment of choice for most PWSs.[3] The argon laser emits light at six different wavelengths, from 457.9 to 514.5 nm, in the blue-green portion of the visible spectrum. This laser produces a continuous beam, although it can be shuttered. The depth of vascular injury is approximately 1 mm, and the wavelengths are absorbed by both oxyhemoglobin and melanin. Because of competition between these two chromophores, there may be less penetration of the laser light to the level of the blood vessel in darkly pigmented or well-tanned patients. As a result of the absorption of the laser light by melanin, hypopigmentation occurs in at least 20% of the patients with PWSs treated with the argon laser.

Unlike the pulsed dye laser, which causes thermal damage that is limited to the blood vessel itself, the argon laser causes nonselective thermal damage to structures surrounding blood vessels. Treatment with the argon laser is also more painful than that with the flashlamp-pumped pulsed dye laser, making anesthesia necessary in patients during the treatment of PWSs. Postoperative wound care is also of greater importance than that for patients who undergo pulsed dye laser treatment, because epidermal and dermal sloughing takes place immediately after the treatment.[4]

The success of treatment with this laser depends primarily on the correct use of the laser, the experience of the user, and appropriate patient selection.[5] The ability to vary technique is substantial compared with the ability to vary the technique used for the pulsed dye laser, which is relatively standardized with fewer modifiable parameters. Results obtained are therefore more variable with the argon laser. Side effects can be limited by using lower energy densities than those originally recommended.

Energy outputs in the range of 0.6 to 0.8 W, versus the 2 to 3 W previously used, have resulted in fewer side effects and good clinical results.[6] A technique described by Scheibner and Wheeland[7] for use with the continuous-wave tunable dye laser can also be adapted for use with the argon laser, with much improved therapeutic results. In this technique, a small spot size and very low power are utilized, with the latter continuously delivered to "heat seal" discrete vessels. Specifically, light is focused to a 100-μm spot and the powers used range from 0.1 to 0.3 W, yielding low power densities of 1000 to 3000 W/cm^2. Use of this technique not only limits thermal damage to the vessels themselves but also minimizes spreading of the heat to surrounding tissue. However, the success of this method depends on the skill of the physician and is very time-consuming relative to other techniques.

Delivery of the continuous-wave laser sources can also be modified through the use of robotized scanning devices, such as the Hexascan. These computerized devices utilize a microprocessor control module and are connected to the argon laser by means of a fiberoptic cable. The handpiece contains a focusing device, electronic shutter, and a power meter, which can deliver a 1-mm-wide beam.[8] A collection of 1-mm spot beams are delivered in a hexagonal shape ranging from 3 to 13 mm in diameter at an increased energy frequency of 16 to 27 J/cm^2. Individual exposures are delivered so that no two adjacent sites are ever exposed one after another. In this way, thermal diffusion may be minimized, and theoretically so is thermal necrosis and resultant scarring. In addition, theoretically, more specific vascular injury can be achieved than that possible with the conventional methods of argon laser delivery. Open trials and early studies comparing the use of the Hexascan with the continuous-wave dye laser (585 nm) to the pulsed dye laser[9] demonstrated the device's effectiveness, but further comparative studies are needed to determine where robotized scanners for the delivery of continuous-wave light fit into the therapeutic armamentarium of treatments for cutaneous vascular disorders.

CONTINUOUS-WAVE TUNABLE DYE LASER

The argon laser–pumped tunable dye laser is a continuous-wave laser that, as its name implies, makes use of an argon laser to pump a dye laser. The argon laser can be uncoupled to emit argon laser light, but any visible wavelength can be produced when it is coupled with the dye laser, depending on the dye chosen. When rhodamine 6G is used as the dye, the peak emission is at 577 nm, but the wavelength can be tuned up or down approximately 20 nm using a computer-controlled prism. The continuous-wave dye laser is used in this way to treat cutaneous vascular disorders at wavelengths of from 577 to 590 nm. The technique used is similar to that used for the argon laser. Studies comparing the continuous-wave tunable dye laser in the yellow light range with the argon laser have not been done to date, but theoretically, treatment with the continuous-wave tunable dye laser should produce slightly better results because of the better absorption of oxyhemoglobin at 577 nm. This laser light is emitted continuously and can be shuttered, as with the argon laser, and the same spot sizes are available for both lasers. Using wavelengths of from 577 to 590 nm, the effect on tissue and the treatment indications are essentially the same as those for argon laser treatment. The lower energy produced by the continuous-wave dye laser may make it less effective than the argon laser for the treatment of deeper vascular lesions, however.

COPPER VAPOR LASER

The copper vapor laser emits light at 578 nm, either alone or in combination with light at 511 nm, with a 6-kHz train (6000 pulses per second) of 30-nsec pulses and a peak power of 80 kW. The train of pulses that are emitted range from 10 to 40 nsec in duration, with 2 mJ of power per pulse, and appear to the human eye to be a continuous beam of light. Its wavelength is well absorbed by oxyhemoglobin, and the beam penetrates relatively deep into the target tissue. Because these pulses cannot be emitted individually, however, the train of pulses results in thermal diffusion from the target vessel and non-selective thermal damage. Clinical studies comparing it with other lasers have not been performed, but there have been reports that the copper vapor laser is effective in the treatment of telangiectases, flat, dark PWSs, and mature, hypertrophic PWSs.

Histologic studies performed by Tan[9] and Walker[10] and their colleagues have shown that a subepidermal blister forms 24 hours after copper vapor laser irradiation of PWSs, and this is accompanied by degeneration of segments of the capillary and reticular dermis. The ectatic blood vessels of PWSs are eventually replaced by fibrous connective tissue within 3 to 6 months after the laser treatment, as shown by electron microscopy. These histologic findings indicate that there is some nonselective damage after copper vapor laser treatment of PWSs and that the possibility of scarring is greater in children with PWSs and in patients with other disorders in which the diameter of the vessels is small.[11]

KRYPTON LASER

The krypton laser also emits at 568 nm in a continuous beam, but no reports have been published regarding the krypton laser in the treatment of vascular lesions. However, on the basis of theoretical considerations and clinical experience, the outcome from krypton laser treatment of PWSs and benign vascular lesions appears to be very similar to that obtained using the continuous-wave dye laser.

CO$_2$ LASER

The CO$_2$ laser emits infrared light at 10,600 nm that is primarily absorbed by water, resulting in the vaporization of tissue during the coagulation of blood vessels. However, the thermal damage produced by the CO$_2$ laser is nonselective, such that treatment of any type of vascular lesion results in the scatter of thermal energy around the cutaneous blood vessel, causing significant epidermal and dermal damage. Despite this nonselective effect, the CO$_2$ laser has been utilized for the eradication of many different types of vascular lesions of the skin.

Patients who undergo CO$_2$ laser treatment routinely require preoperative anesthesia and postoperative care, and the number of treatments depends on the type of lesion being treated. Permanent textural and pigmentary changes are almost always seen after the treatment of cutaneous vascular disorders using the CO$_2$ laser.

Nd:YAG LASER

The Nd:YAG laser is also an infrared laser emitting at 1060 nm. It can be delivered in either a continuous-wave or a pulsed, Q-switched mode. This wavelength is poorly absorbed by all cutaneous chromophores, allowing deep penetration of the beam into the skin to depths of 4 to 6 mm and wide diffusion of the beam. This results in nonspecific thermal damage to skin. This deep penetration has led to use of the Nd:YAG laser in the treatment of thicker PWSs and in the treatment of hemangiomas, but because scarring and permanent pigmentary changes cannot be avoided, its use in the treatment of superficial cutaneous vascular disorders has been less successful.

The continuous-wave, frequency-doubled Nd:YAG laser (KTP laser), emitting at 532 nm, has been used in the treatment of vascular disorders. The 532-nm option of this laser has not been studied in controlled comparative evaluations, but the clinical results appear to resemble those resulting from argon laser treatment, but with less thermal damage than that caused by the continuous-wave Nd:YAG laser emitting at 1064 nm.

The Q-switched Nd:YAG laser is approved for use at a wavelength of 532 nm in the treatment of a variety of vascular disorders. It is effective in the treatment of facial telangiectases and has been shown to be able to lighten PWSs, although not as effectively as the pulsed dye laser. Because the pulse duration (5 nsec) is so much shorter than the thermal relaxation time of vessels in facial telangiectases, the Q-switched Nd:YAG laser ruptures the vessels, causing acute purpura and occasional bleeding.

KTP LASER

Efforts to minimize the thermal exposure of green light for treating cutaneous vascular lesions have been develped with a KTP laser (Laser-scope-Orion), which delivers a train of pulses at energies ranging from 5 to 40 J/cm^2 and a pulsewidth ranging from 2 to 20 milliseconds. The KTP light can also be delivered through a scanning device to minimize further the degree of thermal injury. Clinical data regarding the efficacy of this laser have not yet been published. However, the clinical advantage of this technique would be short-term whitening and crusting of the skin compared to prolonged purpura as seen with the pulsed dye laser.

PULSED GREEN LIGHT LASER

A pulsed green light laser also has been developed by Coherent Laser Co. (Versapulse). This laser has a variable pulsewidth ranging from 2 to 10 milliseconds with a spot size of 2 to 10 mm and energies up to 38 J/cm^2. This laser light is delivered in conjunction with a cooling handpiece that utilizes chilled water through parallel glass plates, which are in contact with the skin surface. The purpose of this handpiece is to protect the epidermis from thermal injury and thus minimize pigmentary changes that occur as a result of the green light absorption by melanin. As with the KTP laser, clinical data are not yet available.

Vascular Abnormalities

PORT-WINE STAINS

Pulsed Dye Laser

The theory of selective vascular injury is well demonstrated by the safety and effectiveness of the treatment of PWSs in infants and children.[12–16] Several studies have shown the effectiveness of the pulsed dye laser in the lightening of PWSs in patients of all ages (Tables 8-1 to 8-3).[12–15,17] Of greatest importance is its unique success in the treatment of children, with minimal risks of scarring and pigmentary alterations.

PWSs in all locations on the body can be effectively treated with the pulsed dye laser, though success is greatest for the treatment of head and neck lesions and slightly less for the treatment of trunk lesions, with lesions on the distal extremities showing a much slower response (see Table 8-3).

Upon the examination of treated PWSs in different anatomic sites above the head and neck, Renfro and Geronemus[18] found that most commonly midline facial PWSs lightened or cleared rapidly, whereas lesions over the second branch of the trigeminal nerve were the slowest to respond. The exact degree of lightening or clearing as reported in the literature has been somewhat confusing. Most studies have shown approximately 75% lightening of all PWSs after three treatment sessions. One study[12] showed 100% clearing in all patients treated, but this finding has not been substantiated in any other clinical evaluations.

Skin types I through III lighten most quickly, with the darker skin types (IV and V) lightening least quickly because of the higher melanin content, which acts as a partial barrier to penetration of the

Table 8-1. Port-wine stain response to laser therapy by type of lesion

| Laser type | Type of lesion | | |
	Macular lesion	Mildly hypertrophic lesion	Very hypertrophic lesion
Pulsed dye	Excellent	Excellent	Poor
Continuous-wave dye, argon, or KTP (conventional technique)	Fair	Good	Good
Continuous-wave dye or argon (Scheibner technique)	Excellent	Good	Good
Continuous-wave dye, argon, krypton, or KTP with Hexascan	Very good	Good	Good
Copper vapor	Good	Very good	Good
CO_2	Poor	Fair	Good
Nd:YAG/continuous-wave	Poor	Poor	Good

laser light. Very dark skin (type VI) does not respond to this treatment. Epidermal sloughing may take place, requiring wound care and resulting in hyperpigmentation.[19]

Mature or hypertrophic PWSs, which have ectatic vessels greater than 100 μm in diameter, often do not respond as well to pulsed dye laser treatment. Occasionally, the vessel size diminishes after repeated treatment sessions, causing some lightening of mature PWSs.

Table 8-2. Port-wine stain response by age to laser therapy

| Laser type | Age of patient | | |
	Infants	Young children and adolescents	Adults
Pulsed dye	Excellent	Excellent	Excellent
Continuous-wave dye, argon, krypton, or KTP (conventional technique)	Poor	Fair	Good
Continuous-wave dye or argon (Scheibner technique)	Fair	Good	Excellent
Continuous-wave dye, argon, or krypton with Hexascan	Data not available	Good	Excellent
Copper vapor	Fair	Fair to good	Excellent
CO_2	Poor	Poor to fair	Good (hypertrophic lesions only)
Nd:YAG	Poor	Poor	Good (hypertrophic lesions only)

Table 8-3.   Port-wine stain response to laser therapy by location

Laser type	Lesion location			
	Face	Neck	Trunk	Extremities
Pulsed dye	Excellent	Excellent	Excellent	Excellent
Continuous-wave dye, argon, krypton, or KTP (conventional technique)	Good	Fair	Fair	Fair
Continuous-wave dye or argon (Scheibner technique)	Excellent	Excellent	Good	Good
Continuous-wave dye, argon, KTP, or krypton with Hexascan	Good	Good	Good	Good
Copper vapor	Good	Good	Fair	Fair
CO_2 (for hypertrophic lesions only)	Good	Good	Good	Good
Nd:YAG (for hypertrophic lesions only)	Good	Good	Good	Good

As a general rule, multiple treatment sessions with the pulsed dye laser are necessary, scheduled at intervals of 1 to 3 months. Although the greatest lightening usually takes place after the first or second treatment, an average of six or more treatment sessions may be necessary before maximal lightening is obtained. A recent study showed that many PWSs that initially appear resistant to treatment continue to lighten with as many as 20 treatments.

Side effects from pulsed dye laser treatment of PWSs are uncommon. In a study of 500 patients, Levine and Geronemus[20] found that no hypertrophic scars had occurred and that the incidence of atrophic scarring was less than 1%. Cutaneous atrophy usually occurs as a result of significant overlapping of the pulses or the use of excessive energy fluences in young children. Transient hypopigmentation and hyperpigmentation have been noted, but neither is permanent in most cases. A chronic dermatitis has also been found in patients with an atopic diathesis who undergo multiple treatments of PWSs.

Cutaneous depressions are sometimes found in patients within 1 to 2 months after pulsed dye laser treatment, but these usually resolve without permanent scarring within 3 to 18 months.

In view of the high degree of efficacy of pulsed dye laser treatment and the low incidence of permanent side effects associated with its use, it is considered the treatment of choice for all macular and slightly raised PWSs.

Argon and Continuous-Wave Dye Laser

Patient selection is particularly important to ensuring the success of the treatment of PWSs with the continuous-wave laser, with the best responses obtained in adult patients with mature, purple hypertrophic lesions located on the head and neck.[4,5] The technique is not difficult to perform, but results can vary, and this depends on the expertise of the operator. The risk of scarring is lowest for patients treated by operators with the greatest experience. PWSs on the lip, angle of the mandible, chest, and upper back are the most prone to scarring in response to argon laser therapy, with hypertrophic scarring the type of scarring that occurs. Permanent loss of pigmentation is particularly common on the neck. The risk of scarring is highest for children 18 years of age or younger. The scarring rate in this age group may be as high as 20% or higher for PWSs in all anatomic locations.

The maximum response of the PWS to argon and continuous-wave dye laser photocoagulation is not seen until 4 to 5 months after treatment. The response is delayed in part because of the fibrosis that occurs around the blood vessel, and it is only after the postoperative wound has healed that additional lightening occurs. A major advantage of these lasers is that, unlike pulsed dye laser treatment which must be performed in multiple sessions, the complete clinical response usually occurs after one treatment session.

Prospective studies in adults and children are necessary to determine the degree to which the technique described by Scheibner and Wheeland[7] and the use of robotized scanning delivery devices can minimize the incidence of scarring and pigmentary change.

Copper Vapor Laser

The copper vapor laser is widely used in the treatment of PWSs and produces results comparable to those produced by the continuous-wave dye and argon lasers. Hypertrophic and nodular PWSs as well as most PWSs in adults respond well to the copper vapor laser, but it has not proved effective in the treatment of children with PWSs. The initial work with the copper vapor laser in the treatment of large PWSs was limited because only very small spot sizes could be used. More recently, with the advent of robotic handpieces, the speed of delivery of the individual pulses has been improved.

Krypton Laser

The krypton laser emits both yellow light at 568 nm and green light at 520 nm. This continuous-wave laser has not been well studied in comparison with other continuous-wave lasers, but it is anticipated that the clinical response will prove comparable to that produced by the argon, continuous-wave dye, and copper vapor lasers.

CO_2 Laser

The primary use of the CO_2 laser in the treatment of PWSs is in patients with hypertrophic and nodular lesions that do not respond particularly well to selective lasers, because they are unable to deliver enough thermal energy to shrink the ectatic vessels.[21,22] Although results have been acceptable in 74% of the adults with PWSs treated with the CO_2 laser, the incidences of scarring and pigmentary change have been dramatically higher in patients treated with this laser than those seen in patients treated with lasers capable of selective vascular damage.[23] The use of the CO_2 laser in the treatment of children and most adults with PWSs is contraindicated in view of the low rates of success and high morbidity.[21]

Nd:YAG Laser

In view of its depth of penetration, the diffusion of its beam, and its nonselective destruction of vascular tissue, the continuous-wave Nd:YAG laser has been used only for the treatment of thick, nodular PWSs.[24] Its use in children has not been reported, but most likely treatment with it would lead to scarring. Its efficacy in the treatment of macular or mildly hypertrophic PWSs in adults has not been well established, and therefore it should be utilized with extreme caution until more is known about its effectiveness in this setting.

TELANGIECTASES AND OTHER SMALL-VESSEL DISORDERS

The treatment of telangiectases may differ depending on the diameter of the vessel, its anatomic location, and the age of the patient. Small-diameter telangiectases of the face may respond well to all of the lasers described in this chapter (Table 8-4). The pulsed dye laser is the least likely to cause scarring; however, because the diameter of its beam is larger than the diameter of a small-diameter telangiecta-

Table 8-4. Response of telangiectases to laser therapy by size of vessels

	Type of telangiectasis				
Laser type	Spider (face and trunk)	Small diameter (face and trunk)	Large diameter (face and trunk)	Small diameter (legs)	Large diameter (legs)
Pulsed dye	Excellent	Excellent	Fair	Fair	Poor
Continuous-wave dye, argon, KTP, or krypton (conventional technique)	Good	Fair	Excellent	Poor	Poor
Continuous-wave dye, argon, KTP, or krypton with Hexascan	Excellent	Good	Excellent	Fair	Poor
Copper vapor	Good	Good	Excellent	Fair	Poor
Nd:YAG	Poor	Poor	Poor	Poor	Poor

sis, treatment results in purpura of the surrounding normal skin that lasts for 7 to 14 days, and this is considered cosmetically unacceptable by some patients. The immediate effects of argon, continuous-wave dye, and copper vapor laser treatment are usually more cosmetically acceptable to patients, because they cause a crust to form over the treated area that lasts for only a few days after treatment and involves an area not much larger than the diameter of the treated vessel. The size of the beam emitted by these lasers can be modified to conform to the diameter of the ectatic vessel, and even a touch less than the diameter. Particular care must be taken when using the continuous-wave or copper vapor lasers in the paranasal areas, however, because transient or permanent atrophy may occur. The flashlamp-pumped pulsed dye laser is preferable for the ablation of fine telangiectases in young children, in view of its high therapeutic safety index.

Telangiectases on the lower extremities, as a rule, do not respond to treatment with any of the lasers, with the exception of small, red telangiectases that are less than 100 μm in diameter. Approximately 60% of patients with these lesions may show a response to treatment with the pulsed dye laser.[25] Although other lasers are occasionally effective, responses are usually inconsistent and unpredictable. Hyperpigmentation is common in patients with mat telangiectases after treatment using any of these lasers.[26]

Spider telangiectases are ideally suited to treatment with the pulsed dye laser because the small diameter of the vessels in this lesion, which takes up a large surface area, often corresponds to the 3- or 5-mm spot size of the pulsed dye laser beam. Spider telangiectases, which are relatively common in children, have been reported to respond after only one or two treatments, without scarring or permanent pigmentary change.[27] The argon, continuous-wave dye, and copper vapor lasers are also effective in the treatment of spider telangiectases, but the risks of pigmentary and textural changes associated with their use are higher than those associated with the use of the pulsed dye laser. Treatment using any of these lasers is also more tedious, because it is necessary to coagulate the central feeding vessels first, after which each of the "legs of the spider" has to be traced.

Large linear vessels, which are often blue, respond least well to the pulsed dye laser treatment but are most appropriately treated with the argon, continuous-wave dye, or copper vapor lasers. However, the large size and greater depth of these lesions often limit their complete eradication. The effective treatment of these vessels often depends on the skill of the physician. Overtreatment can result in atrophy of the treated area.[28]

The red nose syndrome, which is a diffuse redness of the nose or diffuse nasal telangiectasia, is usually secondary to nasal trauma.[29] It may respond well to treatment with any of these lasers, but permanent pigmentary alteration is less likely to occur in response to pulsed dye laser treatment. The continuous-wave and copper vapor lasers are not favored for the treatment of poikiloderma of Civatte because of the permanent depigmentation that is often a sequela of such therapy. The pulsed dye laser may be utilized safely on the neck in the treatment of poikiloderma of Civatte; however, lower energy densities (4.0 to 6.5 J/cm²) are usually required to prevent pigmentary loss.[30]

HEMANGIOMAS AND OTHER LARGE-VESSEL DISORDERS

The treatment of capillary (strawberry) hemangiomas with the pulsed dye, argon, and Nd:YAG lasers has been reported[24,31–35] (Table 8-5). The pulsed dye laser has been used in the treatment of capillary hemangiomas in young infants and children and has been observed to produce lightening and flattening of the lesions as well as to slow their proliferation. However, multiple treatments usually are required to achieve the maximum benefit.[31,32,36] Although the depth of selective vascular injury produced by the pulsed dye laser is limited to 1.2 mm, with multiple treatments the size of these capillary lesions can be reduced. Treatment performed in the first few weeks of life may not, however, prevent progression of the deeper component of the hemangioma.[37] The argon laser is effective in the treatment of strawberry hemangiomas, but textural and pigmentary changes are common side effects. Local or general anesthesia is usually required in patients undergoing treatment with the argon laser, as compared with those undergoing treatment with the pulsed dye laser, who require no anesthesia. In addition, patients treated with the pulsed dye laser require less postoperative wound care, because sloughing usually does occur. The continuous-wave Nd:YAG laser has also been used in the treatment of capillary hemangiomas, but multiple postoperative complications, including some hypertrophic scarring, have been noted in patients so treated.[24,32]

Vascular nodules and tumors, including pyogenic granulomas and tumors with a vascular component, such as Kaposi's sarcoma, respond well to argon laser treatment and similarly should respond well to

Table 8-5. Response of other vascular lesions to laser therapy

Laser type	Vascular lesion		
	Strawberry hemangiomas	Capillary-cavernous hemangiomas	Limited venous malformations
Pulsed dye	Very good	Fair	Fair
Continuous-wave, argon, krypton, or KTP (conventional technique)	Good	Fair	Excellent
Continuous-wave dye or argon (Scheibner technique)	Good	Fair	Good
Copper vapor	Fair	Fair	Good
CO_2	Fair	Fair	Fair
Nd:YAG	Fair	Fair	Good

continuous-wave dye and copper vapor laser treatment.[36–40] The limited depth of vascular injury produced by the pulsed dye laser limits this laser's effectiveness in the eradication of these types of lesions.

Cavernous hemangiomas are very likely to respond to treatment with the continuous-wave dye Nd:YAG laser, but the nonselective injury produced by this laser usually results in scarring.[24] The pulsed dye, argon, continuous-wave dye, krypton, and copper vapor lasers cannot accomplish the appropriate depth of vascular injury to reduce the subcutaneous component of these lesions.

Limited venous malformations (those without an extensive subcutaneous involvement) respond extremely well to argon, continuous-wave, and copper vapor laser photocoagulation. The argon laser is preferable for the ablation of somewhat thicker venous malformations, in view of the higher energy densities it delivers. Because many of these lesions occur on mucosal surfaces (e.g., venous lakes on the vermilion border of the lip), healing often occurs without scarring or pigmentary changes. Venous malformations on nonmucosal skin are more likely to be left with some textural or pigmentary change after treatment with these lasers. Treatment of venous lesions with the pulsed dye laser is often unsuccessful, and recurrences are common.

Cutaneous lymphangiomas benefit most from CO_2 vaporization. This treatment is often effective in controlling lymphorrhea, but recurrences are common if an underlying lymphangioma, with its deeper subcutaneous involvement, is present. In this event, vaporization with the CO_2 laser is not indicated. The subcutaneous aspect of a lymphangioma may sometimes respond to the deeper injury produced by the Nd:YAG laser.[41]

Unlike the low-flow vascular lesions just described, high-flow vascular lesions, which include arterial and arteriovenous malformations, do not respond to laser therapy, because they supply a continuous source of blood within the dermal papillary vessels and this prevents these lasers from having any permanent effect on the vessels. However, pretreatment of the underlying deep component of high-flow lesions by surgical means or by embolization may subsequently allow for laser treatment of the cutaneous component of the lesion to be performed.[42]

References

1. Mulliken JB, Young AE. Vascular birthmarks: hemangiomas and malformations. Philadelphia: Saunders, 1988:77–82.
2. Garden JM, Tan OT, Kerschmann R et al. Effect of dye laser pulse duration on selective cutaneous vascular injury radiation. J Invest Dermatol 1986;87:653–657.
3. Cosman B. Experience in the argon laser therapy of port-wine stains. Plast Reconstr Surg 1980;65:119–129.
4. Finley JL, Barsky SH, Geer DE et al. Healing of port-wine stains after argon laser therapy. Arch Dermatol 1981;117:486–489.

5. Noe JM, Barsky SH, Geer DE, Rosen S. Port-wine stains and the response to argon laser therapy: successful treatment and predictive role of color, age, and biopsy. Plast Reconstr Surg 1980;65:130–136.
6. Silver L. Argon laser photocoagulation of port-wine stain hemangiomas. Lasers Surg Med 1986;6:24–28.
7. Scheibner A, Wheeland RG. Argon-pumped tunable dye laser therapy for facial port-wine stain hemangiomas in adults—a new technique using small spot size and minimal power. J Dermatol Surg Oncol 1989;15:277–289.
8. McDaniel D, Mordon S. Hexascan: a new robotic scanning laser handpiece. Cutis 1990;45:300–305.
9. Tan O, Stafford TJ, Murray S, Kurban AK. Histologic comparison of the pulsed dye laser and copper vapour laser effects on pig skin. Lasers Surg Med 1990;10:551–558.
10. Walker E, Butler P, Pickering JW, Day WA, Fraser R, van Halewyn CN. Histology of port-wine stains after copper vapor laser treatment. Br J Dermatol 1989;121:217–223.
11. Neumann RA, Knobler RM, Leonhartsberger H, Gebhart W. Comparative histochemistry of port-wine stains after copper vapor laser (578 nm) and argon laser treatment. J Invest Dermatol 1992;99:160–167.
12. Tan OT, Sherwood K, Gilchrest BA. Treatment of children with port-wine stains using the flashlamp-pumped pulsed tunable dye laser. N Engl J Med 1989;320:416–421.
13. Reyes B, Geronemus R. Treatment of port-wine stains during childhood with the flashlamp-pumped pulsed dye laser. J Am Acad Dermatol 1990;23:1142–1148.
14. Ashinoff R, Geronemus R. Flashlamp-pumped pulsed dye laser for port-wine stains in infancy: early vs. later treatment. J Am Acad Dermatol 1991;24:467–472.
15. Garden JM, Polla LL, Tan OT. The treatment of port-wine stains by the pulsed dye laser: analysis of pulse duration and long-term therapy. Arch Dermatol 1988;124:889–896.
16. Anderson RR, Parrish JA. Selective photothermolysis: precise microsurgery by selective absorption of pulse irradiation. Science 1983;220:524–527.
17. Holy A, Geronemus R. Treatment of peri-orbital portwine stains utilizing the flashlamp-pumped pulsed dye laser. Arch Ophthalmol 1992;110:793–797.
18. Renfro L, Geronemus R. Anatomical differences of port-wine stains in response to treatment with the pulsed dye laser. Arch Dermatol 1993;129:182–188.
19. Ashinoff R, Geronemus RG. Treatment of a port-wine stain in a black patient utilizing the pulsed dye laser. J Dermatol Surg Oncol (in press).
20. Levine V, Geronemus G. Adverse effects associated with the 577/585 nanometer pulsed dye laser in the treatment of cutaneous vascular lesions: a study of 500 patient (in press).
21. Ratz JL. Current concepts in carbon dioxide laser therapy of port-wine stains. Lasers Surg Med 1983;3:335.
22. Van Gamert M, Welch A, Tan OT, Parrish JA. Limitations of carbon dioxide lasers for treatment of port-wine stains. Arch Dermatol 1987;123:71–73.
23. Lanigan SW, Cotterill JA. The treatment of port-wine stains with the carbon dioxide laser. Br J Dermatol 1990;123:229–231.

24. Lanndthaler M, Haina D, Brunner R et al. Neodymium YAG laser therapy of vascular lesions. J Am Acad Dermatol 1986;14:107.

25. Goldman MD, Martin DE, Fitzpatrick RE, Ruiz-Esparza J. Pulse dye laser treatment of telangiectasia with and without subtherapeutic sclerotherapy. J Acad Dermatol 1990;23:23–30.

26. Goldman M, Fitzpatrick R. Sclerotherapy and laser therapy of leg telangiectasia. J Dermatol Surg Oncol 1990;16:338–344.

27. Geronemus RG. Treatment of spider telangiectases in children using the flashlamp-pumped pulsed dye laser. Pediatr Dermatol 1991;8:61–63.

28. Achauer BN, VanderKam VM. Argon laser treatment of telangiectasia of the face and neck: 5 years' experience. Lasers Surg Med 1987;7:495–498.

29. Noe JM, Finley J, Rosen S, Arndt KA. Post-rhinoplasty "red nose": differential diagnosis and treatment by laser. Plast Reconstr Surg 1988;67:661–664.

30. Geronemus RG. Poikiloderma of Civatte. Arch Dermatol 1990;126:547–548.

31. Ashinoff R, Geronemus RG. Capillary hemangiomas and treatment with the flashlamp-pumped dye laser. Arch Dermatol 1990;22:136–137.

32. Achauer BM, VanderKam VM. Capillary hemangioma (strawberry mark) of infancy: comparison of argon and Nd:YAG laser treatment. Plast Reconstr Surg 1989;84:60–69.

33. Sherwood KA, Tan OT. The treatment of capillary hemangioma with the flashlamp-pumped dye laser. J Am Acad Dermatol 1990;22:136–137.

34. Garden JM, Bakus AD, Paller AS. Treatment of cutaneous hemangiomas by the flashlamp-pumped pulsed dye laser: prospective analysis. J Pediatr 1992;120:550–560.

35. Morelli J, Tan OT, West WL. Treatment of ulcerated hemangiomas with the pulsed tunable dye laser. Am J Dis Child 1991;145:1062–1064.

36. Apfelberg DB, Maser MR, Lash H, Rivers J. The argon laser for cutaneous lesions. JAMA 1981;245:2073–2075.

37. Apfelberg DB, Maser MR, Lash H, Flores J. Expanded role of the argon laser in plastic surgery. J Dermatol Surg Oncol 1983;9:145–151.

38. Apfelberg DB, Druker D, Maser MR et al. Granuloma faciale treatment with the argon laser. Arch Dermatol 1983;119:573.

39. Arndt KA. Adenoma sebaceum: successful treatment with the argon laser. Plast Reconstr Surg 1982;70:91–93.

40. Wheeland RG, Bailin PL, Norris MG. Argon laser photocoagulative therapy of Kaposi's sarcoma: a clinical and histological evaluation. J Dermatol Surg Oncol 1985;11:1180–1184.

41. Dixon JA, Davis BK, Gilbertson J. Laser photocoagulation of malformations of the tongue. Laryngoscope 1986;96:537–541.

42. Fitzpatrick RE, Lowe NJ, Goldman MP et al. Flashlamp-pumped pulsed dye laser treatment of port wine stains. J Dermatol Surg Oncol 1994;20:743–748.

43. Levins P. In: Bungdorf WHC, Katz SA, eds: Dermatology: progress and perspectives. The proceedings of the 18th World Congress in Dermatology. London:Parthenon, 1992.

44. Goldman MP, Fitzpatrick RE, Ruiz-Esparza J. Treatment of port wine stains (capillary malformation) with the flashlamp-pumped pulsed dye laser. J Pediatr 1993;122:71–77.

9 ___ Lasers for the Treatment of Cutaneous Pigmented Disorders

Jeffrey S. Dover
Kay S. Kane

Melanin's broad absorption spectrum (250–1200 nm) makes it a good target for laser light.[1] Virtually any laser that produces ultraviolet, visible, or infrared light can remove unwanted cutaneous pigment to some degree. Even laser light, which is not preferentially absorbed by melanin, can eradicate cutaneous pigment. For example, a CO_2 laser can remove epidermal pigment by simply coagulating the epidermis. In general, epidermal pigment is easier to eradicate than dermal pigment because of its proximity to the skin's surface. The goal in the treatment of epidermal lesions is to remove the unwanted epidermal pigmentation but retain the constitutive pigment. It is more difficult to modify dermal pigmentation, because of its depth in the skin, without causing scarring, vascular injury, hypopigmentation, or hyperpigmentation.

Classification of Pigmented Lesions

From the standpoint of laser therapy, it is convenient to classify cutaneous pigmented lesions into three categories: benign non-nevocellular pigmented lesions, nevocellular processes, and exogenous dermal pigment (tattoos).

Benign cutaneous pigment may be limited to the epidermis or the dermis, or it may be in both locations. Epidermal hyperpigmentation is due either to the presence of an increased number of melanosomes or to an increased rate of melanogenesis. Common epidermal non-nevocellular pigmented lesions include lentigines, ephelides (freckles), café au lait macules, and Becker's nevi. Dermal hyperpigmentation is caused by excess melanin deposition in the dermis. This can result from disruption of the basement membrane, which allows epidermal pigment to drop down into the dermis, where it is retained by macrophages, or it can be due to excess melanin production by the dermal melanocytes. Melasma may be epidermal, dermal, or both, and is caused by an increased amount of melanin in these locations.

Table 9-1.   Pigments used in tattoos

Color	Pigment
Black	Carbon
	Iron oxide
	Logwood
Blue	Cobalt
	Cobaltous aluminate
Green	Chrome oxide
	Hydrous chromium oxide
	Malachite
	Lead chromate
	Ferro-ferri cyanide
	Curcuma
	Phthalocyanine dyes
Red	Mercury sulfide
	Cadmium
	Sienna

Source: Modified from Fisher AA. Dermatitis and discolorations from metals. In: Contact Dermatitis. Philadelphia: Lea & Febiger, 1980:92–93.

Nevocellular processes are classified by the location of the aberrant nevus cells. Nevus cells can be located in the epidermis, dermis, or both, and are termed *junctional, intradermal,* and *compound,* respectively. These lesions may be acquired or congenital; the junctional ones typically appear during the first 40 to 50 years of life and are harmless, the intradermal variety are, by definition, present at birth, and melanomas develop later in approximately 5% of people with smaller congenital nevi and in 6.3% of people with larger congenital nevi.[2,3]

Decorative or accidental (e.g., dirt, carbon, asphalt) tattoos are an exogenously induced form of dermal pigmentation consisting of inks or organometallic dyes which permanently reside within membrane-bound intracellular granules of dermal fibroblasts and macrophages. The amount and composition of the tattoo pigments vary greatly and are sometimes completely unknown (Table 9-1).

Methods of Cutaneous Pigment Removal

The fundamental principle behind the laser removal of cutaneous pigment is the Grothus-Draper law, which states that the absorption of the laser light is necessary for any ensuing mechanical or chemical alteration to occur.[1] Absorption of laser light by cutaneous chromophores depends on the wavelength selected. Wavelengths not absorbed by melanin indiscriminately destroy pigmented as well as nonpigmented structures in the skin in a nonselective manner. However, lasers with wavelengths that are both preferentially absorbed by melanin over other cutaneous chromophores (such as oxyhemoglobin) and penetrate to the depth of the targeted pigment can be utilized to more selectively target cutaneous pigment. As seen in Figure 9-1, a selective window for melanin lies between 630 and 1100 nm, a range of wavelengths that penetrate skin well and that preferentially target melanin over oxyhemoglobin.

The second challenge is to spatially confine the thermal damage to produce selective photothermolysis. By using pulsed laser light of the appropriate duration, heat diffusion and unwanted thermal injury to the adjacent structures after absorption are minimized. By using exposure times that are less than the thermal relaxation time of pigmented particles, the targeted pigmented structures are selectively destroyed and the adjacent nonpigmented cells are spared. In the case of pigmented processes, it is not clear whether the actual laser target is the melanosome, the nevus cell, or the tattoo pigment particle, nor is it clear whether the target differs depending on the type of lesion being treated.

Pulsed lasers emitting appropriate wavelengths have a distinct theoretical advantage over continuous-wave devices, in that they are able to selectively destroy cutaneous pigment.

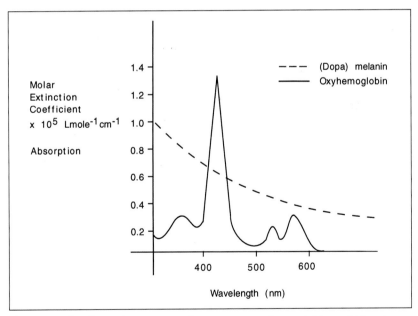

Fig. 9-1. The absorption spectra of cutaneous oxyhemoglobin and (dopa) melanin. (Modified from Dover JS, Arndt KA, Geronemus RG, Olbricht SM, Noe JM, Stern RS. Illustrated cutaneous laser surgery. Norwalk, CT: Prentice-Hall, 1990.)

The History of Laser Treatment of Cutaneous Pigment

MELANIN-BASED PIGMENTED LESIONS

In 1963 Goldman and associates[4] first experimented with a normal-mode (500-μsec pulse duration) ruby laser train of pulses at 649 nm, using it on human skin. They found that the darker the skin color, the more intense was the reaction. On the basis of this observation, they speculated that melanin selectively absorbs laser light. In ensuing studies, in which a Q-switched ruby laser (50-μsec pulse duration) was used, Goldman and colleagues[5-7] found that the exposure threshold for damage was 10 to 100 times less than that associated with the 500-μsec pulse duration and that the damage was independent of skin color, which indicated a more selective effect, perhaps at the level of the melanosome.

Two decades later, Polla[8] and Dover[9] and their co-workers demonstrated by electron microscopy that individual melanosomes are indeed the target of the thermal damage caused by the Q-switched ruby laser. Targeted melanosomes exhibited frank membrane disruption and disorganization of the internal contents (Fig. 9-2). However, the destruction of melanosomes is pulsewidth dependent, in that pulse durations of 40 and 750 nsec disrupt melanosomes, but longer pulse durations such as 400 μsec leave the melanosomes intact. This is consistent with the theory of selective photothermolysis, which states that the pulse duration should be less than the thermal relaxation time of the targeted object for selective photothermolysis to occur. A typical 1.0-μm melanosome has a thermal relaxation time of between 0.5 and 1.0 μsec, as calculated by mathematical modeling.

The mechanism behind melanosomal destruction is unknown. Plasma formation is unlikely, because the peak powers produced are too low for this to occur. Shock wave or cavitation damage, physical effects produced by thermal expansion or as the result of the extreme temperature gradients created within the melanosome, is a more likely explanation. Findings from studies of acoustic waves generated by pulsed irradiation of melanosomes and pigmented cells support this theory.[10] These have shown that melanin absorbs and localizes the high-intensity irradiation from Q-switched lasers, thereby creating a sharp temperature gradient between the melanosome and its surroundings. This gradient leads to thermal expansion and the generation and propagation of acoustic waves, which can mechanically damage the melanosome-laden cells.

During the tissue repair that occurs after laser-induced melanosomal disruption, there is first transient cutaneous depigmentation, followed by repigmentation weeks later.[11] Black guinea pig skin irradiated with 40-nsec Q-switched ruby pulses at radiant exposures of 0.4 J/cm^2 or greater whitens immediately, fades in 20 minutes, depigments 7 to 10 days later, and then repigments 4 to 8 weeks after treatment. After cutaneous repigmentation, guinea pig skin displays persistent leukotrichia, which can last for up to 4 months after laser irradiation (Fig. 9-3). Guinea pig skin exposed to radiant exposures less than that of threshold exposure (<0.3 J/cm²) undergoes paradoxical melanogenesis.[11] This may represent either a sublethal change in the melanosome, which causes interference with the normal feedback inhibition of melanogenesis, or postinflammatory hyperpigmentation. The therapeutic implications of this phenomenon have not been fully explored.

Histologically, melanosomal disruption and the vacuolization of pigment-laden cells in the basal layer occur immediately after laser irradiation.[11] Both keratinocytes and melanocytes exhibit a concentration of

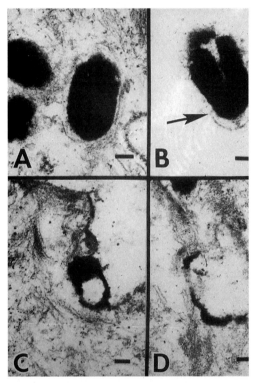

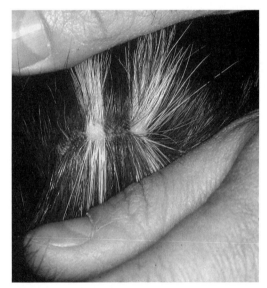

Fig. 9-2.   Electron micrograph obtained immediately after Q-switched ruby laser irradiation. The targeted melanosome shows membrane disruption with disorganization of its internal contents (A) prior to irradiation; (B) immediately after irradiation showing early melanosome disruption; (C) more disruption; (D) almost complete disruption of a melanosome immediately after irradiation.

Fig. 9-3.   Black guinea pig skin irradiated with the Q-switched ruby laser, showing immediate, transient hypopigmentation, followed by delayed cutaneous depigmentation 7 to 10 days after treatment. Despite cutaneous repigmentation, the guinea pig displays persistent leukotrichia up to 4 months after treatment. See Fig. 9-3 in color section.

(Fig 9-2 is reprinted by permission of Elsevier Science Publishing Co., Inc., from Melanosomes are a primary target of Q-switched ruby laser irradiation in guinea pig skin, by Polla LL, Margolis R, Dover JS et al. THE JOURNAL OF INVESTIGATIVE DERMATOLOGY, 89;281–286. Copyright 1987 by The Society of Investigative Dermatology, Inc.)

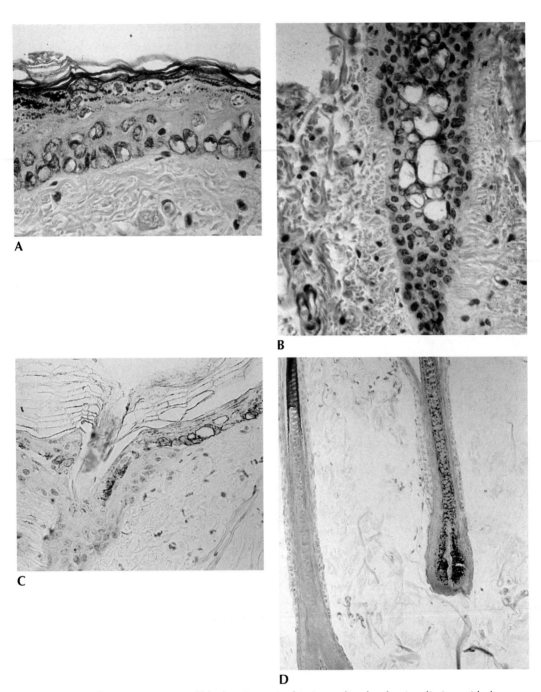

Fig. 9-4. Histologic appearance of black guinea pig skin immediately after irradiation with the Q-switched ruby laser. (A) Characteristic "ring cell" formation in the basal lamina, representing melanocytes and keratinocytes with condensed nuclear and pigment material at their peripheries. (B) Similar changes in a hair follicle. (C) Epidermal changes demonstrated by Fontana-Masson stain. (D) Three months later neighboring irradiated hair shows total irradiation of melanin pigmentation without any structural changes. There is no pigmentary change in the unirradiated hair. See Fig. 9-4 A to C in color section.

pigment and nuclear material at the periphery of the cell, giving them a characteristic "ring cell" appearance (Fig. 9-4). Epidermal necrosis and regeneration of a pigmented epidermis occur over the next 7 days.

Studies of human skin, like studies in guinea pigs, have revealed that the Q-switched ruby laser targets melanosomes, after which the killed pigmented cells are sloughed.[12] This causes transient hypopigmentation, followed by gradual repigmentation back to the patient's normal constitutive color. Other short-pulsed, high-fluence lasers produce similar clinical and histologic changes in human skin.

The ability of pulsed lasers of different wavelengths to disrupt cutaneous pigment has been the subject of three action spectrum studies. Anderson and associates[13] used a Q-switched Nd:YAG laser with a pulse duration of 10 to 12 nsec at three wavelengths (355, 532, and 1064 nm) and tested it on guinea pig skin. They found that the threshold exposures necessary to produce immediate skin whitening (signifying a laser-induced change in the melanosomes) required energy fluences of 0.11, 0.20, and 1.0 J/cm^2 at 355, 532, and 1064 nm, respectively. These results showed that the threshold exposure dose is wavelength dependent and that longer wavelengths (which are less well absorbed by melanin) require higher energy fluences. Electron micrographs revealed that the melanosomes within keratinocytes and melanocytes are disrupted at each wavelength. Histologically the basal cells had the characteristic ring cell appearance secondary to vacuolization and the peripheral concentration of the cellular pigment. It was also found that delayed epidermal depigmentation occurs in the area of the transient immediate whitening, and this is followed by repigmentation back to the constitutive skin color.

In a second action spectrum study, in which a flashlamp-pulsed tunable laser[14] with a pulse duration of 750 nsec was used, the relationship between the wavelength and the whitening threshold was also demonstrated. The threshold fluences at 435, 488, 532, and 560 nm, were found to be 0.44, 0.62, 0.76, and 0.86 J/cm^2, respectively.

In the action spectrum study of guinea pig skin performed by Sherwood and colleagues,[15] a flashlamp-pulsed tunable laser with a pulse duration of 300 nsec at five different wavelengths (504, 590, 684, 720, and 750 nm) was used. These investigators found that the 504-nm wavelength produced the most pigment specific injury, whereas the longer wavelengths caused disruption of the basement membrane with pigmentary incontinence.

TATTOOS

Goldman and associates[4-6] first experimented with lasers and tattoo removal in 1964, but despite their reported success at the time, the method was abandoned until very recently. Clinical research performed in Scotland in the 1980s by Reid and colleagues[16,17] revealed that the Q-switched ruby laser effectively removes both amateur and professional blue-black tattoos without subsequent cutaneous textural change or scarring. Amateur tattoos were found to clear after an average of four to six treatments, whereas professional tattoos required one to three more treatment sessions. The first large U.S. clinical trials in which the Q-switched ruby laser was used to remove amateur and professional tattoos yielded similar results.[18]

Immediately after Q-switched ruby laser exposure, a gray-white circle appears in the treated site, which is more marked in the tattooed areas than in the adjacent normal skin. It is thought to result from the rapid localization of heat-formed steam or gas around pigment particles. A sloughing crust forms over the entire tattoo during the ensuing 2 weeks. Occasionally, tattoo pigment is seen within this crust. After several treatments, there is marked lightening of the tattoo and transient hypopigmentation, but little if any textural change.

Before treatment, tattoo pigment is located within membrane-bound intracellular granules in perivascular fibroblasts, macrophages, and mast cells.[18] After treatment with the Q-switched ruby laser, the usual melanosome-targeted injury to melanocytes and keratinocytes is evident. In addition, there is cellular debris adjacent to altered tattoo pigment particles. A brief neutrophilic response follows, and by day 11 after treatment, all the altered pigment particles are repackaged within the same types of perivascular cells. In the original dose-response study, despite the presence of residual tattoo pigment, 80% of amateur tattoos were found to clear clinically after four to six treatments and 65% of professional tattoos were found to lighten significantly after six to eight treatments.[19]

The mechanism by which the ruby laser removes dermal tattoo pigment without adverse effects is unknown. It is known that the unwanted tattoo pigment is substantially eliminated externally by means of the scale crust as well as by systemic elimination through the rephagocytosis of the altered pigment particles. However, histologic studies of treated tattoos show the presence of considerable residual tattoo pigment. It may be that, after absorption of the laser energy, temperatures sufficiently high to lead to pyrolytic chemical alteration and fragmentation of the pigment particle are attained.[18] This fragmentation may allow some of the pigment particles to be eliminated systemically, with only the lamellated pigment particles remaining. Despite their persistence in the skin, lamellated pigment particles are not as optically apparent as their precursors. Fibrosis that obscures the pigment from view is not a tenable explanation,[18] because biopsy specimens obtained 150 days after treatment have not been found to show any fibrotic changes.

Clinical Results

NONSELECTIVE LASER TECHNIQUES

CO_2 Laser

The CO_2 laser is a continuous-wavelength source that emits infrared light at a wavelength of 10,600 nm, which is completely absorbed by water. Low fluences (<5 J/cm^2 at exposure times of 0.1 second) limit the thermal damage to the epidermis.[20] The thermal damage that does occur in the epidermis occurs in the basal cell layer and consists of vacuolization and the spindling of melanocytes and keratinocytes. This is followed by epidermal necrosis 24 hours later and then dermal-epidermal separation. There is very little superficial thermal damage to the dermis. Sloughing of the damaged epidermis is followed by reepithelialization during the ensuing week, but despite histologic evidence of pigment incontinence (i.e., epidermal pigment-laden macrophages in the dermis), there is no postinflammatory hyperpigmentation. Lentigines have been effectively treated using low fluences. Of 146 solar lentigines so treated, 10% cleared completely and two thirds lightened considerably.[20] However, in a trial comparing low-fluence CO_2 laser treatment with cryotherapy in the elimination of lentigines, liquid nitrogen treatment was found to be four times more likely to achieve lightening of the lentigines than low-fluence CO_2 laser treatment was.[21] Other advantages of cryotherapy are that it is much less expensive and it is quicker and simpler to perform than the laser treatment.

SELECTIVE LASER TECHNIQUES

Continuous-Wave Lasers

The argon laser (488 and 514 nm) and the continuous wave dye laser (577/585 nm) are continuous-wave sources, and the pulse train copper vapor laser (578 nm) is a quasi-continuous-wave laser. All of these lasers have been used to treat cutaneous pigment. However, each emits a wavelength that is well absorbed by melanin but is also absorbed by oxyhemoglobin, so unwanted vessel damage may occur during the treatment of cutaneous pigment. Additionally, if these lasers are used in a freehand mode, the results are not always consistent and the thermal damage is somewhat unpredictable. Robotized scanning devices that can provide uniform energy fluences and ensure rapid and consistent treatments therefore have been devised in an effort to circumvent this problem. The preliminary results from the treatment of café au lait macules and lentigines using these devices are encouraging (Dover JS, Arndt KA, unpublished observations). However, although most epidermal and superficial dermal pigmented lesions lighten or disappear after one or two treatments using a robotized 514-nm argon laser, deeper dermal lesions such as the nevus of Ota may be totally unresponsive.[22]

Q-Switched Ruby Laser

The Q-switched ruby laser is made with a ruby (aluminum oxide) crystal, which has been grown in the presence of chromium so that the crystal lattice forms with the chromium impurity within it. The crystal is surrounded by a helical flashlamp, and the laser naturally produces a train of nonuniform pulses. In the Q-switched mode, very high peak powers can be attained by allowing laser energy to build up in the cavity before discharge. The result is the emission of light at a wavelength of 694 nm, with 28- to 40-nsec pulses generating over 1×10^8 W/cm^2 per pulse.

Ruby laser light penetrates about 1 mm into the skin and is extremely well absorbed by melanin and blue-black tattoo pigment. This deep penetration is clinically advantageous because it can reach pigment-laden cells both in the epidermis and deep in the dermis. Additionally, at a wavelength of 694 nm, the ruby light is minimally absorbed by hemoglobin; it therefore falls within the previously defined therapeutic window for treating pigmented structures but spares vascular structures.

Benign Pigmented Lesions

Epidermal Pigmented Lesions

Most lentigines and ephelides clear after one to four treatments with the Q-switched ruby laser. Taylor and co-workers[23] reported on 29 patients with lentigines that totally cleared after only one treatment. Similar results have been obtained in the treatment of the labial macules of Peutz-Jeghers syndrome.[24] Trials comparing the treatment of lentigines with the Q-switched ruby laser versus the gold standard of therapy, liquid nitrogen cryotherapy, have not been performed. Café au lait macules[22a] (Figs. 9-5 and 9-6), nevus spilus, and Becker's nevi also respond less favorably to treatment with this laser. Ashinoff and

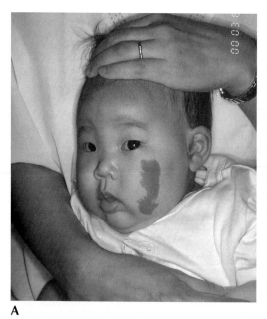 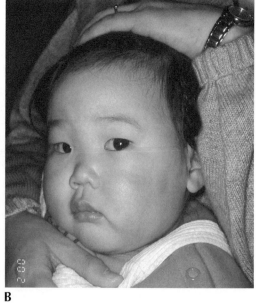

A   **B**

Fig. 9-5. Café au lait macule in an infant before (A) and after (B) five treatments over 8 months with the Q-switched ruby laser. See Fig. 9-5 in color section. (Courtesy Tadashi Tezuka, MD, PhD.)

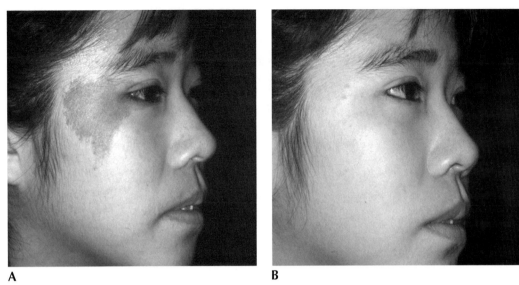

A   **B**

Fig. 9-6.   Café au lait macule on the right temple of a young woman before (A) and after (B) four treatments over 3 months with the 510-nm pulsed dye laser. (Courtesy Tadashi Tezuka, MD, PhD.)

associates[25] treated 15 patients with café au lait macules and found that significant lightening occurred after an average of six treatments. However, café au lait macules, the café au lait background of nevus spilus, and Becker's nevi (Grevelink, verbal communication, 1992) are frequently seen to recur after treatment.[25a]

Dermal Pigmented Lesions
The ruby laser has become a treatment of choice for dermal pigmented lesions such as the nevus of Ito and nevus of Ota (Fig. 9-7). The long wavelength emitted by this laser successfully targets the deep, aberrant dermal melanocytes and destroys them so that histologically there are actually fewer of them after treatment.[26] Geronemus and Ashinoff[27] treated 15 patients with nevus of Ota up to seven times with the Q-switched ruby laser and noted complete clearing in four patients, with significant lightening in the others; only one patient experienced transient hyperpigmentation. Taylor and colleagues[23] treated nine patients with nevus of Ota and noted that hyperpigmentation was a frequent side effect. Monoclonal antibody staining showed this to represent a postinflammatory change rather than to result from the presence of melanin within nevomelanocytes. However, the final results were excellent and the hyperpigmentation was usually temporary. The largest study of the treatment of nevus of Ota using the ruby laser was performed by Watanabe and Takahashi[28] and included over 100 Japanese patients. The degree of lightening was found to be directly proportional to the number of treatments performed. The lesion cleared totally in patients who had at least four treatments. There was little postinflammatory hyperpigmentation, and textural changes developed in no patients. Suzuki[28a]

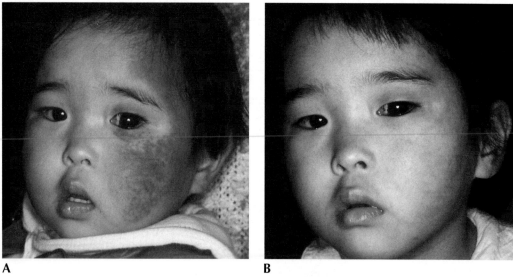

A   **B**

Fig. 9-7.   Nevus of Ota on the left side of the face in an infant before (A) and after (B) 16 treatments over 17 months with the Q-switched ruby laser. (Courtesy Tadashi Tezuka, MD, PhD.)

has demonstrated similar results using the Q-switched Nd:YAG laser. Results of normal mode pulse from ruby laser in the treatment of congenital nevi are encouraging (Fitzpatrick RE, unpublished observation).

Early studies of the treatment of congenital nevi with the Q-switched ruby laser demonstrated that the pigmentation can be reduced significantly after repeated treatments but that it recurs to a significant degree in 90% of those showing good lightening (Fig. 9-8).[29]

Mixed Epidermal and Dermal Lesions
Mixed epidermal and dermal lesions such as postinflammatory hyperpigmentation and melasma respond variably and unpredictably to Q-switched ruby laser treatments.[30] Flat and slightly raised blue nevi are also responsive.[31]

Tattoos
The Q-switched ruby laser is highly effective for the removal of amateur tattoos, moderately effective for the removal of black professional tattoos, and less effective for the removal of brightly colored professional tattoos. In the first North American study[19] to evaluate the treatment of tattoos with the Q-switched ruby laser, 35 amateur tattoos and 22 professional tattoos were treated with a 40-nsec pulsewidth at a fluence of 1.5 to 8 J/cm[2] at a mean interval of 3 weeks. Substantial lightening or total clearing occurred in 78% of the amateur tattoos and 23% of the professional tattoos. Further studies[32] demonstrated even better results using the newer 25-nsec Q-switched ruby laser. However, it has been found that amateur tattoos respond more favorably in fewer treatments (85% are completely removed in

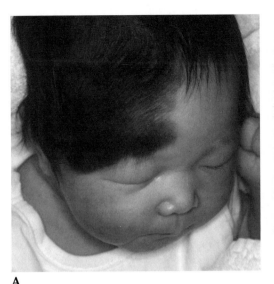
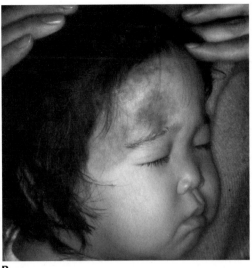

A   B

Fig. 9-8. Congenital nevus involving the right scalp and forehead in an infant before (A) and after (B) 20 treatments over 15 months with the Q-switched ruby laser. (Courtesy Tadashi Tezuka, MD, PhD.)

an average of three treatments[32]) than professional tattoos do (10% are completely removed, 70% are partially removed, and 20% are minimally improved after an average of six treatments[32]). Dark blue and black tattoos respond best. Green tattoos respond variably, with 65% of such tattoos clearing after six to eight treatments.[33] Red tattoos are problematic, because the laser is a red light source and not well absorbed by the pigment particles.[34] Yellow tattoos do not respond because the spectral absorbance of yellow pigment drops dramatically in this range.[33]

Three studies have been performed that compare the efficacy of the Q-switched ruby laser in tattoo removal with that of the other pulsed lasers, specifically the Q-switched Ng:YAG laser and the Q-switched alexandrite laser. Levine and Geronemus[34] compared the Q-switched ruby laser (694-nm wavelength, 25-nsec pulse duration, fluence of 8–10 J/cm^2) with the Q-switched Nd:YAG laser (1064-nm wavelength, 25-nsec pulse duration, fluence of 10–14 J/cm^2) by treating one half of each of 48 tattoos (39 professional, 9 amateur) with one laser and the other half with the other laser. They found that, after one treatment, the Q-switched ruby laser produced more lightening in 18 of the black tattoos and the Q-switched Nd:YAG caused more lightening in 4 of the tattoos; the result was the same in 17 of the tattoos.

McMeekin[35] compared the Q-switched ruby laser (694 nm, 25 nsec, 6 J/cm^2) with the Q-switched alexandrite laser (694 nm, 100 nsec, 6 J/cm^2) in the treatment of 10 black amateur tattoos and found that the Q-switched ruby laser produced better clearing in all of the tattoos.

Zelickson[36] performed a study comparing the three lasers—the Q-switched ruby laser (694 nm), the Q-switched Nd:YAG laser (532 and 1064 nm), and the Q-switched alexandrite laser (755 nm)—in which he injected 14 commonly used tattoo pigments into guinea pig skin and then compared the amount of lightening produced by each. He found that the Q-switched ruby laser was the most efficacious in removing blue-black tattoos, the Q-switched alexandrite laser worked best for blue and green tattoos, and the frequency-doubled Q-switched Nd:YAG laser was useful for removing red tattoos.

Side Effects

In a series of 410 tattoos,[37] hypopigmentation (typically transient) occurred in 184 treated with the Q-switched ruby laser, six treated with the Q-switched ruby and Nd:YAG lasers, and only one treated with the Q-switched Nd:YAG laser. In another series of 212 tattoos,[38] textural changes occurred in 6% of the patients and transient hyperpigmentation in 5%, typically in those with darker skin. Scarring is uncommon (<5% of patients) and appears to occur more often in patients with professional tattoos than in those with amateur tattoos. Incomplete tattoo removal, seen in 20% to 40% of patients, occurs more frequently. Colored tattoos are more refractory to treatment than blue-black tattoos, and professional tattoos are more difficult to remove than amateur ones.

Cosmetic tattoos, which are flesh-colored, white, pink, or varying shades of brown, frequently blacken after laser treatment. Repeated Q-switched ruby laser treatments have occasionally been successful in eradicating these blackened skin-tone tattoos, but surgical excision has been required as a last resort.[38a] This blackening is due to the high temperatures produced by the lasers, which reduce Fe_2O_3 to FeO, which is black and can be produced by any pulsed laser with a pulse duration of 1 nsec or shorter.[38b]

Q-Switched Nd:YAG Laser

The Q-switched Nd:YAG laser is a solid-state, high-fluence, short-pulsed (10–20 nsec) laser that emits at a wavelength of 1064 nm. By placing a doubling crystal in the laser beam's path, the resultant frequency doubling halves the wavelength to 532 nm, which gives the clinician greater flexibility with one laser.

Because melanin, hemoglobin, and water do not absorb the 1064-nm wavelength well, this wavelength is not ideal for the treatment of benign pigmented lesions. The 1064-nm wavelength penetrates deeply (up to 4–6 nm), and although its absorption by tattoo pigment is poor, it is sufficiently preferentially targeted to produce selective damage.[39]

The 532-nm wavelength is well absorbed by melanin and hemoglobin, making it theoretically useful in the treatment of both vascular and pigmented lesions. The inability to selectively target only one of these chromophores, however, limits its utility.

Benign Pigmented Lesions

Epidermal lesions such as lentigines and café au lait macules can be lightened considerably by the frequency-doubled Q-switched Nd:YAG laser.[39a] Eighty-four percent of 17 lentigines were observed to lighten by at least 50% after several treatments using the Q-switched Nd:YAG laser (532 nm, 2–5 J/cm²).[40] Postoperative purpura developed in all patients secondary to vascular injury, and transient hyperpigmentation developed in 25% of the patients.

The Q-switched Nd:YAG laser at 1064 nm is very useful for removing deep dermal pigment, such as occurs in the nevus of Ito and nevus of Ota.[28a,41] Mixed epidermal-dermal lesions are, as they are in response to treatment with the Q-switched ruby laser, often refractory to treatment, recur after early clearing, or worsen with treatment, although no results of studies have been published as yet.[41] The pigmentation of congenital nevi can be diminished using the Q-switched Nd:YAG laser, but recurrence rates approach 100% (Burns AJ, Dover JS, verbal communication, 1995).

The degree of response to laser treatment at either wavelength is proportional to the amount of pigment at the treatment site.[41] Whitening occurs when small spot sizes (1–3 mm) and high impact powers are used. This is followed by pinpoint bleeding, resulting in the formation of a hemorrhagic crust, which then falls off 7 to 10 days later. Unlike treatment with the Q-switched ruby laser,[41] there is no transient hypopigmentation. The 532-nm wavelength causes more whitening, delayed purpura, and hemorrhage with slight crusting. In comparison, the 1064-nm wavelength causes less whitening and purpura but significant hemorrhage in proportion to the amount of tattoo pigment targeted.

Histologically, the effects of the 1064-nm wavelength are identical to those produced by the Q-switched ruby laser.[13] Ring cells described earlier are detected in the epidermal basal cell layer. Unlike the effects of the Q-switched ruby laser, however, the Q-switched laser has been noted to produce the coagulation of erythrocytes within superficial cutaneous vessels.[13]

Tattoos

The Q-switched Nd:YAG laser at 1064 nm clears most amateur blue-black tattoos, with the greatest response occurring after the first treatment (Fig. 9-9).[42] Previously untreated amateur blue-black tattoos fade by 50% after the first treatment and are 95% cleared by the fourth treatment.[38] Twenty-eight patients with blue-black tattoos resistant to treatment with an experimental Q-switched ruby laser using a long pulse duration (approximately 40 nsec) showed 30% lightening of their tattoos after the first treatment with the Q-switched Nd:YAG, and 85% of them showed clearing by the fourth treatment.[43]

In comparative studies, the Q-switched Nd:YAG laser was found to be more effective than the Q-switched ruby laser,[36] and the alexandrite laser.[44] The 1064-nm wavelength of the Q-switched Nd:YAG laser penetrates more deeply and is less absorbed by melanin than the

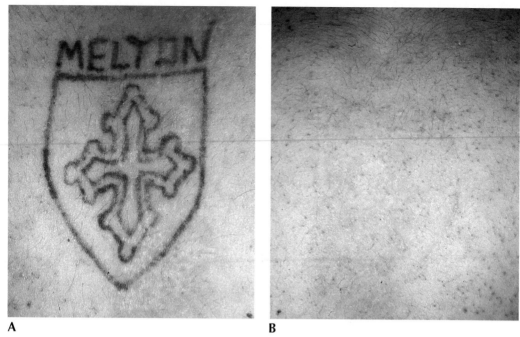

A   **B**

Fig. 9-9. (A) Amateur blue-black tattoo before treatment with the Q-switched Nd:YAG laser. (B) The tattoo has completely cleared after five laser treatments.

694-nm wavelength of the Q-switched ruby laser, making it more efficacious in removing black tattoos.[45] Kaufman and colleagues[44] compared the Q-switched Nd:YAG laser (1064 nm) with the Q-switched alexandrite laser (720 nm) in the treatment of 50 tattoos and saw better initial as well as long-term clearing in response to treatments with the Q-switched Nd:YAG laser.

The 1064-nm wavelength is not highly effective in the clearing of brightly colored tattoos, in that yellow, green, and red tattoos clear less than 25%, even after four treatments.[46] At a wavelength of 532 nm, the frequency-doubled Q-switched Nd:YAG laser is the treatment of choice for red tattoos, which clear up to 75% of the time within three treatments (Fig. 9-10).[46]

Side Effects

Side effects of treatment with the Q-switched Nd:YAG laser at a wavelength of 1064 nm include textural changes (more frequently than occur with Q-switched ruby laser treatment) and hypopigmentation (less frequently than occur with Q-switched ruby laser treatment).[47] In the Massachusetts General Hospital experience, 23% of 410 tattoos treated with the Q-switched ruby, Nd:YAG laser, or both, showed textural changes (more frequently in the Nd:YAG laser–treated tattoos) and 16% exhibited transient hyperpigmentation (again a more frequent side effect of treatment with the Nd:YAG laser).[37]

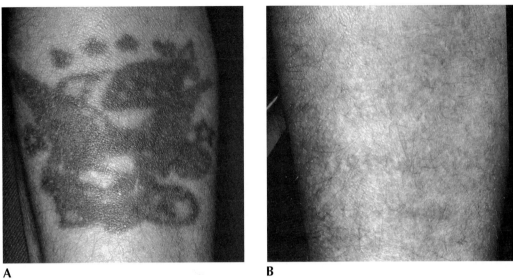

Fig. 9-10.   (A) Professional multicolored tattoo before treatment with the Q-switched Nd:YAG laser. (B) Almost total clearing after six treatments with the Nd:YAG laser, with no textural but slight pigmentary change.

510-nm Pulsed Dye Laser

The pulsed dye laser used for the treatment of pigmented lesions emits at a wavelength of 510 nm (green) with a pulse duration of 300 nsec and was developed on the basis of the findings from Sherwood and associates,[15] action spectrum study, which showed that the 504-nm wavelength produced the most epidermis-specific damage.

Benign Pigmented Lesions

Pulsed dye laser treatments of pigmented lesions result in excellent clearing of epidermal pigmented lesions, such as lentigines, ephelides, seborrheic keratoses, and café au lait macules. In a study of 65 patients (29 patients with lentigines, 16 patients with café au lait macules, 10 with seborrheic keratoses, 10 with postinflammatory hyperpigmentation) with a total of 492 lesions, 50% of the lesions cleared completely after one treatment (2–3.5 J/cm²) and another 33% lightened considerably.[48] Ninety percent of these lesions cleared after three treatments.[49] However, the outcomes of treatment may depend on the anatomic location of the pigmented lesion. One study showed 88% to 89% successful clearing of lentigines on the face and hands, with less favorable outcomes for lesions located on the trunk or legs.[50] Laser treatment causes either purpura (fades in 5 to 7 days) or whitening (fades in 2 to 4 days), followed by darkening of the epidermal lesion and sloughing at 7 to 14 days.[51] The underlying new skin is pink for 2 to 3 days but fades to a normal skin color with no textural changes or scarring. Twenty-five patients with solar lentigines showed an excellent response after one to two treatments.[52] Fourteen patients with café au lait macules showed complete clearing after three to six treatments.[53] Two patients with nevus spilus and two patients with Becker's nevi showed clearing after up to six treatments.[52] Postinflammatory hyperpigmentation of the epidermis has been eradicated by the pulsed dye laser, but other dermal or combined epidermal and dermal pigmented lesions have not responded to such treatment. Epidermal pigmented lesions treated with the pulsed dye laser have been noted to recur 50% of the time.

Tattoos

The 510-nm wavelength of the pulsed dye laser and its shallow depth of penetration into the skin make it less than ideal for the removal of tattoos. However, like the frequency-doubled Q-switched Nd:YAG laser (532 nm), it can effectively remove brightly colored tattoos, such as red, purple, and orange.[49]

Side Effects

The major side effect of pulsed dye laser treatment is purpura, which occurs in most patients and may lead to transient hyperpigmentation as the result of hemosiderin deposition.[15] There are also reports of a more than 50% recurrence rate in patients with café au lait macules treated with the laser. However, the best results in treatment of café au lait macules have been reported with this laser.[22a]

Q-Switched Alexandrite Laser

The Q-switched alexandrite laser is a solid-state laser that emits light at 755 nm with a pulse duration of 100 nsec. The wavelength and pulse parameters are between those of the Q-switched ruby laser and those of the Q-switched Nd:YAG laser, which indicates that it should be effective in the treatment of cutaneous pigmented lesions.[53]

Benign Pigmented Lesions

Early results from the treatment of benign pigmented lesions with the alexandrite laser have shown that epidermal lesions such as lentigines and café au lait macules respond well.[49] Its use in the treatment of dermal pigmented lesions such as nevus of Ota and mixed epidermal-dermal lesions such as melasma and postinflammatory hyperpigmentation has produced results comparable to those of the ruby laser.[54]

Tattoos

Theoretically the alexandrite laser should be similar to the Q-switched ruby laser in its ability to remove tattoos, perhaps with the added advantages that its beam penetrates more deeply and is less absorbed by melanin. Experiments on tattooed pig skin[55] using the alexandrite laser demonstrated that the laser was effective in removing blue-black tattoos.

In human skin, the Q-switched alexandrite laser produces immediate grayish whitening of the skin, followed by the development of erythema and edema. In 25 tattoos (17 professional, 8 amateur) treated with the Q-switched alexandrite laser, the magnitude of the immediate reaction was found to be color dependent, with more whitening and purpura occurring in darker-colored tattoos (black > blue > green > red) than in lighter-colored tattoos (such as yellow).[56] Histologically, fragmentation of pigment granules is observed, with a marked reduction in the amount of pigment by 1 month after treatment. The Q-switched alexandrite laser is best at removing green tattoos,[57,58] but is less effective than either the Q-switched ruby laser or the Q-switched Nd:YAG laser in removing blue, black, or brightly colored tattoos.[35,36,59,60]

Side Effects

Side effects of treatment with the alexandrite laser include transient hypopigmentation, which occurs in about 50% of patients, and textural changes or scarring, which occur in less than 4% of patients.[54]

Table 9-2. Summary of effectiveness of different lasers in treatment of cutaneous pigmented lesions

| Type of laser | Benign nonnevocellular pigmented lesions | | | Tattoos | |
	Epidermal	Dermal	Mixed	Amateur	Professional
Q-switched ruby laser (694 nm)	++++	++++	+	++++	++++ (except red, yellow, and some bright colors)
Q-switched Nd:YAG laser (1064 nm)	++	++++	+	++++	++++ (except red, yellow, and green)
Q-switched Nd:YAG laser (532 nm)	++++	+ to ++	+	++++	+++ (some success with red and other bright colors)
Pigmented lesion pulsed dye laser (510 nm)	++++	++	+	+	++++ (highly successful with red)
Alexandrite laser (755 nm)	+++	+++	+	+++	+++ (except red and yellow)

+ = poor; ++ = fair; +++ = good; ++++ = excellent.

Summary

Cutaneous pigment may be eradicated either nonselectively or selectively. Nonselective lasers (CO_2 laser, 10,600 nm) emit wavelengths that are not preferentially absorbed by melanin but eradicate cutaneous pigmentation by ablation. Continuous-wave selective lasers (argon laser, 488 and 514 nm; continuous-wave dye laser, 577/585 nm, pulse-train copper vapor laser, 578 nm) emit wavelengths that are preferentially absorbed by melanin, thereby destroying pigmented cells rather than other epidermal or dermal constituents. Selective and short-pulsed, high-fluence lasers (Q-switched ruby laser, 694 nm; Q-switched Nd:YAG laser, 1064 nm and 532 nm, pigmented lesion pulsed dye laser: 510 nm, alexandrite laser: 755 nm) achieve selective photothermolysis, in that the wavelengths are preferentially absorbed by the targeted chromophore, and the short pulse durations cause thermal damage to be confined to the pigment-containing organelles. The effectiveness of these various lasers in the treatment of different cutaneous pigmented lesions is summarized in Table 9-2.

References

1. Anderson RR, Parrish JA. The optics of human skin. J Invest Dermatol 1981;77:13–19.
2. Rhodes AR, Melski JW. Small congenital nevocellular nevi and the risk of cutaneous melanoma. J Pediatr 1982;100:219–224.
3. Rhodes AR, Wood WL, Sober AJ, Mihm MC. Nonepidermal origin of malignant melanoma associated with a giant congenital nevocellular nevus. Plast Reconstr Surg 1981;67:782–790.
4. Goldman L, Blaney DJ, Kindel DJ, Richfield D, Franke EK. Pathology of the effect of the laser beam on the skin. Nature 1963;197:912–914.
5. Goldman L, Igelman JM, Richfield DF. Impact of the laser on nevi and melanomas. Arch Dermatol 1964;90:71–75.
6. Goldman L, Wilson RG, Hornby P et al. Radiation from a Q-switched ruby laser. J Invest Dermatol 1965;44:69–71.
7. Goldman L. Optical radiation hazards to the skin. In: Sliney D, Wolbarsht, eds. Safety with lasers and other optical sources: a comprehensive handbook. New York: Plenum, 1983:167–169.
8. Polla LL, Margolis RF, Dover JS et al. Melanosomes are a primary target of Q-switched ruby laser-irradiation in guinea pig skin. J Invest Dermatol 1987;89:281–286.
9. Dover JS, Polla LL, Margolis RJ et al. Pulse width dependence of pigment cell damage at 694 nm in guinea pig skin. Proc SPIE 1987;712:200–205.
10. Ara G, Anderson RR, Mandel KG, Ottesen M, Oseroff AR. Irradiation of pigmented melanoma cells with high intensity pulsed radiation generates acoustic waves and kills cells. Lasers Surg Med 1990;10:52–59.
11. Dover JS, Margolis RJ, Polla LL. Pigmented guinea pig skin irradiated with Q-switched ruby laser pulses. Arch Dermatol 1989;125:43–49.
12. Hruza GJ, Dover JS, Flotte T et al. Q-switched ruby laser irradiation of normal human skin. Arch Dermatol 1991;127:1799–1805.

13. Anderson RR, Margolis RJ, Watenabe S et al. Selective photothermolysis of cutaneous pigmentation by Q-switched Nd:YAG laser pulses at 1064, 532, and 355 nm. J Invest Dermatol 1989;92:28–32.

14. Margolis RJ, Dover JS, Polla LL et al. Visible action spectrum for melanin-specific selective photothermolysis. Lasers Surg Med 1989;9:389–397.

15. Sherwood KA, Murray S, Kurban AK, Tan OT. Effect of wavelength on cutaneous pigment using pulsed irradiation. J Invest Dermatol 1989; 92:717–720.

16. Reid WH, McLeod PJ, Ritchie A, Ferguson-Pell M. Q-switched ruby laser treatment of black tattoos. Br J Plast Surg 1983;36:455–463.

17. Reid WH, Miller ID, Murphy MJ et al. Q-switched ruby laser treatment of tattoos, a 9-year experience. Br J Plast Surg 1990;43:663–669.

18. Taylor CR, Anderson RR, Gange W, Michaud NA, Flotte TJ. Light and electron microscopic analysis of tattoos treated by Q-switched ruby laser. J Invest Dermatol 1991;97:131–136.

19. Taylor CR, Gange RW, Dover JS et al. Treatment of tattoos by Q-switched ruby laser: a dose response study. Arch Dermatol 1990;126:893–899.

20. Dover JS, Smoller BR, Stern RS et al. Low fluence carbon dioxide laser irradiation of lentigines. Arch Dermatol 1988;124:1219–1224.

21. Stern RS, Dover JS, Levin J, Arndt KA. Laser therapy versus cryotherapy of lentigines: A comparative trial. J Am Acad Dermatol 1994;30: 985–987.

22. McDaniel DH. Clinical usefulness of the Hexascan: treatment of cutaneous vascular and melanocytic disorders. J Dermatol Surg Oncol 1993; 19:312–319.

22a. Alster TS. Complete elimination of café-au-lait birthmarks by the 510-nm pulsed-dye laser. Plast Reconstr Surg 1995;96:1660–1664.

23. Taylor CR, Flotte T, Michaud N, Jimbow K, Anderson RR. Q-switched ruby laser treatment of benign pigmented lesions: dermal vs. epidermal. Laser Surg Med 1991;11(suppl 3):65.

24. DePadova-Elder SM, Milgraum S. Q-switched ruby laser treatment of labial lentigines in Peutz-Jeghers syndrome. J Dermatol Surg Oncol 1994; 20:830–832.

25. Ashinoff R, Geronemus RG. Q-switched ruby laser treatment of benign epidermal pigmented lesions. Laser Surg Med 1992;12(suppl 4):73.

25a. Grossman MC, Anderson RR, Farnelli W, Flotte TJ, Grevelink JM. Treatment of café-au-lait macules with lasers: A clinicopathological correlation. Arch Dermatol 1995;131:1416–1420.

26. Goldberg DJ. Benign pigmented lesions: treatment with the Q-switched ruby laser. J Dermatol Surg Oncol 1993;19:376–379.

27. Geronemus RG, Ashinoff R. Q-switched ruby laser therapy of nevus of Ota. Laser Med Surg 1992;12(suppl 4):74.

28. Watanabe S, Takahashi H. Treatment of nevus of Ota with the Q-switched ruby laser. N Engl J Med 1994;331:1745–1750.

28a. Suzuki H, Kobayashi S, Yamamoto K, Kihara T. The optimal age to begin and optimal interval for treatment of nevus of Ota with the Q-switched Nd:YAG laser. Laser Surg Med 1996;(suppl 8):39.

29. Waldorf HA, Kauvar ANB, Geronemus RG. Treatment of small and medium congenital nevi with the Q-switched ruby laser. Arch Dermatol 1996;132:301–304.

30. Taylor CR, Anderson RR. Ineffective treatment of refractory melasma and postinflammatory hyperpigmentation by Q-switched ruby laser (see Comments). J Dermatol Surg Oncol 1994;20:592–597.

31. Milgraum S, Cohen M, Auletta M. Treatment of blue nevi with the Q-switched ruby laser. J Am Acad Dermatol 1995;32:307–310.

32. Wheeland RG. Q-switched ruby laser treatment of tattoos. Laser Surg Med 1991;11(suppl 3):64.

33. Goyal S, Arndt KA, Stern RS, O'Hare D, Dover JS. Laser treatment of tattoos: a prospective, paired, comparison study of the Q-switched Nd:YAG (1064 nm), frequency-doubled Q-switched Nd:YAG (532 nm), and Q-switched ruby lasers. J Am Acad Dermatol 1997;36:122–125.

33a. Kilmer S, Anderson R. Clinical use of the Q-switched ruby and the Q-switched Nd:YAG (1064 nm and 532 nm) lasers for treatment of tattoos. J Dermatol Surg Oncol 1993;19:330–338.

34. Levine V, Geronemus RG. Tattoo removal with the Q-switched ruby laser and the Nd:YAG laser: a comparative study. Cutis 1995;55:291–296.

35. McMeekin TO. A comparison of the alexandrite laser (755nm) with the Q-switched ruby laser (694nm) in the treatment of tattoos. Laser Surg Med 1993;13(suppl 5):54.

36. Zelickson BD, Mehregan D, Zarrin A et al. Clinical, histological, and ultrastructural evaluation of tattoos treated with three laser systems. Laser Surg Med 1994;15:364–372.

37. Grevelink JM, Casparian JM, Gonzalez E et al. Undesirable effects associated with treatment of tattoos and pigmented lesions with Q-switched lasers at 1064nm and 694nm—the MGH experience. Laser Surg Med 1993;131(suppl 5):53.

38. Levins PC, Anderson RR. Q-switched ruby laser treatment of pigmented lesions and tattoos. Clin Dermatol 1995;13:75–79.

38a. Tope W, Tsoukas M, Farinelli W, Anderson R. Tattoo ink darkening: the effect of wavelength, fluence, and pulsed duration. Laser Surg Med 1996;(suppl 8):40.

38b. Anderson R, Geronemus R, Kilmer S, Farinelli W, Fitzpatrick R. Cosmetic tattoo ink darkening: A complication of Q-switched and pulsed laser treatment. Arch Dermatol 1993;129:1010–1014.

39. DeCoste SD, Anderson RR. Comparison of Q-switched ruby and Q-switched Nd:YAG laser treatment of tattoos. Laser Surg Med 1991;11(suppl 3):64.

39a. Kilmer SL, Wheeland RG, Goldberg DJ, Anderson RR. Treatment of epidermal pigmented lesions with the frequency-doubled Q-switched Nd:YAG laser. A controlled, single-impact, dose-response, multicenter trial. Arch Dermatol 1994;130:1515–1519.

40. Goldberg DJ. Treatment of pigmented and vascular lesions of the skin with the Q-switched Nd:YAG laser. Laser Surg Med 1993;13(suppl 5):55.

41. Kilmer SL. Q-switched Nd:YAG laser treatment of tattoos. Presented at the American Academy of Dermatology, December 1992.

42. Kilmer SL, Lee MS, Grevelink JM, Flotte TJ, Anderson RR. The Q-switched Nd:YAG laser (1064 nm) effectively treats tattoos: a controlled, dose-response study. Arch Dermatol 1993;129:971–978.

43. Kilmer SL, Lee M, Farinelli W, Grevelink JM, Anderson RR. Q-switched Nd:YAG laser (1064 nm) effectively treats Q-switched ruby laser resistant tattoos. Laser Surg Med 1992;12(suppl 4):72.

44. Kaufman R, Boehncke WH, Konig K, Hibst R. Comparative study of Q-switched alexandrite laser treatment of tattoos. Laser Surg Med 1993;13(suppl 5):54.

45. Kilmer SL, Anderson RR. Clinical use of the Q-switched ruby and the Q-switched Nd:YAG (1064nm and 532nm) lasers for treatment of tattoos. J Dermatol Surg Oncol 1993;19:330–338.

46. Kilmer SL, Lee MS, Anderson RR. Treatment of multi-colored tattoos with the Q-switched Nd:YAG laser (532nm): a dose response study with comparison to the Q-switched ruby laser. Lasers Surg Med 1993;13 (suppl 5):54.

47. Levine V, Geronemus R. Tattoo removal with the Q-switched ruby laser and the Nd:YAG laser: A comparative study. Cutis 1995;55:291–296.

48. Grekin RC, Shelton RM, Geisse JK, Frieden I. 510-nm pigmented lesion dye laser. J Dermatol Surg Oncol 1993;19:380–387.

49. Fitzpatrick RE, Goldman MP, Ruiz-Esparza J. Laser treatment of benign pigmented lesions using a 300 nanosecond pulse and 510 nm wavelength. J Dermatol Surg Oncol 1993;19:341–346.

49a. Stafford T, Tan O. 510-nm pulsed dye laser and alexandrite crystal laser for the treatment of pigmented lesions and tattoos. Clin Derm 1995; 13:69–73.

50. Fitzpatrick RE, Goldman MP, Ruiz-Esparza J. Laser treatment of benign pigmented epidermal lesions using a 300 nsecond pulse and a 510 nm wavelength. J Dermatol Surg Oncol 1993;18:341–347.

51. Tan OT, Morelli JG, Kurban AK. Pulsed dye laser treatment of benign cutaneous pigmented lesions. Laser Surg Med 1992;12:538–542.

52. Alster TS. Treatment of benign pigmented epidermal lesions with the 510nm pulsed dye laser: further clinical experience and treatment parameters. Laser Surg Med 1993;(suppl 5):55.

53. Kaufmann R, Boehncke WH, Konig K, Hibst R. Comparative study of the Q-switched Nd:YAG and alexandrite laser treatment of tattoos. Lasers Surg Med 1993;13(suppl 5):54.

54. Alster TS, Williams CM. Treatment of nevus of Ota by the Q-switched alexandrite laser. Dermatol Surg 1995;21:592–596.

55. Fitzpatrick RE, Goldman MP, Ruiz-Esparza J. The use of the alexandrite laser (755nm, 100 nsec) for tattoo pigment removal in an animal model. J Am Acad Dermatol 1993;28(5):745–750.

56. Fitzpatrick RE, Goldman MP. Tattoo removal using the alexandrite laser. Arch Dermatol 1994;130:1508–1514.

57. Fitzpatrick RE, Ruiz-Esparza J, Goldman MP. Alexandrite laser of tattoos; a clinical and histological study. Lasers Surg Med 1993;13(suppl 5):54.

58. Stafford T, Lisek R, Tan O. Role of the alexandrite laser for removal of tattoos. Laser Surg Med 1995;17:32–38.

59. Alster T. Q-switched alexandrite laser treatment (755nm) of professional and amateur tattoos. J Am Acad Dermatol 1995;33:69–73.

60. Stafford TJ, Lisek R, Tan OT. Role of the alexandrite laser for removal of tattoos. Lasers Surg Med 1995;17:32–38.

10 —— Tissue Cutting: Traditional Lasers, Solid-State Devices, and Diode Laser

Joseph T. Walsh, Jr.

The development of new laser-based surgical procedures is in part dependent on the discovery of new sources of laser radiation. The purpose of this chapter is to describe the new events taking place in the development of tissue-cutting lasers. The chapter is divided into three sections. The basic concepts of laser-tissue interactions are reviewed in the first section, with an emphasis on those interactions most vital to the development of new laser sources. This section also includes a discussion of some of the technical issues that shape the development of new laser sources. The lasers used to cut tissue are discussed in the second section, with a particular focus on the infrared light–emitting lasers. Diode lasers and the promise they hold for the cutting of tissue, as well as a description of some current diode laser applications, are presented in the third section.

Laser technology has developed rapidly, such that it has reached a point where it is now possible to develop a laser that can meet almost any specification in terms of the wavelength, pulse duration, energy, and power, as long as price is not an issue. In fact, we are now entering an era in which the development of new laser-based medical applications will not be limited so much by technological factors as much as by our relatively limited understanding of acute and delayed laser-tissue interactions.

Laser-Tissue Interactions

SELECTION OF WAVELENGTH

A laser is really just a source of energy, albeit one with some unique properties. One property of this energy source is that the energy emitted can be deposited quickly in a very small, well-defined volume of tissue. Alternatively, one can choose to have the light absorbed by a large volume of tissue. The key to controlling this deposition is the selection of an appropriate wavelength of light. Figure 10-1 shows a plot of absorption versus wavelength for the major tissue chromophores. For example, there is strong absorption by proteins and

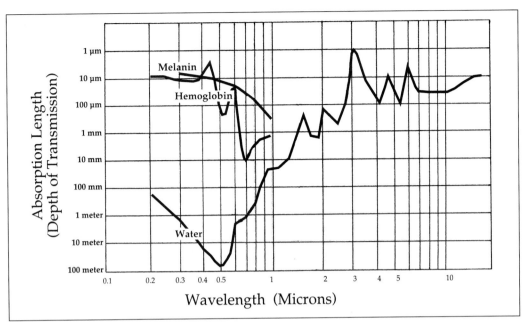

Fig. 10.1. The absorption coefficients of major tissue chromophores in the ultraviolet, visible, and infrared portions of the spectrum.

nucleic acids in the ultraviolet (UV) light portion of the electromagnetic spectrum, whereas melanin and hemoglobin preferentially absorb light in the visible light region of the spectrum. In the 600- to 1000-nm range, intrinsic chromophores only weakly absorb the incident radiation. This red to near-infrared (NIR) region of the visible spectrum has been dubbed the *therapeutic window*, because such light can penetrate deeply into tissue and be absorbed, for example, by exogenous dyes, which in turn induces a therapeutic effect.[1] Water is the major absorber of IR light.[2] Recent evidence indicates, however, that the data shown in Figure 10-1 only just begin to describe laser-tissue interactions, in that they were derived using low-intensity radiation, whereas lasers emit high-intensity radiation that rapidly heats tissue. This means that, even during nanosecond-long pulses, the absorption coefficient of tissue can change by several orders of magnitude.[3–5] Continued investigations of the dynamics of tissue chromophores are therefore necessary in order to arrive at a more full understanding of laser-tissue interactions.

If a particular structure must be destroyed, then one needs a laser that emits light strongly absorbed by that structure (see Chapter 3). If deeply penetrating light is required, then one needs a laser that emits light in the therapeutic window. A variety of dye lasers emit such radiation; however, the solid-state and diode lasers that have been developed recently allow adequate tuning throughout this range and are burdened by few of the maintenance-related disadvantages of the dye lasers. If tissue is to be cut, then one needs a laser that emits strongly absorbed UV or IR radiation. The excimer laser, which emits UV radiation, is discussed in Chapter 14; the IR light–emitting continuous-wave CO_2 laser is discussed in Chapters 11 and 12. Mid–IR light–emitting lasers and short–pulse duration CO_2 lasers are discussed in this chapter.

SELECTION OF PULSE DURATION

After the wavelength has been selected, the duration of irradiation must be selected. This problem has been discussed in other chapters. In brief, however, the longer the pulse duration, the more thermal energy diffuses from the site of absorption. If the goal is to control bleeding, then thermal damage is desired, which requires a long pulse duration. If, however, thermal damage is to be limited, then a short pulse of strongly absorbed radiation is necessary. In general, if absorption of the incident radiation is strong, then the width of the thermal damage zone can be limited to approximately the optical penetration depth $(1/\mu_a)$.[6] More sophisticated models for predicting the width of the thermal damage zone are discussed in the literature.[6–8] This limited width is only achieved if the pulse is shorter in duration than the thermal relaxation time of the initially heated layer of tissue. The initially heated layer has a width of $1/\mu_a$, and the thermal relaxation time (τ_R) of that width is given by the following equation:

$$\tau_R = \frac{(1/\mu_a)^2}{4\kappa} \qquad\qquad \text{Eq. 1}$$

where κ = the thermal diffusivity of the tissue (typically $\kappa \approx 1.3 \times 10^{-3}$ cm^2/sec).[9]

Thus, if the radiation is absorbed in the first 1 μm of tissue, the thermal relaxation time is approximately 2 μsec. Ten times deeper absorption depths lead to one hundred times longer thermal relaxation times. The thermal damage produced by the CO_2 laser, which emits 10.6-μm radiation that is absorbed in approximately the first 20 μm of tissue, is limited if the pulse is less than approximately 0.5 msec long. For a laser emitting at the peak of the water absorption curve (i.e., at 2.94 μm), the laser pulse must be less than approximately 1 μsec long to limit thermal damage.

It has recently been suggested that one can cut tissue and leave even less thermal damage if the pulse duration is less than the "stress relation" time.[10] This concept follows from data indicating that short pulses of strongly absorbed laser radiation do not vaporize tissue in the traditional sense. That is, instead of a phase transition from water to vapor that requires the addition of the heat of vaporization to the water, the temperature at the site of absorption greatly exceeds the critical temperature for water (647°K). The resultant pressure can exceed 1000 atm. Thus, material explodes out of the ablation crater.[11] The velocity of the resultant plume has been measured and found to exceed the speed of sound in air.[12–15] Consequently, not only is it important to confine the thermalized optical energy to the site of absorption but it is also important to confine the pressure rise to the site of absorption. Pressure waves travel at the speed of sound (c_{sound}). Thus, the pulse duration should be shorter than the stress relation time ($\tau_{acoustic}$) required for a pressure wave to traverse an optical penetration depth ($1/\mu_a$). That is:

$$\tau_{acoustic} = \frac{1}{\mu_a c_{sound}} \qquad\qquad \text{Eq. 2}$$

The speed of sound in tissue is approximately equal to the speed of sound in water, or approximately 1500 m/sec. At a wavelength of 308 nm, the absorption coefficient is approximately 90 cm^{-1},[10] thus the stress relaxation time is 6.7 μsec and the pulse duration, τp, should be less than approximately 7 μsec. A requirement that stress be confined during a laser pulse is more stringent than that thermal energy be confined during the pulse. Although data are not available verifying the importance of stress confinement to the ablation efficiency in tissue, such data are available for tissue phantoms.[16] The pertinence of this restriction to tissue cutting will remain unclear until further basic research is completed.

There are some practical limits to how short the pulse duration can be. If a constant energy pulse is shortened to the point where the incident irradiance is approximately 10^8 W/cm^2, then plasma formation is likely. Plasma formation decreases ablation efficiency during the pulsed laser ablation of tissue.[17] Shortening of the laser pulse also plays a role in causing fiber damage. In brief, optical fiber damage is irradiance dependent. Thus, if a certain energy per pulse is needed to achieve efficient ablation, then the pulse must be long enough so that the irradiance producing fiber damage is not exceeded.[18]

SELECTION OF OTHER PARAMETERS

Once the wavelength and pulse duration necessary for the desired application have been specified, one must determine the energy or power necessary for the desired task. When using a pulsed laser, one typically desires both sufficient energy per pulse, so that each pulse is effective, and sufficient average power, so that the task is completed in a reasonable time. (The average power emitted by a pulsed laser equals the energy emitted per pulse times the pulse repetition rate, e.g., 1 J/pulse ×10 Hz =10 W.) The average power is the key parameter for a continuous-wave laser, or a laser in which the pulse is much longer than the thermal relaxation time.

Other irradiation parameters affect the interaction of laser radiation with tissue; these parameters include the spot size, peak irradiance, and the pulse repetition rate and are discussed in the context of particular applications.

It should be reiterated, however, that the photophysics of laser-tissue interactions serve as the design parameters in the development of new medical lasers. Thus a discussion of new lasers and their medical applications must be based on an understanding of the photophysics involved. Further, the biologic response of the tissue to the initial photophysical intervention must also be considered. Fortunately, most of the interactions described in the present chapter are largely photothermal, and thus the biologic response is not typically dependent on the wavelength but rather dependent on the extent of the residual thermal damage zone. The photophysical and photobiologic responses specific to these systems are discussed for each of the laser systems described.

Tissue-Cutting Lasers

Numerous lasers can effectively cut tissue. The most important of these lasers are listed in Table 10-1. The systems fall into three broad categories: UV, with a wavelength of 200 to 380 nm; visible, with a wavelength of 380 to 780 nm; and IR, with a wavelength of 780 nm to 1 mm.

EXCIMER LASERS

The 193-nm excimer laser is well known for its ability to cut tissue, leaving as little as 1 μm of altered tissue at the cut edge.[13,19,20] Experimental evidence suggests that the 193-nm excimer laser cuts tissue by means of the direct photodecomposition of the tissue matrix. The photon energy of a 193-nm photon is sufficient to break C-C bonds; thus tissue ablation is possible without vaporization of the tissue water.[13] The 193-nm excimer laser was recently approved by the U.S. Food and Drug Administration for use in corneal sculpting. However use of the excimer laser for the ablation of cutaneous lesions has been limited to experimental studies. Studies of short- and long-term healing have demonstrated that lesions induced with the 193-nm excimer laser heal rapidly, with minimal inflammation.[21] The 193-nm radiation also does not appear to be mutagenic.[22,23] Such a system would therefore be very good for the precise removal of cutaneous lesions, although one must use a fairly high pulse repetition rate to cut through a blood-filled field.[20] At low pulse-repetition rates the blood fills the ablation crater between pulses and the laser energy is then invested in clearing the blood rather than ablating the tissue.[20]

The 248-nm excimer laser also produces clean cuts in tissue.[20,24] However, the mutagenic effects of 248-nm radiation are quite pronounced and the inflammation induced during healing is considerable.[22] Thus, it is unlikely that the excimer laser emitting at 248 nm would be considered for clinical use. However, there are excimer lasers that can emit radiation at other wavelengths. For example, 308-nm ra-

Table 10-1. Lasers capable of effectively cutting tissue

Name	Wavelength	Thermal damage*
Excimer	193 nm	1 μm[19]
	248 nm	20 μm[20]
Quadrupled Ti:sapphire	≈210 nm	1 μm
Quintupled Nd:YAG	213 nm	1 μm[25]
Nd:YAG	1.44 μm	450 μm[27]
Co:MgF$_2$	1.7–2.2 μm	100–400 μm[42]
Tm:YAG	2.0 μm	100 μm
Ho:YAG	2.1 μm	100 μm
HF	2.7–3.3 μm	5–20 μm[43]
Er:YSGG	2.78 μm	10 μm[44–46]
Raman-shifted Nd:YAG	2.80 and 2.92 μm	10 μm[11]
Er:YAG	2.94 μm	10 μm[46]
CO	6 μm	50 μm
CO$_2$ (continuous-wave and pulsed)	10.6 μm	35–50 μm[35]
FEL	<200 nm–>100 μm	Varies
OPOs	Tunable in IR	Varies

*Approximate minimal width of the thermal damage zone in collagen-based tissues such as skin and cornea. Selected references are given; if good references were not found, the author's best estimate is given.

diation is used for laser angioplasty because it can be transmitted via an optical fiber. The cutaneous applications of such short-pulse, high-energy UV radiation are not likely to be widespread, however.

OTHER UV-EMITTING LASERS

The disadvantages of the excimer lasers include the size of the system, the need to use toxic gases, the purchase price of the system, and the maintenance costs. Thus, only a few solid-state systems that emit in the far-UV region are being considered. Of these systems, the quintupled Nd:YAG laser is the only one to have been used in tissue studies. The output from this laser is achieved in the following way. The 1.06-μm output from a Q-switched Nd:YAG laser is first doubled to 532 nm using a type I CD*A crystal. The 532-nm radiation is then doubled to 266 nm using a BBO crystal. Finally, using another BBO crystal, the 1.06-μm radiation is frequency mixed with the 266-nm radiation to generate the fifth harmonic, or 213 nm.[25] The 213-nm radiation effectively cuts tissue, leaving zones of thermal damage similar to those produced by the 193-nm excimer laser. Improvements in crystal-growing technology that have led to increases in the energy generated by the laser system may result in the development of a clinically useful system.

Yet another approach to the generation of far-UV laser radiation for tissue cutting is the quintupling of the output from a pulsed Ti:sapphire laser system. Ti:sapphire lasers are pumped by an argon laser and tunable from about 700 to 975 nm. By quintupling the output from the Ti:sapphire laser system, it is possible to obtain 10-nsec-long pulses of 220-nm radiation with sufficient energy (e.g., 10 mJ per pulse) to cut tissue. Ti:sapphire laser systems are popular and useful for spectroscopic studies conducted in physical chemistry laboratories, but the quintupling of such systems is a relatively recent development. A clinically useful system may be developed once more research has been done.

Finally, rapid advances in "bandgap engineering" have led to the expectation that UV-emitting diode lasers may be produced before the next century.[26] These lasers are discussed in detail at the end of this chapter.

VISIBLE LIGHT–EMITTING LASERS

There are no lasers emitting light in the visible region of the spectrum that can effectively cut tissue without leaving a several-millimeter-wide zone of thermal damage at the cut edge. Such a wide zone of thermal damage is known to impede healing, lead to an unacceptable clinical result, and interfere with the histologic evaluation of excised specimens.

ND:YAG LASERS

There are several laser systems emitting light in the IR region of the spectrum that can effectively cut tissue. The 1.44-μm Nd:YAG laser* emits radiation at a local peak in the tissue absorption curve (see Fig. 10-1) as much as 2 J per pulse with approximately 650-μsec-long pulses. Such pulses rapidly cut tissue, leaving approximately 450 μm of thermal damage at the cut edge.[27] Such damage is comparable to that left by a continuous-wave CO_2 laser. Thus, the 1.44-μm Nd:YAG laser cuts like a CO_2 laser. However, its radiation can be delivered through standard silicon-based optical fibers, whereas CO_2 laser radiation can be delivered only through an articulated arm.

The 1.44-μm Nd:YAG laser has been investigated recently, in part because the absorption of 1.44-μm radiation by water is nearly identical to that of 2.1-μm radiation. Several years ago it was reported

---

*The Nd:YAG laser most commonly used in the clinical arena emits at 1.06 μm and is often called a "YAG" laser. The radiation from such a laser is very poorly absorbed by tissue, and cutting with the 1.06-μm Nd:YAG laser results in considerable thermal damage.

that similar cuts could be obtained using a holmium (Ho):YAG laser*
emitting 2.1-μm radiation with a similar amount of energy per pulse
and a similar pulse duration.[28,29] Nd:YAG crystals are somewhat less
expensive than Ho:YAG crystals, and Nd:YAG laser systems have
been better characterized than Ho:YAG laser systems, thus there may
be some technical advantages to using neodymium instead of holmium. The transmission of 1.44-μm radiation through traditional
silicon-based optical fibers also gives the neodymium-based system
an advantage over the holmium-based system, which requires special
low-OH fibers to deliver the optical radiation to the tissue site. It is
likely that noncutaneous (e.g., orthopedic[30]) applications will drive
the development of these two laser systems in the near future.

THULIUM AND HOLMIUM LASERS

Several other lasers emit radiation near the 1.9-μm band in the water
absorption curve. The thulium:YAG laser, emitting at the peak of the
1.94-μm band, has been shown to produce somewhat less thermal
damage during tissue cutting than the Ho:YAG laser.[31] Both systems,
however, require the use of low-OH fibers. Thulium and holmium
laser systems cause slightly different tissue effects; however, these differences have yet to be exploited for the purpose of specific clinical
indications. Further, given the dynamic optical properties of water,
major differences in the effects of lasers emitting near 1.94 μm are
not expected.[11]

ERBIUM LASERS

There are also several lasers that emit radiation in the 3-μm band of
the water absorption spectrum. The erbium (Er):YAG laser emits at
the peak of the band, at 2.94 μm. The Er:YSGG laser emits at 2.79
μm, where the low-intensity absorption is about a factor of 3 less
than the absorption at the peak. It had been proposed that a laser
emitting less than 1-μsec-long pulses of 2.94-μm radiation could
cut tissue, leaving as little as 1 μm of thermal damage at the cut
edge. Such small zones of damage have, however, never been observed; only zones as small as 5 μm in width have been observed.[6,11]
There are several reasons for these observations, the most important one being that, during an ablative laser pulse, the absorption
coefficient of the water in tissue decreases by as much as a factor of

---

*Ho:YAG lasers are sometimes co-doped with thulium and/or chromium to im-
prove the lasing efficiency. The thulium, holmium, chromium:YAG laser has
been dubbed the THC:YAG. The wavelength emitted remains at approximately
2.1 μm, however.

100.[3-5] Thus the incident laser radiation penetrates much deeper into the tissue than one would predict on the basis of the low-intensity spectrum shown in Figure 10-1. If one considers the dynamic absorption coefficient, then one expects little difference between the effects of 2.79- and 2.94-μm radiation. Indeed, both wavelengths produce typically 10 to 15 μm of thermal damage when the laser is operated in the Q-switched mode (≈100-nsec-long pulses) and 25 to 50 μm of thermal damage when the laser is run in the normal-spiking mode (≈250-μsec-long pulses).[6] Both the Er:YAG and Er:YSGG lasers can be relatively compact systems. The radiation cannot, however, be transmitted through a standard optical fiber, and thus an articulated arm or coated flexible waveguide must be used to deliver the radiation to the target tissue. Currently such erbium lasers emit up to 1 J per pulse and 15 to 20 W of average power, thus cutting rapidly and effectively; however, as one would expect, hemostasis is not achieved with such a small zone of thermal damage at the cut edge.

Two potentially significant applications of the erbium laser are being developed. Several companies are supporting clinical trials in which erbium lasers are being used for skin resurfacing. Normal-spiking mode erbium lasers, as well as short-pulsed and scanned CO_2 lasers, leave 25- to 150-μm zones of thermal damage following ablation in a collagenous tissue such as the dermis. Such a zone of damage is known to result in diminution of rhytids. Is is hoped that an erbium laser can be less expensive and cause fewer complications than the CO_2 laser systems. In particular, there is hope that the erbium laser will cause less thermal damage than the CO_2 lasers and thus decrease the incidence of long-term facial redness.

The other emerging application of erbium lasers is in blood drawing. A single pulse from an erbium laser can induce bleeding from within the dermis. It is hoped that such a system will replace cost-effectively the lancets currently used to draw small volumes of blood. Use of such a system would decrease disposal costs of sharp biohazardous instruments and be safer for hospital personnel.

CARBON MONOXIDE LASERS

The CO laser is being considered for tissue-cutting purposes because it emits near the peak of the 6-μm absorption band of water. However, the CO laser suffers the same problems as the erbium laser, in that the radiation cannot be transmitted through an optical fiber. Additionally, a pulsed CO laser is more difficult to engineer than a solid-state erbium laser. Given that the tissue optics of the CO laser do not give it much of an advantage over an erbium laser, it is unlikely that such a system could induce a tissue effect that cannot be achieved by lasers that are already available.

PULSED CO_2 LASERS

Continuous-wave CO_2 lasers have been used as medical tools for many years. When focused to a spot on the order of a few hundred micrometers in diameter, it can be used to effectively cut soft tissues, leaving a zone of thermal damage in collagenous tissues such as skin that is typically a few hundred micrometers in width. Until recently, the only clinically available pulsed CO_2 lasers were those created either by chopping the laser output or by "superpulsing" the system. Chopping the output results in pulses that are typically tens to hundreds of milliseconds in duration. Superpulsed systems typically produce pulses that are several hundred microseconds in duration, but the definition of "superpulsed" varies from manufacturer to manufacturer, and thus the pulse-duration characteristics of the lasers vary as well. The goal of these pulsing schemes was to provide cuts with less thermal damage at the cut edge; that is, if the laser energy is delivered to the tissue quickly, then there is little time for thermal energy to penetrate deeper into the tissue. As a result, the lasers emitting pulses of shorter duration do not damage as large a volume of tissue as the longer–pulse duration and continuous-wave lasers. However, the goal of thermal damage confinement is only partially achieved with these pulsing schemes.

To minimize the thermal damage produced by an ablative pulse of laser radiation, three major criteria must be satisfied: (1) the pulse must be shorter than the thermal relaxation time of the layer of tissue in which the optical energy is deposited; (2) each pulse must be energetic enough to effectively ablate the tissue; and (3) the time between pulses must be long enough for the thermal energy deposited by the first pulse to dissipate before the next pulse arrives. The pulsing schemes for the CO_2 laser just described typically satisfy none of these criteria. Namely, for the CO_2 laser to satisfy these criteria, the pulse duration must be less than about 500 μsec in duration; there should be at least 5 J/cm^2 per pulse incident on the tissue (for a 100-μm-diameter spot size, this means 400 μJ incident per pulse); and the time between pulses should be on the order of tens of milliseconds.[33,34] Current continuous-wave CO_2 lasers used for clinical applications do not emit radiation that meets these criteria, thus pulsing only lessens, but does not minimize, the thermal damage. A transversely excited, atmospheric pressure (TEA) CO_2 laser does, however, emit radiation with the desired output. Using 2-μsec-long pulses of 10.6-μm radiation from a TEA CO_2 laser operating at 2 pulses per second, the damage zone in skin is typically 50 μm wide.[35]

Unfortunately, although the TEA CO_2 laser could be adapted for surgical uses, the gas-handling requirements and the large power supply needed have made the cost of such an adaptation prohibitive. In addition, there are currently no clinical applications for which it is needed.

OPO cavity of two new beams of light, both at a longer wavelength than the pump wavelength. These new wavelengths can be tuned by rotation of the crystal. OPOs are being developed that can emit radiation near the 2-μm and 3-μm absorption band of water and in the 4- to 5-μm region. The pump lasers currently being considered for use in this system are the Nd:YAG, Co:MgF$_2$, and Er:YAG lasers. Crystals being used include KTP, KTA, BBO, and ZnGeP. For further details about OPOs, the reader is referred to more technical sources.[39,40] However, it should be noted that, with the advent of diode lasers (see later discussion), it is now possible to pump Nd ions embedded in an OPO crystal that thus emits tunable radiation in the IR region. Such a system can be low cost (e.g., $1000 to $5000), lightweight (e.g., approximately 10 pounds), and portable. Such a system can be tuned as simply as by turning a dial; thus a laser that can cut and coagulate can readily be made. The production of such systems is currently under way.[41]

As was stated at the beginning of this chapter, if the desired wavelength, energy, and average power can be specified for a particular application, an OPO can, with but a few constraints, be developed to meet these specifications. On the basis of the foregoing discussion, it should be clear that the OPOs offer some tremendous advantages over other tunable sources of infrared radiation. In particular, an OPO is relatively inexpensive (all the electronics and optics can be purchased for only several thousand dollars), easy to construct, and maintenance free (i.e., there are no dyes to change). The output from an OPO can be fairly powerful (e.g., 10 W or more) (A. Geiger, personal communication, 1994). Currently the OPOs are limited by the inability of the crystals to handle high peak power, but this problem will gradually be overcome as crystal growers become more proficient at eliminating impurities from the crystals. Interestingly the crystals used in OPO systems were first developed in China. It seems that crystal growth was considered acceptable art, not technology—the latter largely being forbidden after the cultural revolution. Thus crystal growth was one of the few fields that the technically oriented Chinese could pursue. Now crystal growth is being done worldwide. As more optical materials are developed for use in OPOs, the tuning range in the IR region should continue to increase, as should the pulse energy and the average power these devices are capable of generating.

Diode Lasers

Diode lasers are devices that operate by the conversion of electrical energy into electrons (negatively charged mobile particles) and holes (positively charged mobile particles analogous to electrons) that drift into the active region of a semiconductor diode junction, where they recombine to emit light.[39] The conversion of electrical energy into light within such a device can be very efficient; typical diode lasers convert more than 50% of the electrical power into light. By contrast, an argon laser converts less than 1% of incoming electrical power to light. Thus, diode lasers do not need large power supplies or large cooling systems. In brief, diode lasers can be small. However, although diode lasers can be battery operated, diode laser pointers being a good example, it is unlikely that battery-operated laser systems capable of cutting tissue will be available in the near future. If, however, the market for diode lasers is sufficient to justify mass production, such as that for the diode lasers used in compact disk players, then the cost per diode can drop as considerably, as the cost for most semiconductor materials (e.g., computer chips) has.

When diode lasers are fabricated into arrays, one can achieve tens of watts of output power. For example, one diode laser manufacturer (SDL, Inc., San Jose, CA) will bundle several diode arrays to create a system producing 60 W of output at approximately 910 nm. Most diode lasers emit in the 795- to 830-nm range, although new diode lasers emitting at shorter and longer wavelengths are being developed. For example, hundreds of milliwatts of power at about 2 μm have been obtained from diode lasers being developed at Lincoln Laboratories, and at least one diode manufacturer (SDL, Inc., San Jose, CA) has advertised a 500-mW continuous-wave diode laser emitting in the 1.9- to 2.1-μm region. The potential medical applications of such a laser are clear, because previous work with a continuous-wave Ho:YAG laser, which emits radiation at 2.01 μm, showed that such a laser could cut tissue in a manner very similar to a continuous-wave CO_2 laser. A continuous-wave Ho:YAG laser is very impractical, however, because it must be cooled with liquid nitrogen. However, a diode laser that can cut like a continuous-wave CO_2 laser could compete very effectively with electrocautery. In particular, it is quite likely that a continuous-wave 2-μm diode laser could cut and coagulate tissue without the need for patient grounding and without concerns about the electrical current tracking along unspecified pathways within the tissue. Further, issues of sterility would be moot, because the laser would function in a noncontact mode.

The future of diode lasers currently seems unbounded. The race to build diode lasers that emit in the UV and IR region is quite intense and is fueled largely by the telecommunications, optical storage, and industries. The technical challenge is to manipulate the composition of a semiconductor so that the energy gap between the conduction band and the valance band within the semiconductor is set at the energy of the desired photons. Such manipulations have been dubbed "bandgap engineering." The continued success of bandgap engineering is the key to further developments in the diode laser field. Current researchers are not limited by fundamental physics, however, but by the purity of their products and the ability to creatively manipulate the semiconductor composition. The end of new developments is not in sight, and medicine is likely to be a major beneficiary of these developments.

Diode laser arrays that can emit sufficient power for cutting are just coming on the market; however, it has already been shown that one can pump standard solid-state materials using a diode laser array and obtain very efficient lasers that can readily cut tissue. This is possible because a diode laser array is used that emits radiation directly into the absorption band of a solid-state medium. Thus, unlike the flashlamp-pumped systems, in which much of the pump energy is transformed into heat, little of the pump energy in the diode laser-pumped systems that pump into the absorption band is lost in the form of heat and most is converted into light of the desired wavelength. For example, one can use a diode laser emitting at 785 nm to efficiently pump a thulium-based system. The advantages of diode laser array–pumped lasers are that the conversion of electrical energy into the desired optical energy is more efficient; the power supply can be smaller; the heat load and thus the cooling system are smaller; and such a system has the potential to be more reliable and less expensive. Lap-top–sized systems capable of efficient tissue cutting are likely to become available in the next few years.

Summary

As already stressed, it is our knowledge of laser-tissue interactions and the identification of clear applications of lasers for cutaneous surgery, not technology, that are imposing limits on the development of new, smaller, and more effective lasers for cutaneous applications. In addition, despite all the money being supplied to fund medical laser research and development, no laser-based treatment will be acceptable until the treatment is proved efficacious, the laser system can be operated in a medical and surgical environment, and the product is acceptably priced and meets the needs of the nonresearch clinician.

References

1. Parrish JA, Deutsch TD. Laser photomedicine. IEEE J Quant Electron 1984;20:1386–1396.
2. Hale GM, Querry MR. Optical constants of water in the 200-nm to 200-μm wavelength region. J Opt Soc Am 1972;12:555–563.
3. Vodopyanov KL. Saturation studies of H_2O and HDO near 3400 cm^{-1} using intense picosecond laser pulses. J Chem Phys 1991;94:5389–5393.
4. Cummings JP, Walsh JT. Erbium laser ablation: the effect of dynamic optical properties. Appl Phys Lett 1993;62:1988–1990.
5. Staveteig PT, Walsh JT. Dynamic 193-nm optical properties of water. Applied Optics (in press).
6. Walsh JT, Flotte TJ, Deutsch TF. Er:YAG laser ablation of tissue: effect of pulse duration and tissue type on thermal damage. Lasers Surg Med 1988; 9:314–326.
7. McKenzie AL. Physics of thermal processes in laser-tissue interactions. Phys Med Biol 1990;35:1175–1209.
8. Frenz M, Romano V, Zweig AD, Weber HP, Chapliev NI, Silenok AV. Instabilities in laser cutting of soft media. J Appl Phys 1989;66:4496–4503.

9. Welch AJ. The thermal response of laser irradiated tissue. IEEE J Quant Electron 1984;20:1471–1481.

10. Dingus RS, Scammon RJ. Gruneisen-stress induced ablation of biological tissue. Proc SPIE 1991;1427:45–54.

11. Walsh JT, Cummings JP. The effect of dynamic optical properties of water on mid-infrared laser ablation. Lasers Surg Med 1994;15:295–305.

12. Srinivasan R, Dyer RE, Braren B. Far-UV laser ablation of cornea: photoacoustic studies. Lasers Surg Med 1984;6:524–527.

13. Srinivasan R. Ablation of polymers and biological tissue by ultraviolet lasers. Science 1986;234:559–565.

14. Walsh JT, Deutsch TF. Measurement of Er:YAG laser ablation plume dynamics. Appl Phys [B] 1991;52:217–224.

15. Izatt JA, Sankey ND, Partovi F et al. Ablation of calcified biological tissue using pulsed hydrogen fluoride laser radiation. IEEE J Quant Electron 1990;26:2261–2270.

16. Jacques SL, Gofstein G, Dingus RS. Laser-flash photography of laser-induced spallation in liquid media. Proc SPIE 1992;1646:284–294.

17. Walsh JT, Deutsch TF. Er:YAG laser ablation of tissue: measurement of ablation rates. Lasers Surg Med 1989;9:327–337.

18. Pascala TJ, McDermid IS, Laudenslager JB. Ultranarrow linewidth, magnetically switched, long pulse, xenon chloride laser. Appl Phys Lett 1984;44:658–660.

19. Puliafito CA, Steinert RF, Deutsch TF, Hillenkamp F, Dehm EJ, Adler CM. Excimer laser ablation of the cornea and lens. Exp Stud Ophthalmol 1985;92:741–748.

20. Morelli J, Kibbi A, Farinelli W, Boll J, Tan OT. Ultraviolet excimer laser ablation: the effect of wavelength and repetition rate on in vivo guinea pig skin. J Invest Dermatol 1987;88:769–773.

21. Walsh JT, Hruza G, Flotte TJ. The healing of laser induced skin wounds. (submitted for publication).

22. Green HA, Margolis RJ, Boll J, Parrish JA, Oseroff AR. Unscheduled DNA synthesis in human skin after in vitro ultraviolet-excimer laser ablation. J Invest Dermatol 1987;89:201–204.

23. Green HA, Boll J, Parrish JA, Kochevar IE, Oseroff AR. The cytotoxicity and mutagenicity of low intensity 248 and 193 nm excimer laser radiation in mammalian cells. Cancer Res 1987;47:410–413.

24. Lane RJ, Linsker R, Wynne JJ, Torres A, Geronemus RG. Ultraviolet-laser ablation of skin. Arch Dermatol 1985;121:609–617.

25. Ren Q, Gailitis RP, Thompson KP, Lin JT. Ablation of the cornea and synthetic polymers using a UV (213 nm) solid-state laser. IEEE J Quant Electron 1990;26:2284–2288.

26. Razeghi M. The MOCVD challenge. Philadelphia: Hilger, 1989.

27. Hambley R, Hebda PA, Abell E, Cohen BA, Jegasothy BV. Wound healing of skin incision produced by ultrasonically vibrating knife, scalpel, electrosurgery, and carbon dioxide laser. J Dermatol Surg Oncol 1988; 14:1213–1217.

28. Nishioka NS, Domankevitz Y, Venugopalan V, Bua DP. Tissue ablation with a pulsed Nd:YAG laser operating at 1.44 μm wavelength. Lasers Surg Med 1992;(suppl 4):7.

29. Treat MR, Trokel SL, Reynolds RD et al. Preliminary evaluation of a pulsed 2.15-μm laser system for fiberoptic endoscopic surgery. Lasers Surg Med 1988;8:322–326.

30. Nishioka NS, Domankevitz Y, Flotte TJ, Anderson RR. Ablation of rabbit

liver, stomach and colon with a pulsed holmium laser. Gastroenterology 1989;96:831–837.

31. Sherk HH. The use of lasers in orthopedic procedures. J Bone Joint Surg 1993;75:768–776.

32. Nishioka NS, Domankevitz Y. Comparison of tissue ablation with pulsed holmium and thulium lasers. IEEE J Quant Electron 1990;26:2271–2275.

33. Stern DA, Puliafito CA, Dobi ET, Reidy WT. Infrared laser surgery of the cornea. Ophthalmology 1988;95:1434–1441.

34. Walsh JT, Cummings JP. The effect of pulse repetition rate on the erbium laser ablation of soft and hard tissue. Proc SPIE 1990;1202:12–21.

35. Welch AJ, van Gemert MJC. Time constants in thermal laser medicine. Lasers Surg Med 1989;9:405–421.

36. Walsh JT, Flotte TJ, Anderson RR, Deutsch TF. Pulsed CO_2 laser tissue ablation: effect of tissue type and pulse duration on thermal damage. Lasers Surg Med 1988;8:108–118.

37. Stellar S, Levine N, Ger R, Levenson SM. Laser excision of acute third-degree burns followed by immediate autograft replacement: an experimental study in the pig. J Trauma 1973;13:45–53.

38. Green HA, Burd EE, Nishioka NS, Compton CC. Skin graft take and healing following 193-nm excimer, continuous-wave carbon dioxide (CO_2), pulsed CO_2, or pulsed holmium:YAG laser ablation of the graft bed. Arch Dermatol 1993;129:979–988.

39. Brau CA. Free-electron lasers. Boston: Academic, 1990.

40. Yariv A. Optical electronics. New York: Holt, Rinehart and Winston, 1985.

41. Advanced solid-state lasers technical digest, 1992. Washington, DC: Optical Society of America. 1992.

42. Chadra S, Ferry MJ, Daunt G. 115 mJ, 2-micron pulses by OPO in KTP. In: Advanced solid-state lasers technical digest. Washington, DC: Optical Society of America, 1992:271–273.

43. Schomacker KT, Domankevitz Y, Flotte TJ, Deutsch TF. Co:MgF_2 laser ablation of tissue: effect of wavelength on ablation threshold and thermal damage. Lasers Surg Med 1991;11:141–151.

44. Seiler T, Marshall J, Rothery S, Wollensak J. The potential of an infrared hydrogen fluoride (HF) laser (3.0 μm) for corneal surgery. Lasers Ophthalmol 1986;1:49–60.

45. Walsh JT, Cummings JP. The effect of pulse repetition rate on the erbium laser ablation of soft and hard tissue. Proc SPIE 1990;1202:12–21.

46. Kermani O, Lubatschowski H, Asshauer T et al. Q-switched CTE:YAG (2.69μm) laser ablation: basic investigations on soft (corneal) and hard (dental) tissues. Laser Surg Med 1993;13:537–542.

47. Ren Q, Venugopalan V, Schomacker K et al. Mid-infrared laser ablation of the cornea: a comparative study. Laser Surg Med 1992;12:274–281.

11 — The CO_2 Laser: Use as an Excisional Instrument

Ronald G. Wheeland

The ability to operate the CO_2 laser in two entirely different modes accounts for its being the most widely used medical laser system today. These modes consist of an excisional mode, involving the use of a focused beam, and an ablative mode, involving the use of a defocused beam.[1,2] The CO_2 laser emits infrared energy with a wavelength of 10,600 nm, which results in a unique type of tissue interaction, because it is selectively absorbed by water but lacks color specificity. When CO_2 laser energy strikes living soft tissue, which has a water content of from 70% to 90%,[3] there is instantaneous vaporization through the conversion of intracellular and extracellular water to steam at 100°C.[4] This process occurs so rapidly that the thermal conduction to adjacent tissue is minimized.[5] The zone of thermal injury created by the CO_2 laser in soft tissue is between 60 and 130 μm, because 99% of this energy is absorbed within two extinction lengths.[6,7] This permits the performance of very precise surgery without significant thermal damage.

Irradiance

To properly use the CO_2 laser in its excisional mode of operation, it is important to understand how the irradiance can be varied to improve control, speed, and hemostasis. The irradiance, or power density, represents the intensity of the energy of the light beam, which in turn determines the ability of the CO_2 to incise tissue.[8–10] This laser parameter is expressed in terms of watts per square centimeter and is calculated using the following formula:

$$\text{Irradiance (W/cm}^2) = \frac{\text{Power output (W)} \times 100 \text{ (mm}^2/\text{cm}^2)}{\text{Effective spot size (mm}^2)}$$

When the CO_2 laser is used in lieu of a scalpel, its beam is minutely focused to a diameter of 0.1 or 0.2 mm and a relatively high laser output of 20 to 35 W is used. This combination results in a very high irradiance of between 50,000 and 100,000 W/cm², which is sufficient to incise tissue.

Delivery Systems

The laser energy is delivered to the patient by a system that consists of an articulating arm with mirrored joints. The beam passes through an optical lens and is focused appropriately for use in excisional surgery. Reliable and reusable fiberoptics have not as yet been developed for the delivery of high-power CO_2 laser energy. However, several quartz-based and crystalline halide fiberoptic delivery systems are being investigated.[11-14] A 30-cm, flexible, hollow, rectangular wave guide was developed as an alternative delivery system for the CO_2 laser, but because the beam was distorted when the tube was flexed, causing the device to be unreliable, it was subsequently withdrawn from the market. Researchers are working on the development of a Teflon tube with an inner wall coated with a metal layer and a dielectric overlayer.[15] However, once reliable optical fibers are perfected for use with the CO_2 laser, they should afford substantially greater flexibility in the performance of incisional CO_2 laser surgery by eliminating reliance on the cumbersome articulated arm to deliver the energy.

Although some excisional CO_2 laser surgical procedures are performed using an operating microscope and a joystick manipulator, the laser is most often used in a freehand fashion. This is done by holding a small sterilizable handpiece with a built-in focusing lens. To precisely position the CO_2 laser beam before actual discharge of the laser energy, a coaxial, biologically inactive, helium-neon laser that emits red light is used as an aiming beam.

Advantages of CO_2 Laser Surgery

The main reason the CO_2 laser is used for incision surgery is because of the excellent degree of *hemostasis* obtained.[15] Blood vessels 0.5 mm in diameter and smaller are routinely sealed as the incision is made, minimizing blood loss and improving visibility in the surgical field. There are also other benefits to this technique. First, *lymphatic channels* are also closed in a similar fashion, which has proved beneficial in the treatment of certain malignant tumors.[16] In addition, sensory nerves are sealed by the laser, so most patients report *minimal pain* after many of the procedures done with the CO_2 laser.[17] Each of these benefits is discussed separately in greater detail.

Incisional Depth and Hemostatic Technique

The depth of the incision made by the CO_2 laser is both a function of the irradiance used and the speed with which the incision is made. Laser incisions tend to be made more slowly than those made with a scalpel. However, with practice, the operator can use the laser as precisely as the scalpel and produce wounds of identical quality. This has been shown for certain delicate cosmetic surgery procedures, including blepharoplasties.[18-20] In addition, the improved hemostasis generally makes up for this slowness and in some cases may actually make it possible to perform laser surgery faster than conventional surgery. For safety reasons, an electrocoagulating device should always be available to control any bleeding from large vessels that may occur. The quality of hemostasis is a function of both the irradiance used and the speed with which the beam of light is moved along the incision line; specifically, lower irradiance and faster movement result in less hemostasis. The laser parameters chosen for a given procedure are determined by the anatomic location and vascularity of the surgical site.

The defocused CO_2 laser beam can be used in some cases to stop bleeding from larger blood vessels that were not sealed by the focused incising laser beam. In this technique, brief (0.2–0.5 second) pulses of laser energy are delivered to the cut ends of the blood vessel, which are being held with forceps. Bleeding from large, low-flow blood vessels can typically be well controlled using this technique, even in patients taking aspirin or nonsteroidal antiinflammatory agents. When the CO_2 laser is used for incisional surgery, immediate primary repair or closure of a wound with a local flap or graft[21] can be performed without the risk of complications or a significant risk of postoperative bleeding.

Tensile Strength

Although the final appearance of a CO_2 laser–incised wound is indistinguishable from that of a wound made using a scalpel,[22] there has been some controversy over the subsequent tensile strength of the wound. It was initially reported that scalpel incisions heal with a greater tensile strength than laser incisions, until approximately 3 weeks, at which time the tensile strength of both wounds becomes equal. This delay in the development of tensile strength was thought to be the direct result of the high-quality hemostasis achieved by the CO_2 laser energy, which causes the formation of the fibrin clot, a vital preliminary step in wound healing, to be reduced. However, this may also stem from the direct inhibition of fibroblasts by the CO_2 laser, a topic discussed later in the section on the treatment of keloids.

However, there have been recent reports of CO_2 laser incisions actually healing faster and with greater tensile strength than scalpel incisions.[23–26] Regardless of which is the case, ultimately this issue does not appear to be clinically significant. However, because of the many and varied procedures being performed using the CO_2 laser, it is important for all users of the CO_2 laser to be aware of this controversy, so they can take the necessary precautions to ensure a safe operation.

Limitation of Blood Loss

There are several indications for use of the CO_2 laser, and these include the excision of highly vascular tumors[27,28] and of nonvascular lesions in highly vascular anatomic locations, such as the oral cavity,[29] scalp,[30,31] genital area, and digits. Laser excision can be performed safely and successfully, even in anticoagulated patients. Laser excisions can also be performed in patients with cardiac pacemakers in whom electrosurgical devices might be contraindicated. The CO_2 laser can be used as well for those procedures done in an operating room, without interfering with the electronic monitoring instruments.

Conventionally performed partial matrixectomy for the treatment of ingrown toenails (Fig. 11-1) can be associated with significant operative bleeding because of the abundant blood supply to the site. Bleeding may occur, even if a tourniquet is employed, because epinephrine is contraindicated. This may cause much anxiety on the part of both the patient and the physician, as well as interfere with visibility at the site, which could compromise the results because, if the matrix is obscured, the surgeon's ability to identify and remove the imbedded nail plate fragments is limited.

In addition, the CO_2 laser can be used to incise the granulation tissue (Fig. 11-2) at the site of an ingrown nail in a relatively bloodless fashion (Fig. 11-3). Further, the focused beam can be used to quickly incise through the nail plate without difficulty (Figs. 11-4 and 11-5). If partial matrixectomy is desired, after the proximal nail fold has been incised using the focused beam, the defocused beam can then be used to precisely vaporize the matrix. This precise vaporization is possible because of the excellent visibility afforded by the high degree of hemostasis.

Oncology

Additional benefits of the CO_2 laser surgical technique have been observed in the treatment of various malignant tumors.[32,33] Specifically, because the CO_2 laser seals lymphatic channels as it incises tissue, this has the effect of reducing the widespread dissemination of breast

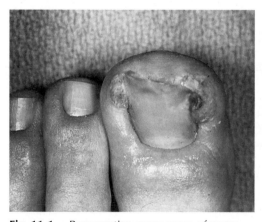

Fig. 11-1. Preoperative appearance of recurrent ingrown toenail.

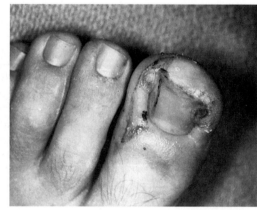

Fig. 11-2. Planned excision is marked preoperatively.

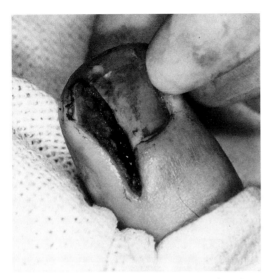

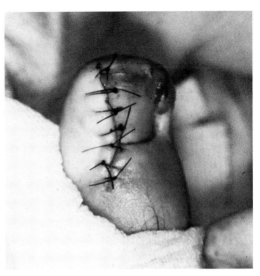

Fig. 11-3. Intraoperative appearance, showing the nearly bloodless excision performed using the CO$_2$ laser.

Fig. 11-4. Primary closure of partial matricectomy wound immediately after laser surgery.

cancer cells after mastectomy. In a similar fashion, this technique may also prove useful in the management of squamous cell carcinomas[34] and melanomas[34,35] (Fig. 11-6).

The typical scalpel procedure used for the removal of primary (stage I) cutaneous melanomas (Fig. 11-7) is modified slightly to permit use of the CO$_2$ laser. Using the focused beam and a power setting of 20 to 25 W (irradiance, 50,000 to 75,000 W/cm^2), the incision is made down into the subcutaneous fat (Figs. 11-8 to 11-10). Because of the differences in the vaporizing and melting points of adipose

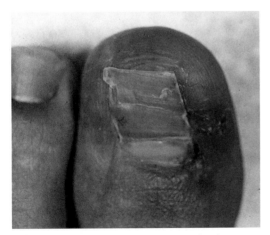

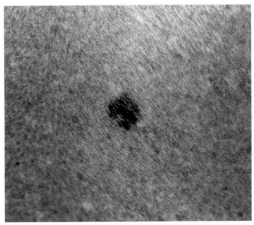

Fig. 11-5. Appearance of the completely healed matricectomy site 3 months postoperatively.

Fig. 11-6. Clinical appearance of a superficial spreading melanoma of the trunk.

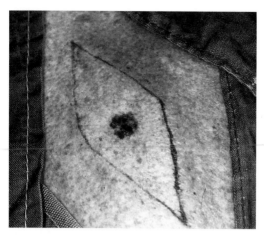

Fig. 11-7. Wet surgical towels surround site of planned laser excision of melanoma.

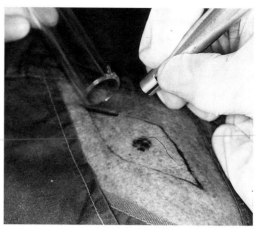

Fig. 11-8. A focused CO_2 laser beam is used to incise the skin; note proximity of smoke evacuator nozzle to wound.

tissue,[36] this tissue acts as an insulator and protects against inadvertent deeper injury by the laser beam. However, it also is responsible for slowing the incisional process. Once the incision has been made, the specimen is easily removed by severing the deep soft-tissue attachments (Fig. 11-11), again with the focused beam. With the assistance of angled mirror attachments, placed on the end of the laser handpiece, the beam can be deflected either 90 or 120 degrees to aid in the incision. Alternatively, the handpiece can be held horizontally to the skin surface and the specimen completely removed using sweeping back-and-forth motions. Once the specimen has been excised, the adjacent tissue can be undermined in a similar fashion in preparation for wound closure using the angled-mirror technique

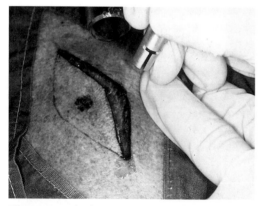

Fig. 11-9. The laser incision is made bloodlessly into the subcutaneous fat on one side of the ellipse.

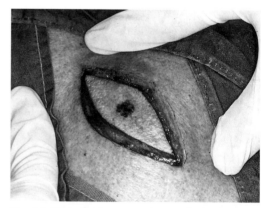

Fig. 11-10. Appearance of wound after incision has been completed, showing complete hemostasis.

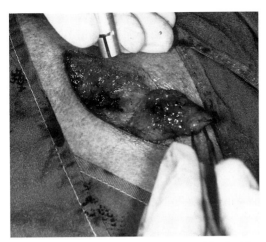

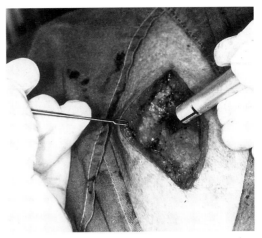

Fig. 11-11. The specimen is removed by holding the laser handpiece horizontally to the skin surface and severing the soft-tissue attachments.

Fig. 11-12. Undermining of adjacent tissue using the laser and a skin hook to lift the edge of the wound.

and a skin hook to lift the edge of the incised tissue and provide better exposure (Fig. 11-12).

Pain Reduction

Just as the CO_2 laser seals blood vessels and lymphatic channels, it also, as mentioned earlier, seals sensory nerve endings as an incision is made.[17] This has the effect of reducing postoperative pain.[5] Those patients who have had two identical procedures performed, one with the scalpel and one with the CO_2 laser, typically report that the postoperative discomfort after the laser procedure is less than that after the scalpel procedure. Although CO_2 laser surgery is certainly not painless, as many patients wish to believe it is, it does appear to be associated with a substantial reduction in postoperative pain compared with conventional surgery because of its unique ability to seal nerve endings, minimize inflammation,[37] and reduce edema.[5]

Histologic Interpretation

Tissue excised with the laser can be studied pathologically without difficulty because the CO_2 laser energy can be focused so precisely and absorbed so selectively that little damage is done to the surrounding tissue. This preserves the histologic detail of laser-excised specimens, unlike tissue harvested with electrosurgical instruments, which can cause extensive thermal coagulation of the tissue. An excellent example of how this ability has been put to use clinically is the microscopically controlled surgical excision of cutaneous malignant lesions (Mohs' surgical technique)[38] performed with the CO_2 laser for the management of skin cancer in anticoagulated patients. In this technique, tissue is removed horizontally and processed immediately into frozen sections, which can be interpreted histologically without difficulty. Once a tumor-free plane has been reached the wound can then be immediately and easily repaired.

Safety Issues Pertaining to CO_2 Laser Excisional Surgery

FIRE

When the CO_2 laser is to be used for excisional surgery in lieu of a scalpel technique, the technique must be modified slightly to minimize the risk of fire resulting from the laser beam igniting dry surgical drapes,[39] flammable surgical skin preparation agents, and certain general anesthetic gases. For this reason, it is best that no flammable materials be allowed in the laser operating room. If sterile cloth surgical drapes are to be placed around the surgical site, they should be kept moist with sterile saline or sterile water throughout the procedure to minimize the risk of ignition should the laser beam inadvertently come in contact with them (see Fig. 11-7). In addition, the disposable, nonflammable anesthetic gases that have been recently developed must be used, and, if oral or laryngeal surgical procedures are being performed, foil-wrapped endotracheal tubes or other endotracheal tubes specially developed for laser procedures must be employed.

EYE INJURY

Probably the greatest safety concern is potential ocular injury to the patient, surgeon, or operating room personnel. For this reason, the eyes of all must always be adequately protected during CO_2 laser surgery. Because CO_2 laser energy cannot pass through plastic, glass, or a polycarbonate material, simple prescription lenses can provide adequate protection, as long as protective plastic side shields are placed on the bows of the glasses. Wet gauze can be taped over the patient's eyes to absorb the CO_2 laser energy and prevent inadvertent injury. Special laser eyeshields made of stainless steel[40,41] or methylmethacrylate can be placed on the cornea of patients undergoing laser surgery near the orbit.

REFLECTION OF LIGHT

The reflection of laser energy[42] off of standard, flat, metallic surgical instruments poses yet another potential risk to the patient, surgeon, and operating room personnel. For this reason, anodized or burnished tools have been developed that reflect less incident light.

However, because the reflected energy diverges as it travels through space, causing it to decrease rapidly in amount, the risk of being injured by reflected laser light appears to be relatively small.

LASER PLUME

The CO$_2$ laser produces a great deal of smoke and steam as it incises tissue, and this constitutes another hazard. Although it was once thought that the plume was sterile,[16] it has now been shown that some bacteria are able to survive within it.[43,44] Fragments of papillomavirus DNA have also been recovered from the CO$_2$ laser plume produced during the treatment of human warts.[45] For reasons of both safety and comfort, this noxious, malodorous material should therefore be removed with an approved laser smoke evacuating system (see Fig. 11-8).[46–48] Very efficient smoke evacuation systems are now readily available that can efficiently filter particles as small as 0.01 μm and minimize the potential risk resulting from inhaling this material.

LASER TATTOOING

After the laser skin incision has been completed and the wound is ready for closure, the incision line should be carefully inspected to see whether any carbon particles have been deposited in it.[49] These particles are occasionally produced during excisional surgery when the beam becomes slightly defocused, leading to some inadvertent vaporization. This vaporized tissue is black or brown, and if it is not removed before wound closure, brown pigmentation along the incision may be visible. Although this pigmentation usually disappears spontaneously within 6 to 8 weeks as the result of removal by tissue macrophages, it does result in the formation of a more obvious, unsightly scar and it may also delay wound healing. Removal is accomplished very easily by simply wetting a sterile cotton-tipped applicator in normal saline and lightly swabbing it along the incision line to remove the carbonized particles and produce a clean incision line ready for surgical closure.

Clinical Uses for CO$_2$ Laser Excision

Besides using the CO$_2$ laser to make incisions in anticoagulated patients and patients with vascular lesions and to remove vascular lesions, there are further appropriate uses for the CO$_2$ laser, and these include its use in the treatment of keloids, rhinophyma, malignant melanoma, and squamous cell carcinoma. It can also be used to perforate cranial bone to promote the development of granulation tissue, and it can be used as well in patients with cardiac pacemakers and in patients connected to cardiac monitors.

KELOIDS

One promising application of the CO_2 laser is its use for the removal of keloids (Fig. 11-13).[50,51] In this procedure, local anesthesia is employed and the focused CO_2 laser beam is used to remove the palpable keloid using a high irradiance of approximately 50,000 W/cm^2. Once most of the keloid has been removed (Figs. 11-14 to 11-16), the edges and base of the wound are carefully palpated (Fig. 11-17). Any residual fibrotic material is subsequently removed in a stepwise fashion until the grossly identifiable keloid is totally removed.

To further reduce the risk of recurrent keloid formation, possibly stimulated by the tension produced during immediate primary repair of the defect, these wounds are almost always allowed to heal by second intention (Fig. 11-18). Healing may take 3 to 6 weeks, depending on the size of the wound, its location, and the quality of wound care provided by the patient. There is also a high risk of recurrence of keloids that have recurred after conventional therapy and subsequently removed with the laser. In these cases, the base and edges of the wound may be injected with intralesional steroids immediately after laser excision to retard regrowth of the keloid. A compression dressing or garment may also be applied during the initial phases of wound healing to further reduce the risk of recurrence.

In keloids resulting from the piercing of ears,[50] a through-and-through defect may be produced when the dumbbell-shaped translobular fibrotic material is surgically removed. This may be best managed by partially violating the general rule of allowing all keloid-removal wounds to heal by second intention. Good functional and cosmetic results generally occur.

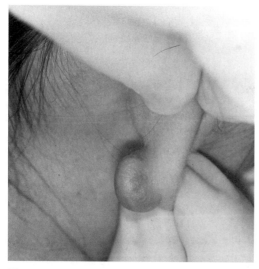

Fig. 11-13.   Preoperative appearance of recurrent keloid on posterior aspect of the earlobe.

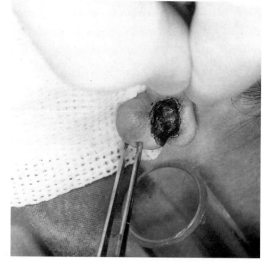

Fig. 11-14.   The focused CO_2 laser is used to remove the keloid without bleeding.

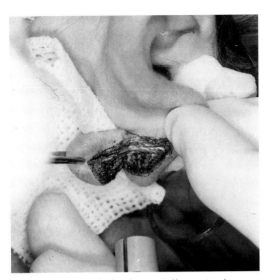

Fig. 11-15. The keloid is initially excised so that it is flush with the surrounding skin surface.

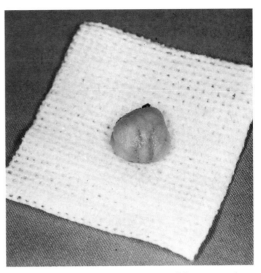

Fig. 11-16. Gross appearance of the excised keloidal mass.

Good results and healing without recurrent keloid formation occur in approximately 50% of patients with keloids removed with the CO$_2$ laser, though a higher cure rate of 80% to 100% is seen for the laser removal of keloids from certain anatomic sites, such as the earlobes and nape of the neck (acne keloidalis nuchae).[51] The reason for the effectiveness of the CO$_2$ laser in the removal of keloids is unclear but may partially result from the fact that it causes minimal injury to the adjacent tissue. It may also partially be due to the lack of tension asso-

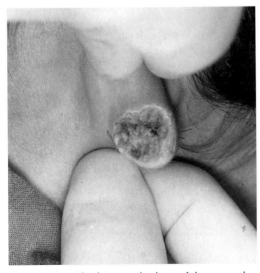

Fig. 11-17. The base and edges of the wound are carefully palpated and inspected for evidence of residual keloid tissue.

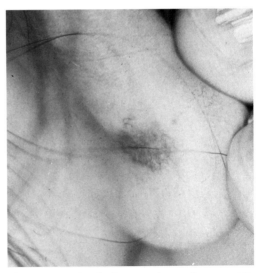

Fig. 11-18. A soft, flat, supple scar is present 8 months after laser excision of earlobe keloid.

ciated with primary wound closure, because all of the lasered wounds are allowed to heal by second intention. Or, it may result from the direct inhibition of fibroblasts by the infrared radiation from the CO_2 laser. With regard to the latter, it has been observed that the low-energy radiation emitted by another infrared laser, the Nd:YAG laser, inhibits collagen synthesis and fibroblast proliferation in tissue culture,[52–57] and perhaps the CO_2 laser works in a similar fashion. Additional laboratory investigations should help to clarify the mechanism by which this therapeutic modality exerts its beneficial effect. Meanwhile, extensive clinical evidence from several different laser centers has shown that this technique is effective for the treatment of keloids.

RHINOPHYMA

Although many techniques have been used in the management of rhinophyma, the bloodless procedure offered by the CO_2 laser affords significant advantages.[58–60] The precise tissue removal without significant bleeding permits complete visualization throughout the procedure. Healing is uneventful, without significant postoperative pain or swelling, and the final cosmetic results compare favorably with those from standard forms of treatment; in fact, laser treatment may cause less scarring than electrosurgery.[61]

PERFORATION OF EXPOSED CRANIAL BONE

The focused energy from the CO_2 laser has also been used successfully to stimulate the growth of granulation tissue over exposed cranial bone by perforating the bone with laser light.[62] Traditional methods previously used to promote the development of granulation tissue over bone denuded of its periosteum (Figs. 11-19 and 11-20) have included boring with a drill, scoring with a chisel, and abrading with a burr. The CO_2 laser can also be used to perforate the outer table of the skull using focused, brief pulses of high-energy light. The technique is rapid and causes minimal patient anxiety and has proved to be very successful. As with the older techniques, however, care must be taken when working with irradiated bone or over the frontal sinuses because of the deeper penetration possible.

The technique involves the delivery of short, 0.1- or 0.05-second pulses of high irradiance (50,000–60,000 W/cm²) in a gridlike fashion every 2 to 3 mm over the surface of the exposed bone. Usually only one or two pulses are required to perforate through the outer table of the skull. Upon perforation, a tiny drop of blood flows through the perforation from the central vascular diploë (Fig. 11-21). Granulation tissue then forms at these perforations, which allows epithelial cells to migrate from the wound margins across the exposed bone (Fig. 11-22). The time it takes for this to occur is both a function of the area of the exposed bone and the quality of wound care provided by the patient.

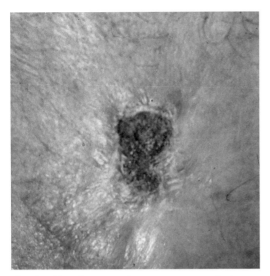

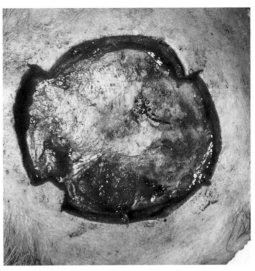

Fig. 11-19. Preoperative appearance of a large, recurrent, morpheaform basal cell carcinoma of the forehead.

Fig. 11-20. The appearance of defect immediately after Mohs' micrographic surgery, showing removal of the periosteum centrally.

Superpulsed CO$_2$ Laser Surgery

Superpulsing may permit CO$_2$ laser excisional surgery to be performed with even less thermal damage to the surrounding tissue than is normally possible.[63] When the CO$_2$ laser is initially activated, a very brief, high-power energy is generated within the optical cavity.

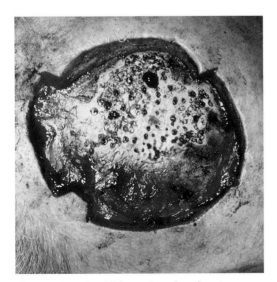

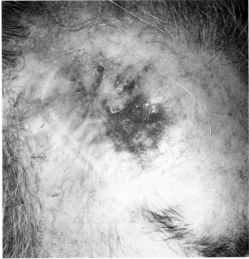

Fig. 11-21. A gridlike series of perforations have been made through the outer table of the skull, resulting in a minute amount of bleeding at each hole.

Fig. 11-22. Nearly complete reepithelialization has occurred by 8 weeks postoperatively.

This is known as a *superpulse*. Some laser systems have been modified to deliver continuous series of superpulses with a high peak energy and short duration.

Conventional CO_2 lasers differ significantly from superpulsed CO_2 lasers, in that they have a much lower peak power and the pulses created by mechanical shutters are consequently of much longer duration, from 0.05 to 0.5 second. Using sophisticated electronic techniques, the superpulsed laser can generate peak powers two to ten times greater than the same laser can ordinarily produce in its continuous mode of operation (Fig. 11-23). The pulses produced by the superpulsed CO_2 lasers are of very short duration, typically from 0.1 to 0.9 msec. Depending on the manufacturer, the repetition rates and pulsewidths in laser systems may be individually selected or they may come preset. Typical repetition rates vary from 200 to 500 Hz, but higher repetition rates are possible, up to 4 or 5 kHz.

Ideally, every laser surgical procedure would involve the use of the shortest energy pulse possible to minimize thermal conduction to adjacent tissues (Fig. 11-24).[64] It has been shown that a temperature rise of only 8°C above normal body temperature is lethal to cells. Consequently, heating results in a zone of thermal necrosis surrounded by an even larger zone of sublethal thermal damage. Both of these zones of damage must undergo repair before the wound can heal.

Because the amount of laser energy required to ablate a given volume of tissue is constant, it would be best to use the highest irradiance that can be precisely controlled and expose the tissue for the shortest time possible to limit inadvertent thermal damage. In conventional CO_2 laser excisional surgery, to rapidly make incisions using high irradiances without heating tissue excessively, the laser must

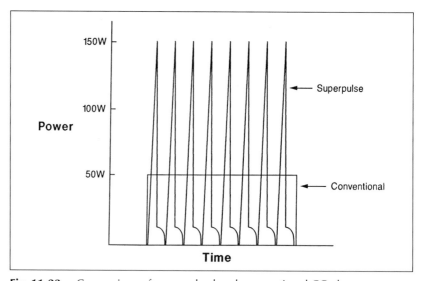

Fig. 11-23. Comparison of superpulsed and conventional CO_2 lasers.

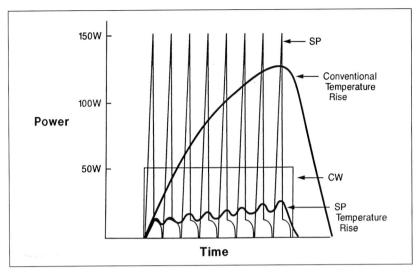

Fig. 11-24. Comparison of thermal injury produced by superpulsed (*SP*) and conventional (*CW*) CO$_2$ lasers.

be moved very quickly to avoid making too deep an incision. However, this results in an obvious reduction in precision. Although both control and precision are improved with the use of lower irradiances, the drawback to this is that there is then significant thermal conduction to adjacent tissue, because the required exposure time is significantly increased[65] and the quantity of heat transferred is primarily a function of the length of exposure.[66]

The precision necessary is possible with the superpulsed laser because of its ability to produce high peak power pulses with short cooling pauses in between. Superpulsing differs from the mechanical technique known as *chopping,* in which short pulses are created using a revolving fenestrated disk. Although chopping can produce very short pulses of laser energy, the peak power levels generated are typical of those generated by conventional CO$_2$ lasers. Superpulsed lasers also differ from Q-switched lasers, which produce high peak powers and pulses of exceeding short duration (often only a nanosecond long), a combination that can result in cellular ionization and the production of thermoacoustic waves in tissue, both of which can have adverse effects.

Part of the control and precision possible with a superpulsed CO$_2$ laser is a function of reducing the total amount of energy delivered to the tissue to only a third of that delivered by a conventional continuous-wave CO$_2$ laser. This is a function of the duty cycle, or the percentage of time the laser is actually emitting energy, and is calculated as the product of the pulse duration times the repetition rate. A standard duty cycle for a superpulsed CO$_2$ laser is 10%, but this may range from 2% to 50%. The prime advantage of delivering these high-energy, short-duration superpulses is that the target tissue can cool during the off phase, or pause cycle, between each pulse. This simultaneously minimizes inadvertent thermal damage by reducing the average power delivered (Fig. 11-25) and improves precision. Even finer precision can be achieved by reducing the duty cycle of a superpulsed laser further by pulsing the superpulses. This causes an interruption in the usual delivery of superpulses at regular intervals by introducing additional pauses in the chain of pulses.

The pulse duration and repetition rate selected depend on the type of surgery being performed, the anatomic location, its associated vascularity, and the surgeon's preference. If the pulses are too closely spaced, there may be insufficient time for tissue to cool and the resultant thermal damage may be identical to that produced by conventional continuous-wave CO_2 lasers. On the other hand, if the pulses are too short or the repetition rate too low, the quality of the hemostasis obtained will be markedly reduced. The incision will also proceed even more slowly, because only a small amount of energy is then being delivered.

Although it is well known that minimizing thermal damage and reducing inadvertent wound edge necrosis during excisional surgical procedures are best accomplished through the use of a superpulsed laser generating high peak power with short pulse durations, the ideal surgical parameters for superpulsed lasers have not been scientifically determined. However, employing the shortest possible pulse duration at the lowest possible frequency theoretically seems sound as a way to limit thermal conduction to surrounding tissue. In summary, the major advantage to using superpulsed lasers to incise tissue surgically is the precise and controlled way in which they do it, and this is because they deliver only a fraction of the energy delivered by a continuous-wave laser. Additional benefits of superpulsing have also been demonstrated for the incision of noncutaneous tissues, and these include more rapid wound healing, less inflammation, and a quantitative reduction in scarring.

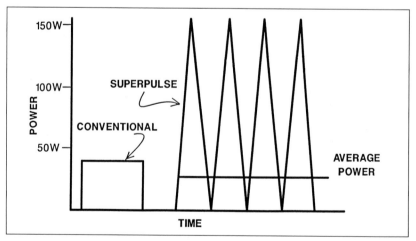

Fig. 11-25.   Comparison of average power of superpulsed and conventional CO_2 lasers.

Combined Laser Excision and Vaporization

In certain situations the CO_2 laser can be used to greatest effect by employing both the incisional and the vaporizational modes. In this way, the focused, high-irradiance CO_2 laser energy can be used first to bloodlessly debulk excess soft tissue, such as in the treatment of rhinophyma or large, benign appendageal tumors (Figs. 11-26 and 11-27).[67] Then the defocused, low-irradiance CO_2 laser energy can be used precisely to more superficially ablate residual areas of persistent excess soft tissue or small residual foci of appendageal tumors (Fig. 11-28). The wounds created are allowed to heal by second intention (Fig. 11-29), and the cosmetic result obtained is excellent because of the minimal thermal injury involved.

Recent Advances in Excisional Laser Surgery

TISSUE WELDING

When a lower level of laser energy, in the range of 50 to 150 W/cm^2, is delivered to the edges of an incised wound, the thermal effect is sufficient to cause protein coagulation. The coagulum is of sufficient strength to weld the wound together.[68] This laser welding technique has been performed successfully on small blood vessels,[69,70] nerves, urethras, fallopian tubes, and skin.[71,72]

The technique involves first the approximation of the wound edges with forceps or absorbable sutures and then irradiation of the edges with brief pulses of lower-energy laser light. Several different

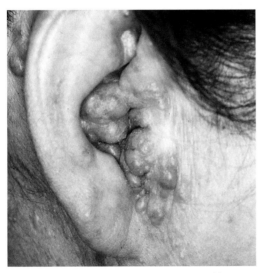

Fig. 11-26. Pretreatment appearance of large trichoepitheliomas that occlude external auditory canal.

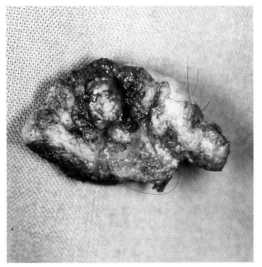

Fig. 11-27. Gross appearance of pathologic tissue excised with laser to debulk the treatment site in a bloodless fashion.

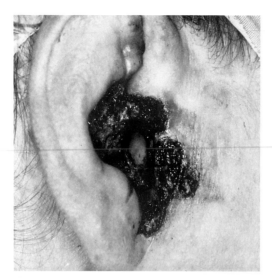

Fig. 11-28. Superficial laser vaporization has reopened ear canal and removed small foci of trichoepitheliomas from concha and preauricular area.

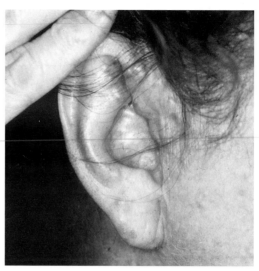

Fig. 11-29. Final appearance 4 months after combined laser excision and vaporization.

lasers have been used to weld cutaneous wounds, but four in particular are capable of creating a functional tissue weld when used in this fashion. These include the argon laser,[73] CO_2 laser,[73] Nd:YAG laser[73,74] at 1060 nm, and the Nd:YAG laser at 1320 nm. It certainly appears that the CO_2 laser could be used to not only bloodlessly incise skin and soft tissue at a high irradiance but then subsequently to weld the wound edges together at a low irradiance.

NEAR-INFRARED LASER INCISIONS

Recently, synthetic sapphire tips have been coupled to optical fibers from a Nd:YAG laser to enable the delivery of near-infrared laser energy to tissue in a direct-contact fashion.[75] These tips come in a variety of sizes and shapes[76] and enable the precise focusing of the Nd:YAG laser energy so that the Nd:YAG laser can be used as another type of light scalpel to excise tissue in a relatively bloodless fashion. The biggest advantage of this instrumentation over CO_2 laser systems is the ease with which fiberoptics can be used, in comparison with articulating arms. However, much additional work showing other potential benefits of the technique is necessary before the CO_2 laser can be relegated to a secondary status in the performance of cutaneous surgery. Until then, it is anticipated that many more useful applications of the CO_2 laser as a cutting tool will be found.

References

1. Bailin PL, Ratz JL, Wheeland RG. Laser therapy of the skin: a review of principles and applications. Dermatol Clin 1987;5:259–285.
2. Wheeland RG, Walker NPJ. Lasers—twenty-five years later. Int J Dermatol 1986;25:209–216.
3. Kaplan I. Current CO$_2$ laser surgery. Plast Reconstr Surg 1982;69:552–555.
4. Fisher JC. The power density of a surgical laser beam: its meaning and measurement. Lasers Surg Med 1983;2:301–315.
5. Koranda FC, Grande DJ, Whitaker DC et al. Laser surgery in the medically comprised patient. J Dermatol Surg Oncol 1982;8:471–474.
6. Ben-Bassat M, Ben-Bassat M, Kaplan I. An ultrastructural study of the cut edges of skin and mucous membrane specimens excised by carbon dioxide laser. In Kaplan I, ed. Laser surgery. New York: Academic Press, 1976:95–100.
7. Ben-Bassat M, Ben-Bassat M, Kaplan I. A study of the ultrastructural features of the cut margin of skin and mucous membranes specimens excised by carbon dioxide laser. J Surg Res 1976;21:77–84.
8. Arndt KA, Noe JM, Northam DBC, Itzkan I. Laser therapy: basic concepts and nomenclature. J Am Acad Dermatol 1981;5:649–654.
9. Huether SE. How lasers work. AORN J 1983;38:207–215.
10. Sliney DH. Laser-tissue interactions. Clin Chest Med 1985;6:203–208.
11. Rontal M, Rontal E, Fuller T, Jacob HJ. Flexible nontoxic fiberoptic delivery system for the carbon dioxide laser. Ann Otol Rhinol Laryngol 1985;94:357–360.
12. Fuller TA. Mid-infrared fiber optics. Lasers Surg Med 1986;6:399–403.
13. Katzir A, Weiss R. Advances in infrared fibers. Laser Optronics 1988;7:29–37.
14. Shenfeld O, Ophir E, Goldwasser B et al. Silver halide fiber optic radiometric temperature measurement and control of CO$_2$ laser–irradiated tissues and application to tissue welding. Lasers Surg Med 1994;14:323–328.
15. Gannot I, Dror J, Calderon S et al. Flexible waveguides for IR laser radiation and surgery applications. Lasers Surg Med 1994;14:184–189.
16. Apfelberg DB, Maser MR, Lash H, Druker D. CO$_2$ laser resection for giant perineal condyloma and verrucous carcinoma. Ann Plast Surg 1983;11:417–422.
17. Ascher PW, Ingolitsch E, Walter G et al. Ultrastructural findings in CNS tissue with CO$_2$ laser. In: Kaplan I, ed: Laser surgery II. Jerusalem: Jerusalem Academic Press, 1978:81–90.
18. Baker S, Muenzler WS, Small RG, Leonard JE. Carbon dioxide laser blepharoplasty. Ophthalmology 1984;91:238–243.
19. David LM, Sanders G. CO$_2$ laser blepharoplasty: a comparison to cold steel and electrocautery. J Dermatol Surg Oncol 1987;13:110–114.
20. David LM. The laser approach to blepharoplasty. J Dermatol Surg Oncol 1988;14:741–746.
21. Goldman L. Surgery by laser for malignant melanoma. J Dermatol Surg Oncol 1979;5:141–144.
22. Norris CW, Mullarky MB. Experimental skin incision made with the carbon dioxide laser. Laryngoscope 1982;92:416–419.
23. Hall RR. The healing of tissues incised by a carbon dioxide laser. Br J Surg 1971;58:222–225.

66. Mihashi S, Jako GJ, Incze J et al. Laser surgery in otolaryngology: interaction of CO_2 laser and soft tissue. Ann NY Acad Sci 1976;267:264–294.
67. Wheeland RG, Bailin PL, Kronberg E. Carbon dioxide (CO_2) laser vaporization for the treatment of trichoepitheliomata. Dermatol Surg Oncol 1984;10:470–475.
68. Garden JM, Robinson JK, Taute PM et al. The low-output carbon dioxide laser for cutaneous wound closure of scalpel incisions: comparative tensile strength studies of the laser to the suture and staple for wound closure. Laser Surg Med 1986;6:67–71.
69. Quigley MR, Bailes JE, Kwaan HC et al. Microvascular anastomosis using the milliwatt CO_2 laser. Lasers Surg Med 1985;5:357–365.
70. White RA, Abergel RP, Klein SR et al. Laser welding of venotomies. Arch Surg 1986;121:905–907.
71. Robinson JK, Garden JM, Taute PM et al. Wound healing in porcine skin following low-output carbon dioxide laser irradiation of the incision. Ann Plast Surg 1987;18:499–505.
72. Rooke CT, Dix PP, Choma TJ et al. CO_2 laser welding versus conventional microsuture repair in patch-graft urethroplasty. Urology 1993; 41:585–589.
73. Abergel RP, Lyons R, Dwyer R et al. Use of lasers for closure of cutaneous wounds: experience with Nd:YAG, argon and CO_2 lasers. J Dermatol Surg Oncol 1986;12:1181–1185.
74. Abergel RP, Lyons R, Dwyer R et al. Skin closure by Nd:YAG laser welding. J Am Acad Dermatol 1986;14:810–814.
75. Rockwell RJ Jr, Moss CE. Hazard zones and eye protection requirements for a frosted surgical probe used with an Nd:YAG laser. Lasers Surg Med 1989;9:45–49.
76. Hukki J, Krogerus L, Castren M, Schroder T. Effects of different contact laser scalpels on skin and subcutaneous fat. Lasers Surg Med 1988;8: 276–282.

12 —— The CO_2 Laser: Use as an Ablative Instrument

Suzanne M. Olbricht

In the treatment of cutaneous disorders, the CO_2 laser is used as a surgical tool for cutting or ablation, that is, the removal of tissues. As discussed in the previous chapter, to cut tissue, the energy of the CO_2 laser is emitted as a tightly focused beam with very high power densities, which produces highly localized thermal destruction that can be precisely directed using a terminal attachment. If the CO_2 laser beam is unfocused and of a lower power density, it can be directed with precision to ablate through the processes of vaporization and coagulative necrosis. As an ablating tool, the CO_2 laser is used primarily when a very thin, localized, superficial strip of tissue destruction is desired and healing by second intention is assumed. Wound healing results in the formation of a scar that may be nonapparent, minimal, atrophic, or hypertrophic, depending on the depth and volume of the damage attained and the body location of the thermal injury. The purpose of this chapter is to review the characteristics of the CO_2 laser and the laser energy-tissue interactions that effect ablation and to describe the technique of ablation, plus its indications and complications.

Instrumentation

The construction of the CO_2 laser is similar to that of other lasers. The components consist of the main laser resonating cavity, auxiliary laser systems such as a helium-neon (He-Ne) laser, an energy source, a delivery system, and a control panel. The resonating cavity contains the gain medium, composed of a mixture of CO_2, nitrogen, and helium gases. The CO_2 molecules are the active component; the other gases are added to improve energy transfer within the CO_2 molecule. The He-Ne laser is mounted with the same axis as the CO_2 laser. It serves as an aiming beam, because the CO_2 laser beam is invisible. The energy source is either an electrically or radio-frequency–stimulated system, depending on the type of waveform to be produced. Transmission of the laser beam from the resonating cavity to the tissue is provided by an articulated arm system, consisting of a series of hollow rigid tubes with reflecting mirrors at each connection. At the end of the rigid tubes is either a handpiece or a microscope with a micromanipulator. The beam is focused through a lens in the terminal attachment, and a large variety of focal lengths and spot sizes at the focal point can be supplied. Handpieces often have removable guides that mark the focal point. The spot size, focal length, and focusing and unfocusing of the beam are therefore controlled at the terminus. The power output and beam type are adjusted on the control panel on the main unit. The length of time the beam is delivered is controlled at several sites. All lasers have several on-off switches for safety purposes; generally these include a lock, a mechanism on the control panel, another mechanism to regulate shutter duration on the control panel, a switch on the articulated arm, and, as a final control, a foot pedal or an off-on button on the terminal end of the delivery system.

At one time, CO_2 lasers were the size and weight of refrigerators, with cumbersome articulated arms, fragile mirror systems, and large handpieces. However, recent technological advances have made it possible to produce small, relatively inexpensive, dependable, low-power desktop models supplying 15 to 25 W of power and floor models supplying 30 to 100 W of power, but taking up less than 2 square feet of floor space. Delivery systems have also evolved, such that now the articulated arms and small handpieces are less bulky, more mobile, more easily manipulated, and less susceptible to misalignment. Some low-power lasers deliver the beam through a semiflexible thin tube, called a *waveguide,* which is somewhat similar in size and shape to fiberoptic delivery systems. One manufacturer has produced a desktop model that has the main resonating cavity within the handpiece itself. Controls are now computerized and involve the use of light-touch keypads instead of awkward knobs. These allow instantaneous, precise determinations of the power output and the theoretical power density at tissue level. New handpieces have also been devised, the most unique of which transmits an unfocused beam with a spot size of 3 mm. The beam has also been coupled to computer-driven scanners, which produce precise geometric patterns.

The CO_2 laser produces a beam of energy in the far-infrared portion of the electromagnetic spectrum at 10,600 nm. This beam of energy may be emitted as a continuous wave, a shuttered continuous wave, or a pulsed wave (Fig. 12-1). A continuous-wave beam is one that has little or no variation in the power output over time. The laser operator controls the duration of the beam with shutters, which may be opened or closed to either permit the beam to exit from the laser cavity or to obstruct it. An internal shutter with an electronic control is usually provided; it may be set to open for 0.01 second to several seconds, depending on the model. A repetitive series of shuttered beam exposures may also be produced. Sometimes the shuttered beam is referred to as a *pulse,* but technically this is a misleading term. A true pulse has a much higher energy peak within a much briefer emission and affects tissue differently from a shut-

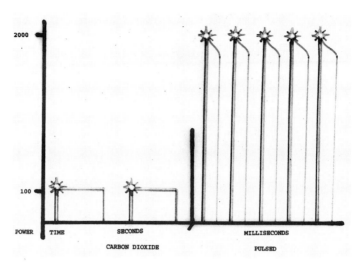

Fig. 12-1. Waveforms of CO$_2$ laser beams.

tered beam of constant, albeit brief, energy, even if the average powers are the same. In another mechanical technique, called *chopping*, fanlike devices are used that revolve at different frequencies to produce very short bursts of continuous-wave energy.

Pulsed CO$_2$ lasers produce a train of very short pulses with a high peak power by means of radio-frequency excitation. The superpulse waveform was the first pulsed CO$_2$ laser beam to be engineered for medical purposes. Pulse durations typically range from 0.1 to 0.9 millisecond with repetition rates of 1 to 5000 pulses per second. Some models allow the pulsewidth and repetition rate to be selected; in others the duration is preset to vary with the average power desired. The peak powers achieved are two to ten times those achieved by a continuous-wave beam; the average powers are similar. Duty cycles, or the time in which the laser beam is produced, range from 2% to 50%. A second duty cycle, created mechanically with a shutter, can, however, also be superimposed to create a short burst of 10 or more pulses. A modification of the superpulsed CO$_2$ laser, the Ultrapulse, has pulse energies five to seven times higher than those of conventional superpulsed lasers, with a peak pulse power of greater than 450 W, an energy per pulse of up to 250 mJ, and an average power of up to 100 W. The pulsewidth is less than a millisecond. Even with a pulse spot size as large as 2.5 mm, it can deliver 5 J/cm^2 per pulse. The transversally excited atmospheric (TEA) CO$_2$ laser has been used for industrial purposes and in medical research to study the tissue effects of pulsed energy. Its peak pulse power is similar to those of other pulsed CO$_2$ lasers, but it produces extremely brief pulses of 2 to 10 µsec in duration, with the initial energy peak occurring in less than half of a microsecond. The pulse repetition rate may be set from 1 to 100 pulses per second.

Principles of Laser-Tissue Interactions

Tissue injury begins when the CO_2 laser energy is absorbed by water in the tissue, producing heat. With a pulse energy of more than 5 J/cm², tissue water is heated instantaneously to a temperature greater than the boiling point. This rapid heating causes tissue structures to explode as the result of the effects of shock waves, cavitation, and rapid thermal expansion, and thereby vaporizes tissue into a plume containing tissue components and water (see Chap. 3). The heat also diffuses through the adjacent tissues. Tissue immediately adjacent to the site of vaporization heats to between 50°C and 100°C. Either denaturation or the irreversible coagulation of proteins may occur, depending on the duration of exposure to heat at these temperatures. Epidermal components respond uniformly to heating, but the dermal components respond variably, with type I collagen fibers, the major architectural element, being the most sensitive. Tissue heated to less than 50°C generally recovers completely. If the energy used is below the minimum necessary to induce vaporization, tissue coagulates and desiccates. With prolonged exposure, heat accumulates slowly and temperatures of 300° to 600°C may result,[1] creating extensive peripheral thermal damage secondary to thermal diffusion. Char results from the burning of tissue at greater than 300°C. Therefore, grossly and microscopically, three zones of damage may be identified around the site of vaporization: carbonized eschar, coagulative necrosis, and a sheath of edema (Fig. 12-2).[2] Beyond the edema, there is a sharp transition to normal tissue. Although CO_2 laser energy may produce other phenomena in tissues adjacent to the site of vaporization, such as mechanical (flow of hot liquefied materials)[3] or photochemical effects, thermal damage appears to be the most significant. Tissue affected by coagulative necrosis is either

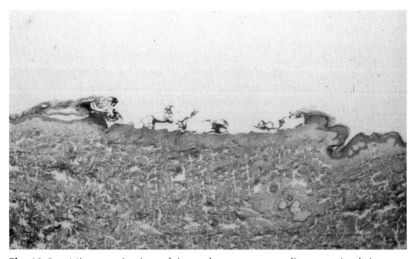

Fig. 12-2. Microscopic view of tissue damage surrounding vaporized site.

sloughed or resorbed and remodeled during wound healing. The repair processes are similar to those occurring after other thermal injuries. Clinically speaking, ablation of tissue occurs through the processes of vaporization as well as coagulative necrosis and subsequent repair.

CO$_2$ laser energy penetrates only about 20 μm into water (see Chap. 3). In tissue, however, penetration is affected by scattering (minimal at this wavelength), the exposure spot size, the duration of exposure, and the proportion of water within the tissue.[3] Accurate direct measurements of penetration profiles inside living skin are not available and have only been approximated on the basis of in vitro measurements and theories regarding the optical properties of the skin. It is commonly quoted that the energy of the CO$_2$ laser penetrates less than 0.2 mm into the skin.[4–6] More precise calculations have been determined on the basis of the tissue damage that has been seen in response to a total energy dose in a guinea pig model. This has yielded the finding that a beam with a power density of 10 kW/cm^2, easily obtained by a 30-W, commercially available CO$_2$ laser, takes 12.5 msec to penetrate 1 mm of skin in vivo and a beam with a power density of 1 kW/cm^2 takes 125 msec to do so.[3] These speeds cannot be controlled manually, so for most clinical uses, it is assumed that the laser energy penetrates more than 1 mm.

The volume of tissue vaporized varies directly with the power density at the tissue level. The width of the zone of thermal damage of adjacent tissue, however, is directly proportional to the duration of the exposure. If exposure times are shorter than the time it takes the heated tissue to cool, adjacent thermal damage is minimized, because there is no excessive heat energy available for diffusion.[7] Therefore, a short laser exposure time with a high-power density vaporizes the same volume of tissue as a longer exposure at a lower power density, but with much less adjacent thermal damage (Fig. 12-3). This has been confirmed in a study utilizing a guinea pig model in which the width of the histologically evident tissue damage was found to be relatively constant over a wide range of power densities administered in the same exposure time but shorter exposure times were found to lead to diminished tissue damage.[3] The tissue damage observed ranged from 50 μm (2-μsec pulse) to 750 μm (50-msec pulse) from the crater.[8] Continuous-wave lasers, moved manually across the skin, have been found to produce tissue damage ranging from 100 μm to 2 mm beyond the incision.[9–11] In addition, tissue-damaging temperature elevations have been recorded as far as 2 mm from the wound edge.[9]

Tissue effects, both vaporization and adjacent tissue damage, are therefore related to absorption, heat diffusion, and the continuing process of vaporization and dehydration, allowing more absorption and diffusion. These factors relate to the power density and duration of exposure. In practical terms the control of ablation, as well as control of the residual wound and partial control of the resulting scar, depend on a variety of factors within the command of the surgeon. A

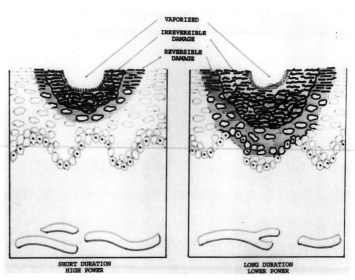

Fig. 12-3. Comparison of thermal damage varying with power and duration for same power density at tissue level.

knob or touchpad control on the main laser unit is used to vary the power output. The spot size may be altered by changing the handpiece and focusing lens or by modifying the distance the handpiece is held from the skin surface (Fig. 12-4). The duration of exposure to the laser beam may be adjusted by shuttering, moving, or both, the handpiece more or less quickly across the skin surface. The true pulsed waveforms represent further ways to modify the duration of exposure, such that, for any given average power, laser energy is pro-

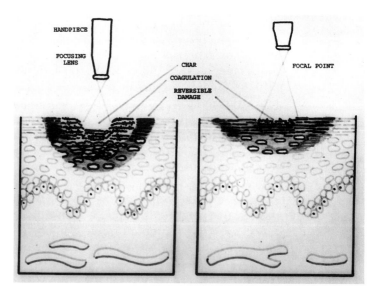

Fig. 12-4. Comparison of thermal damage varying with spot size and distance of handpiece from the skin for the same power output.

duced for a shorter time. The surgeon therefore has many ways of exerting delicate control over the type and amount of destruction produced.

Wound Healing

As already noted, the ablation produced by the CO$_2$ laser occurs through the processes of vaporization and coagulative necrosis and is modified by the process of wound healing. Wound healing can be divided into three distinct phases: inflammatory, proliferative, and maturational. The inflammatory phase occurs within the first 3 to 10 days after wounding and is characterized by vasodilatation and increased vascular permeability and by white blood cell migration, first polymorphonuclear leukocytes, then monocytes and macrophages, and then lymphocytes. The molecular biologic events that occur during healing have been relatively well characterized.[12] The proliferative phase overlaps with the inflammatory phase and generally begins 1 to 2 days after wounding and lasts a minimum of 10 to 14 days. After this, reepithelialization, neoangiogenesis, and fibroblast proliferation occur, and granulation tissue becomes clinically evident. As early as 2 days after injury, fibroblasts produce type III collagen in a gel-like consistency, together with proteoglycans and elastin. Collagen eventually constitutes more than 50% of the newly formed scar. As the proliferative phase comes to an end, the tensile strength of the scar may be only 5% of its original strength.[13] Also during this phase, the wound contracts as a result of the production of specialized contractile proteins by modified myofibroblasts. During the maturational phase, which begins 2 to 3 weeks after wounding and continues lifelong to some extent, the type III collagen gel is replaced by a more stable interwoven form and then by type I collagen. Water and glycosaminoglycans are lost from the wound, leading to the compression of collagen fibers, which may then cross-link more effectively. The tensile strength continues to improve, although it is never more than 80% as strong as the original skin. This phase is a continuing process of remodeling, involving the synthesis of new collagen and the degradation of old collagen by tissue-specific collagenases. Wound healing therefore constitutes a series of processes that produce a scar, which shares many of the features of preexisting normal skin.

The wound healing occurring after laser surgery differs somewhat from that occurring after conventional scalpel surgery. As previously noted, at the conclusion of surgery, three zones of damage may be present: carbonized eschar (char), coagulation necrosis, and a sheath of edema. Grossly visible eschar is usually removed manually at the time of surgery by wiping the area with a wet gauze. The zone of coagulation necrosis widens over the first few days,[14] then begins to slough. Within 6 to 7 days, the wound has a bed of granulation tissue and reepithelialization begins. The onset of epidermal migration is somewhat delayed, as opposed to that which occurs in scalpel-created wounds, but the rate of epidermal migration is not decreased.[15–19] Laser-, scalpel-, and electrosurgically created wounds all begin to contract at the same time.[20] The tensile strength of laser incisions made using a continuous-wave CO_2 laser has been noted to be less than that of scalpel incisions during the first 1 to 3 weeks, but both types of wounds reach a maximal strength around 3 months, and this is not significantly different between the two.[18,21,22]

Of note, in most studies of the wound healing that occurs after either incision or ablation by the CO_2 laser, either the power density or duration of delivery has not been specified or controlled. In addition, in reports of some studies, it has not been noted whether eschar was removed manually at the conclusion of the procedure, even though it is known that the presence of scab retards reepithelialization.[22] Two studies performed using gynecologic tissues have demonstrated more rapid healing of superpulsed CO_2 laser–created incisions than incisions created using continuous-waveform lasers or electrosurgery.[24,25] A comparison of the epithelialization of middermal wounds created by ablation with a superpulsed CO_2 laser controlled by a mechanical scanning device with wounds produced by a dermatome showed a significant reduction in the reepithelialization of laser-created wounds as opposed to dermatome-cut wounds on day 3, but complete recovery by day 14.[26] Of note, the surface of the laser-created wound was dry and remained dry under the dressing, while the dermatome wound was moist and probably remained moist under the dressing, despite the known retarding effect of dryness on reepithelialization.[22] No comparison was made with a similar wound created by controlled continuous-wave energy. Although it seems apparent that the use of optimal treatment parameters would improve healing in wounds created by ablation with the CO_2 laser, studies documenting this have not been done yet. Likewise, no improvement in the tissue healing of wounds created with a superpulsed CO_2 laser as opposed to a continuous-wave beam has been adequately demonstrated, even though a strong case can be made for this on theoretical grounds.[1,27]

Technique

The basic technique for using the CO_2 laser as an ablative instrument is given in Table 12-1. Tissue vaporization is occurring when an opalescent bubbling of the skin surface is seen. This bubbling is associated with a crackling or popping sound. Although these phenomena are said to indicate that epidermis has been ablated,[28] they probably represent the initial explosion of any tissue lying on the surface. Subsequent passes over the same site with the laser beam may not be accompanied by as much bubbling or noise, because the tissue has by then been heated and desiccated somewhat and explodes with less vigor. When the tissue fragments and thin coagulum are wiped away, an intact pinkish white base may be found in the epi-

Table 12-1. Technique for ablation

1. Surgical plan: determine desired end-point.
2. Preparation of site: lesion and necessary margins may be outlined with surgical marking pen and cleaned with normal saline.
3. Anesthesia: local, regional, or general.
4. Draping: wet sponges for prevention of inadvertent burns.
5. Power output setting: 4 to 30 W, depending on lesion and site.
6. Waveform: continuous-wave, shuttered, or superpulsed beam.
7. Spot size at the tissue surface: 0.5- to 5-mm-diameter defocused beam, depending on distance of handpiece from tissue surface.
8. Vaporization with beam defocused:
   a. Continuous-wave or superpulsed beam used with airbrushlike movements, or
   b. Shuttered beam directed to single site.
9. Debridement: wipe with wet sponge (saline, sterile water, hydrogen peroxide) to clean off tissue fragments, char, or coagulum.
10. Repeat treatment: vaporization and debridement repeated as necessary to achieve desired end-point.
11. Surgical dressing: appropriate for size and site of wound.
12. Postoperative instructions for wound care: appropriate for size and site of wound.

dermis if the lesion is thick or within the superficial dermis with normal dermatoglyphic markings if the lesion is thin. Visible contraction of the tissue occurs when the dermis is vaporized or heated. When a coarse, woven pattern of collagen bundles is seen, this indicates that the base of the crater is in the deep dermis. If this plane is penetrated, grapelike globules of yellowish fat will protrude. Charring should usually be avoided, because, as already noted, it denotes slow tissue burning at very high temperatures, producing heat diffusion to surrounding tissues, rather than vaporization.

The surgeon depends on visual feedback, either accomplished by gross inspection or through an operating microscope, to gauge the depth of vaporization and the degree of surrounding tissue damage and may continuously vary the power density by changing the power output, spot size, duration of delivery, or speed of movement. He or she therefore has an instrument that can be easily and rapidly adjusted to meet the conditions posed by each specific site, lesion, or wound, even as the wound changes throughout the procedure. Limitations to this technique include its dependence on the ability of the surgeon to accurately judge the depth of the lesion, the inability to precisely calculate power densities and the duration of exposure for each treatment, and the inability of the same surgeon to reduplicate precisely the treatment at another time, much less the readers of the surgeon's description of the procedure. Two investigators[29] attempted to rectify the situation by biopsying several different small lesions in three different patients, judging the depth of the lesions histologically, and calibrating the laser to produce craters of a precise width and depth in a single pulse. The power output of the laser was kept constant, but the duration of the pulse was varied. The maximum depth of the crater was studied histologically, but the amount of adjacent thermal damage was not mentioned. Although the results appeared to be satisfactory and this approach may be more reproducible, it is also cumbersome and is not used widely in clinical practice.

Efforts to control the volume of tissue ablated initially led to the use of low-power densities, and it was documented that the scar is indeed smaller when a single pulse of laser energy at a lower power density is delivered, as opposed to a single pulse of laser energy of the same duration but at a higher power.[30] However, this is not relevant clinically, because low power densities used for longer durations produce more thermal damage to adjacent tissues, leading to more pain postoperatively and slower wound healing. Because the endpoint of any ablative procedure is eradication of the lesion, the optimal power density is that which is just high enough to achieve rapid vaporization of the complete lesion but low enough for the surgeon to control. An experienced surgeon who applies this principle, using a laser model which he or she is accustomed to, with manual control of the handpiece, is likely to achieve good, consistent results. The empiric technique with this modification has become standard, despite its limitations, primarily because of its ease and flexibility.

The CO_2 laser has been used to selectively damage normal epidermis, using very low fluences (low power densities delivered in a brief, shuttered beam) less than the vaporization threshold of 5 J/cm2.[31,32] However, this epidermal damage is not a laser-specific injury but instead results from heat transfer and can be reproduced by a hot water bath or heated copper template.[33,34] Because the therapeutic range for this type of injury is narrow, delivery of low fluence requires an attention to detail. The power output, spot size, duration of exposure, and distance from the cutaneous surface must be precisely controlled, taking into account the focal length and beam profile of the model being used. Overlapping pulses produce cumulative effects.[3,35] This technique is not a freehand procedure. Treatment produces a brief erythematous flare and sometimes a gray cast to the surface, but no vaporization, char, or coagulum is appreciable. It produces sharp but brief pain, and anesthesia is not required, unlike all other procedures in which the CO_2 laser is used.

If extremely superficial ablation is desired, lateral damage is limited and the technique improved by utilizing a pulsed CO_2 laser and a handpiece in which the beam is not focused or a computerized pattern is generated (see Chap. 13). As noted previously, a pulsed CO_2 laser beam may deliver the same power density as a continuous-wave beam but the train of pulses produces a high peak power, which maximizes tissue vaporization, and a short pulse duration, which minimizes thermal injury. Beam parameters must be set carefully, however. If repetition rates of more than 1000/sec are set, the pulsed laser then duplicates the tissue effects of a continuous-wave laser. Conversely, if the repetition rate is too low, the threshold for vaporization is not reached. The ideal repetition rate for producing vaporization without unwanted thermal damage has been calculated to be between 50 and 100/sec.[36] The Ultrapulse can deliver enough energy for vaporization to occur in a single pulse with a spot size of 2.5 mm and is easiest to control if delivered with a low repetition rate and shuttered into brief bursts of energy.[27] A pulsed laser causes much less charring but does produce pinkish white discoloration of the surface. Pulsing has been shown to allow better control of the thermal damage in animal models,[25,37] and the Ultrapulse has its proponents,[27] but improvement in the clinical results from ablative surgery has been described only in isolated case reports.[27,38,39] Improved results are certainly not guaranteed, because few cutaneous processes have a uniform depth throughout and ablation still depends on visual inspection by the surgeon.

Three different types of lesions can be used to illustrate the varying ways in which the principles of laser-tissue interaction are applied in laser surgical procedures. For instance, the treatment of actinic cheilitis requires superficial tissue injury—coagulative necrosis of the mucosa is enough, because the ensuing tissue slough removes the atypical cells and they are then replaced with clinically and histologically normal mucosa during normal wound healing (Table 12-2; Fig. 12-5).[40] Brief pulses of energy are used to precisely remove syringomas located in a critical area, the eyelid (Table 12-3; Fig. 12-6). The treatment of thick plantar warts, however, sometimes requires vigorous deep and wide destruction to prevent recurrence (Table 12-4; Fig. 12-7). The precise techniques for ablating a variety

Table 12-2.   Technique for treatment of actinic cheilitis

1. Surgical plan: end-point desired is coagulation or white discoloration of entire external lower mucosal lip.
2. Preparation of site: vermilion border may be outlined with surgical marking pen.
3. Anesthesia: mental block with 2% lidocaine, plain. Additional 3 ml of 1% lidocaine with epinephrine injected into superficial submucosa, paying particular attention to lateral commissures.
4. Draping: wet sponge over teeth and cutaneous lower lip.
5. Power output setting: 10 to 12 W.
6. Waveform: continuous-wave or superpulsed beam.
7. Spot size: defocused beam with spot size of 4 to 5 mm at tissue surface.
8. Vaporization: move quickly with airbrushlike movements along lower lip, beginning within mouth and working toward vermilion. One or two slightly overlapping passes are generally sufficient. If char is seen, the beam is being moved too slowly.
9. Debridement: wipe with wet sponge if required.
10. Repeat treatment: any thick or particularly scaly areas can be retreated.
11. Dressing: bacitracin ointment.
12. Postoperative instructions: clean twice a day with mild soap and water. Apply bacitracin ointment multiple times throughout the day.

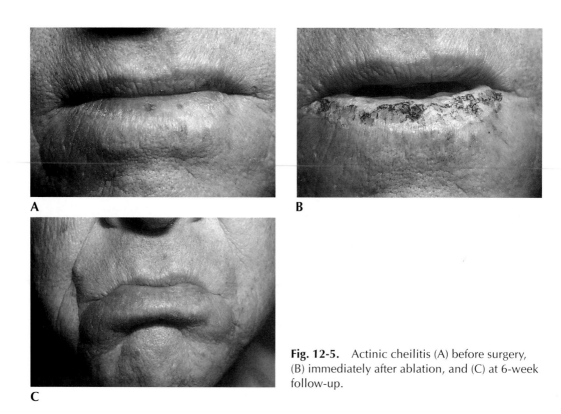

Fig. 12-5.   Actinic cheilitis (A) before surgery, (B) immediately after ablation, and (C) at 6-week follow-up.

Table 12-3.   Technique for treatment of syringomas

1.   Surgical plan: end-point desired is to ablate each lesion to a depth just below the normal skin.
2.   Preparation of site: wipe eyelids clean with normal saline.
3.   Anesthesia: local instillation of small amounts of 2% lidocaine with epinephrine in the superficial subcutaneous tissue. Inject enough to raise a bleb under each lesion.
4.   Draping: protect eye with gauze soaked in saline and/or place plastic corneal shield.
5.   Power output: 10 to 12 W.
6.   Waveform: shuttered continuous-wave beam or shuttered superpulsed beam at 0.1 to 0.2 second.
7.   Spot size: defocused beam with spot size of 2 to 3 mm at tissue surface. Spot size can be adjusted manually to fit the diameter of the lesion.
8.   Vaporization: direct shuttered beam to lesion with one or two "pulses."
9.   Debridement: wipe clean with normal saline.
10.   Repeat treatment: vaporization and debridement as necessary to achieve desired end-point.
11.   Surgical dressing: bacitracin ointment.
12.   Postoperative instructions: clean twice a day with mild soap and water. Apply bacitracin ointment after cleaning.

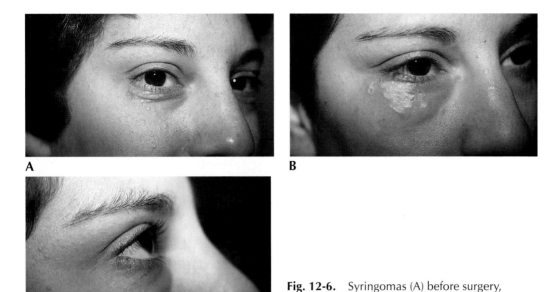

Fig. 12-6. Syringomas (A) before surgery, (B) immediately after surgery, and (C) at 6-month follow-up.

Table 12-4. Technique for treatment of a thick plantar wart

1. Surgical plan: end-point desired is ablation of wart and 5 to 10 mm of surrounding epidermis.
2. Preparation of site: mark margins with surgical marking pen.
3. Anesthesia: local instillation of 2% lidocaine with epinephrine in the superficial cutaneous tissue. Regional anesthesia may be helpful.
4. Draping: protect normal adjacent skin with saline- or water-soaked gauze.
5. Power output: 25 to 30 W.
6. Waveform: continuous-wave or superpulsed beam.
7. Spot size: defocused beam with spot size of 3 to 5 mm at tissue surface.
8. Vaporization: move beam with airbrushlike movements over wart and margins.
9. Debridement: wipe with wet sponge or curette.
10. Repeat treatment: vaporization and debridement as necessary until normal tissue markings in deep dermis are identified. Debridement by scissors may be helpful, because large steam pockets may develop after three or four passes.
11. Surgical dressing: bacitracin ointment, Telfa, and tape.
12. Postoperative instructions: elevation of foot for several days; minimize trauma to the site for several weeks; clean once to twice a day with mild soap and water. Keep covered with bacitracin ointment and dressing.

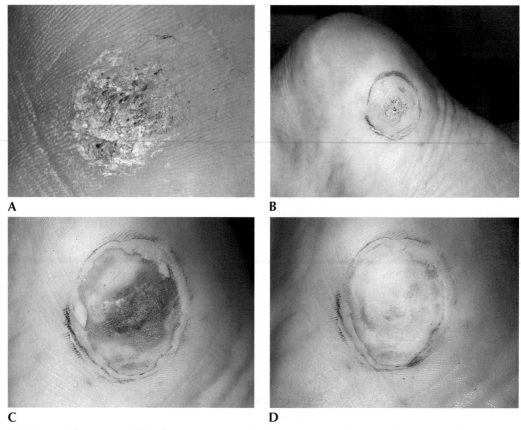

Fig. 12-7. Plantar wart (A) before surgery, (B) after first pass, (C) after several passes, and (D) at conclusion of surgery.

of cutaneous lesions using the CO_2 laser are well described in a recently published atlas and practitioners' guide.[41]

Clinical Applications

Numerous applications of the CO_2 laser in the treatment of cutaneous disorders have been described during the past 20 years. The disorders that can be ablated using a CO_2 laser, either as observed in our laser unit or as reported in the literature, are listed in Table 12-5. Laser treatment is the treatment of choice for some of the disorders, because of its effectiveness, the minimal amount of unwanted adjacent tissue damage produced, and the ease with which it is accomplished. It is used as an alternative tool in the treatment of other disorders, because it can achieve treatment results similar to those of standard surgical modalities, but it facilitates the procedure, making it easier for both the patient and the surgeon. The CO_2 laser also offers an additional therapeutic option for some patients with lesions that have been difficult to treat or responded poorly to standard medical or surgical therapies. A few disorders treated in the 1980s

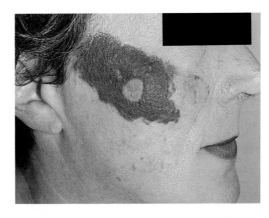

▶**Fig. 5-1.** Test spot within a purple, cobble-stone-surface port-wine stain on the cheek of a woman. The port-wine stain color within the test spot has completely disappeared, leaving a flat, slightly erythematous surface at the same level as that of the normal surrounding skin. The erythema will fade with time. The port-wine stain surrounding the purple area has subsequently been treated. The extensive port-wine stain on the forehead and cheeks is covered with cosmetics. See Fig. 5-1 on p. 74. (Courtesy Joel M. Noe, MD.)

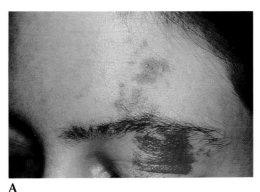
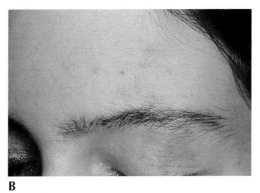

A   B

Fig. 5-2. (A) Red port-wine stain on the eyelid and forehead before treatment with the argon laser. (B) Fading of port-wine stain several months after treatment with the argon laser. There is no textural change. See Fig. 5-2 on p. 75.

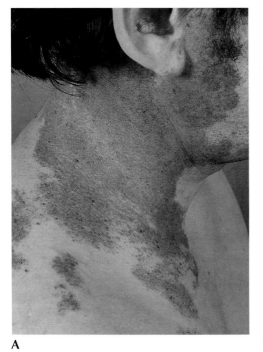
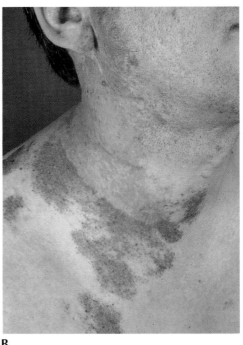

A   B

Fig. 5-3. (A) Port-wine stain on the neck and side of the face before treatment with the argon laser. (B) Results of treatment. There is significant fading with no textural changes. See Fig. 5-3 on p. 76.

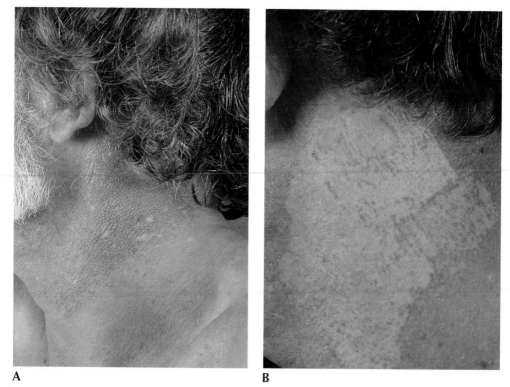

A   B

Fig. 5-5. (A) Poikiloderma of Civatte on the left side of the neck of a fair-skinned man, with considerable photodamage. (B) Striking hypopigmentation at the sites treated with the argon laser. See Fig. 5-5 on p. 77.

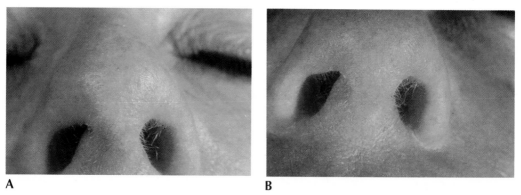

A   B

Fig. 5-6. (A) Spider ectasia on a patient's nose before treatment with the argon laser. (B) Complete disappearance of lesion after therapy. See Fig. 5-6 on p. 82.

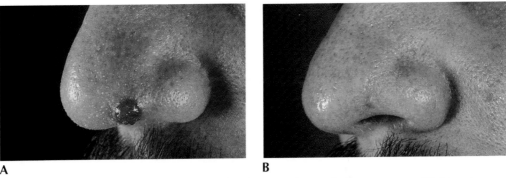

A

B

Fig. 5-8. (A) Kaposi's sarcoma on the left side of a patient's nose before treatment. (B) Almost complete disappearance of the lesion after therapy. See Fig. 5-8 on p. 84.

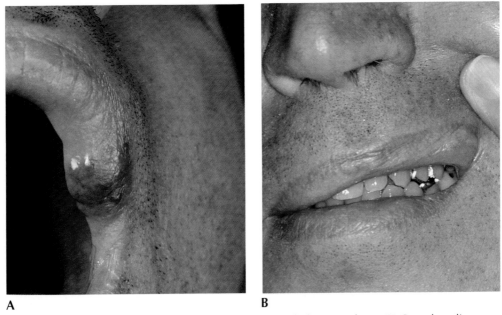

A

B

Fig. 5-9. (A) Large venous lake on lips before therapy with the argon laser. (B) Complete disappearance of the lesion after therapy. See Fig. 5-9 on p. 84.

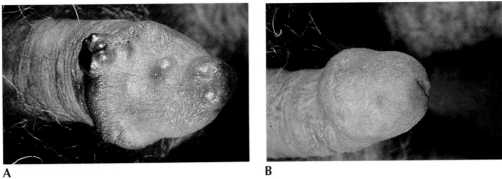

A

B

Fig. 5-10. (A) Vascular malformation on the glans penis before treatment with the argon laser using 1.0-W power with a 1-mm spot size. (B) Complete disappearance of the lesions 6 months after therapy. See Fig. 5-10 on p. 85.

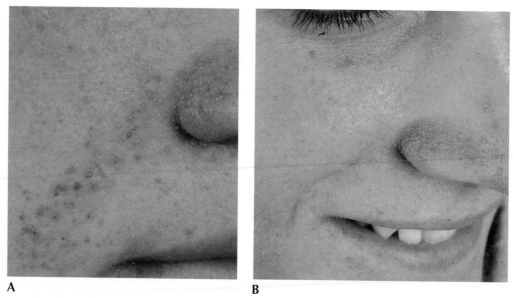

A   B

Fig. 5-12. (A) Papules typical of adenoma sebaceum associated with tuberous sclerosis before argon laser therapy. (B) Complete subsidence of lesions 6 months later. See Fig. 5-12 on p. 87.

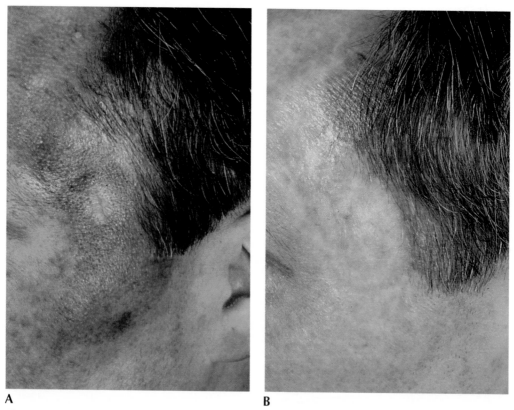

A   B

Fig. 5-13. (A) Nevus of Ota on the left side of a patient's face, showing a marked decrease in pigmentation at the site of an argon laser test site. (B) Appearance after treatment of the entire lesion. There was a striking decrease in pigmentation associated with slight hypopigmentation and atrophy. See Fig. 5-13 on p. 88.

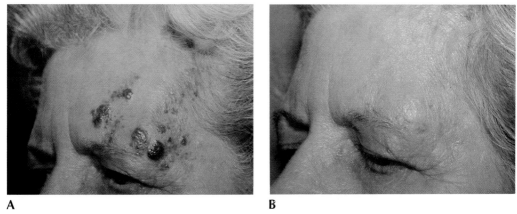

Fig. 5-14. (A) Papular and nodular, purple port-wine stain on the left forehead of a woman before treatment with the copper vapor laser. (B) Good to excellent result when assessed several months later. See Fig. 5-14 on p. 95. (Courtesy of Milton Waner, MD.)

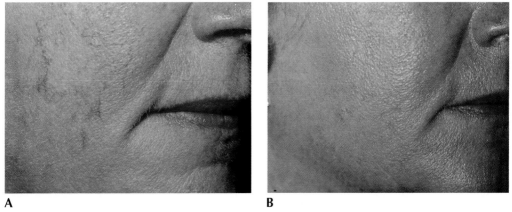

Fig. 5-15. (A) Telangiectasia on the right cheek of a woman before copper vapor laser treatment. (B) Complete disappearance of lesions postoperatively. See Fig. 5-15 on p. 96. (Courtesy of Milton Waner, MD.)

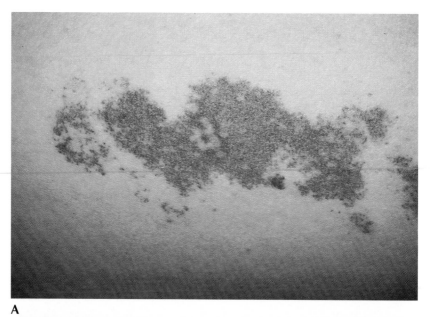

A

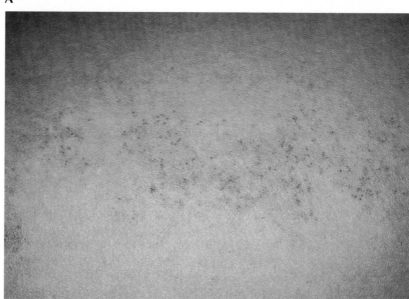

B

Fig. 6-1. (A) Port-wine stain on left thigh of 25-year-old woman. (B) Site after nine treatments with the flashlamp-pumped, pulsed dye laser. See Fig. 6-1 on p. 114.

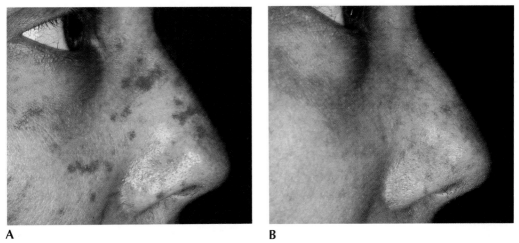

A **B**

Fig. 6-2. (A) Matted telangiectasia on right nose of 35-year-old woman. (B) Site after two treatments with the flashlamp-pumped, pulsed dye laser. See Fig. 6-2 on p. 117.

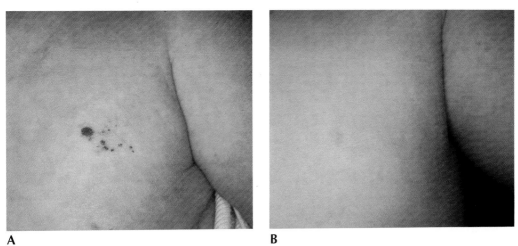

A **B**

Fig. 6-3. (A) Capillary hemangioma, superficial and deep type, in a 2-month-old female infant. (B) Site after five treatments with the flashlamp-pumped, pulsed dye laser. There has been resolution of the superficial component only. See Fig. 6-3 on p. 118.

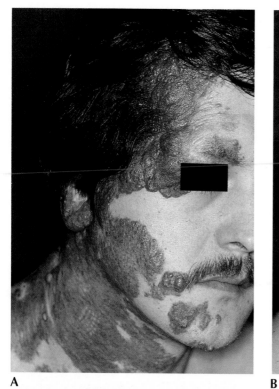

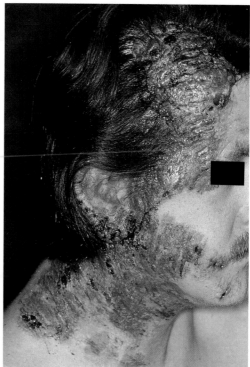

A

B

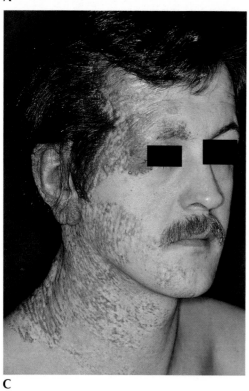

C

Fig. 7-4. Nd:YAG laser treatment of an extensive port-wine stain with angiomatous nodules in a 28-year-old man. (A) Before treatment. (B) Crusting 7 days after treatment. (Spot size, 2 mm; exposure time, 0.5–1.0 second; output power, 30 W.) (C) Result of one treatment with patient under general anesthesia. See Fig. 7-4 on p. 130.

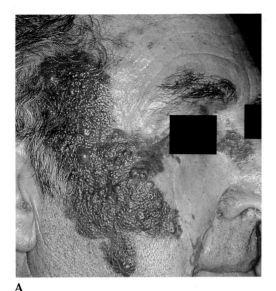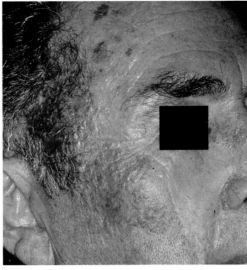

A   B

Fig. 7-5. Combined Nd:YAG laser and argon laser treatment of a port-wine stain with a nodular surface in a 50-year-old man. (A) Before therapy. (B) Result of five treatments with patient under local anesthesia. (Nd:YAG laser irradiations: spot size, 2 mm; exposure time, 0.5 second; output power, 30 W. Argon laser irradiations: spot size, 2 mm; exposure time, 0.3 second; output power, 3 W.) See Fig. 7-5 on p. 131.

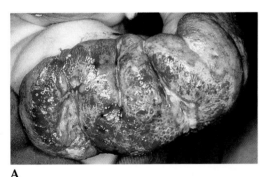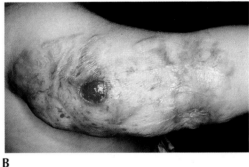

A   B

Fig. 7-9. Extensive ulcerated and bleeding, mixed hemangioma in a 4-month-old female infant. (A) Before treatment. (B) Regression after four Nd:YAG laser treatments. See Fig. 7-9 on p. 135. (Reproduced with permission from Landthaler M, Hohenleutner U, Abd El-Raheem T. Laser therapy of childhood haemangiomas. Br J Dermatol 1995;133:275–281.)

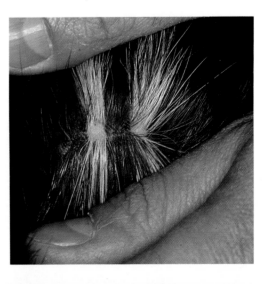

Fig. 9-3. Black guinea pig skin irradiated with the Q-switched ruby laser, showing immediate, transient hypopigmentation, followed by delayed cutaneous depigmentation 7 to 10 days after treatment. Despite cutaneous repigmentation, the guinea pig displays persistent leukotrichia up to 4 months after treatment. See Fig. 9-3 on p. 169.

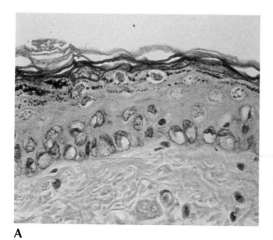

A

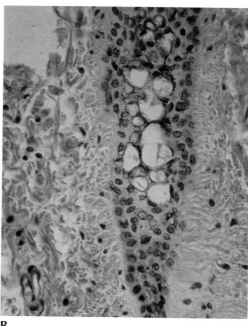

B

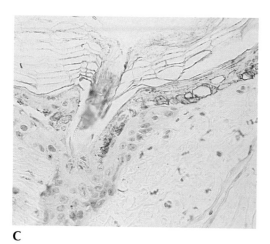

C

Fig. 9-4. Histologic appearance of black guinea pig skin immediately after irradiation with the Q-switched ruby laser. (A) Characteristic "ring cell" formation in the basal lamina, representing melanocytes and keratinocytes with condensed nuclear and pigment material at their peripheries. (B) Similar changes in a hair follicle. (C) Epidermal changes demonstrated by Fontana-Masson stain. See Fig. 9-4 on p. 170.

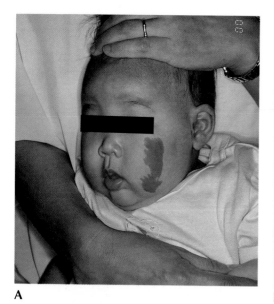

A

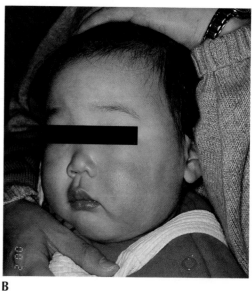

B

Fig. 9-5. Café au lait macule in an infant before (A) and after (B) five treatments over 8 months with the Q-switched ruby laser. See Fig. 9-5 on p. 174. (Courtesy Tadashi Tezuka, MD, PhD.)

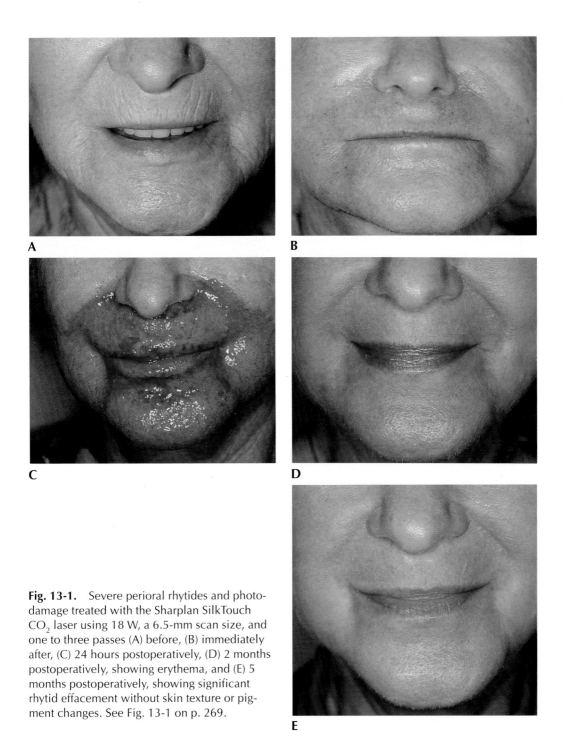

Fig. 13-1. Severe perioral rhytides and photo-damage treated with the Sharplan SilkTouch CO_2 laser using 18 W, a 6.5-mm scan size, and one to three passes (A) before, (B) immediately after, (C) 24 hours postoperatively, (D) 2 months postoperatively, showing erythema, and (E) 5 months postoperatively, showing significant rhytid effacement without skin texture or pigment changes. See Fig. 13-1 on p. 269.

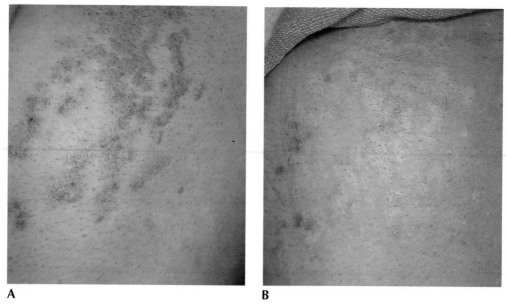

A   **B**

Fig. 13-8.   Inflammatory linear epidermal nevus treated with the Sharplan SilkTouch CO_2 laser for severe pruritus using 20 W and a 6.5-mm scan size in the painting mode. (A) Before and (B) 7 months after the procedure, showing hypopigmentation. The injury has to extend into the dermis with resulting dermal fibrosis to prevent lesion recurrence. See Fig. 13-8 on p. 279.

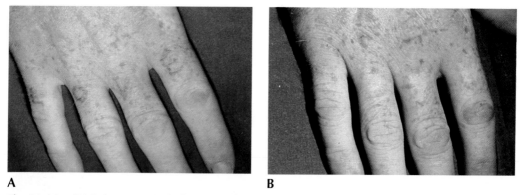

A   **B**

Fig. 16-14.   Digital tattoos. (A) Before coagulation. (B) Depigmentation 1 year later. See Fig. 16-14 on p. 340.

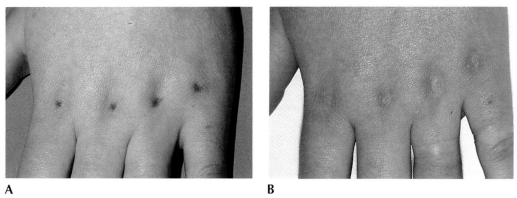

Fig. 16-15. Tattoos on knuckles. (A) Before coagulation. (B) 6 months later. See Fig. 16-15 on p. 341.

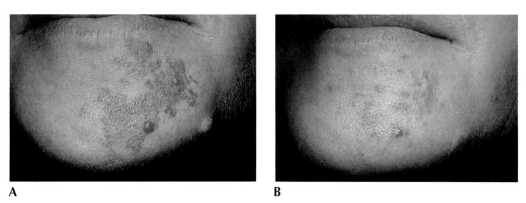

Fig. 16-16. Port-wine stain on chin. (A) Before coagulation. (B) 12 months after last treatment (four sessions). See Fig. 16-16 on p. 343. (Reproduced with permission from Colver GB. The infrared coagulator in dermatology. Dermatol Clin 1989;7:165.)

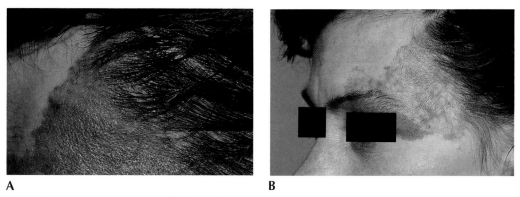

Fig. 16-17. Port-wine stains on left temple. (A) Before coagulation. (B) 3 months after last treatment (six sessions), but treatment not yet completed. See Fig. 16-17 on p. 343.

Photodynamic Therapy for Cancer

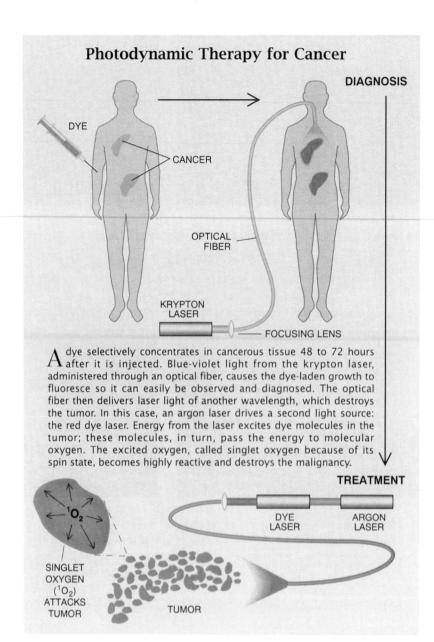

DIAGNOSIS

DYE

CANCER

OPTICAL FIBER

KRYPTON LASER

FOCUSING LENS

A dye selectively concentrates in cancerous tissue 48 to 72 hours after it is injected. Blue-violet light from the krypton laser, administered through an optical fiber, causes the dye-laden growth to fluoresce so it can easily be observed and diagnosed. The optical fiber then delivers laser light of another wavelength, which destroys the tumor. In this case, an argon laser drives a second light source: the red dye laser. Energy from the laser excites dye molecules in the tumor; these molecules, in turn, pass the energy to molecular oxygen. The excited oxygen, called singlet oxygen because of its spin state, becomes highly reactive and destroys the malignancy.

TREATMENT

$^1O_2$

DYE LASER

ARGON LASER

SINGLET OXYGEN ($^1O_2$) ATTACKS TUMOR

TUMOR

Fig. 17-1. Photodynamic therapy for cancer. See Fig. 17-1 on p. 352. (Reproduced from Scientific American 1991;June.)

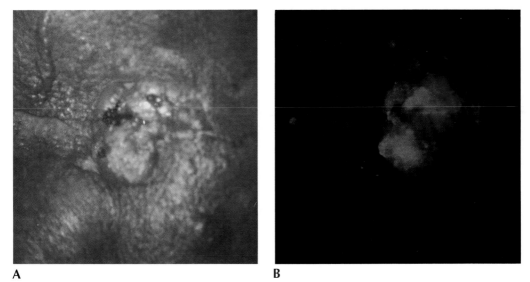

A   B

Fig. 17-5. Patient with dermal recurrence of breast cancer on anterior chest wall injected previously with Photofrin. Excitation with blue light (A) from a krypton-ion laser (λ = 405 nm) is used, and red fluorescence can be observed in the malignant cells (B) with appropriate filters. See Fig. 17-5 on p. 357.

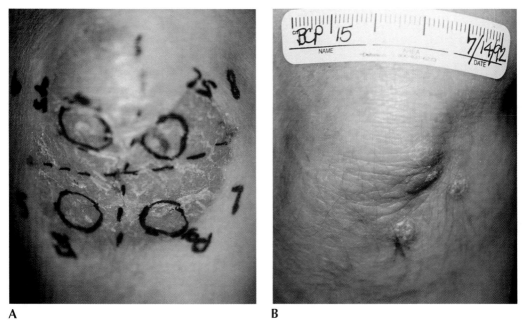

A   B

Fig. 17-10. Patient with psoriasis on elbow injected previously with Photofrin (A) before PDT and (B) 3 months after PDT. See Fig. 17-10 on p. 371.

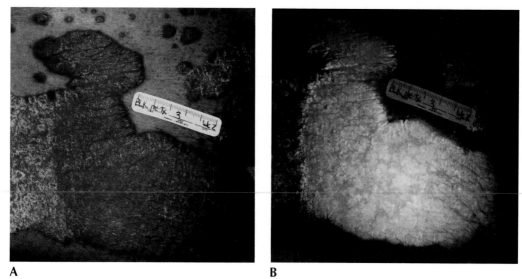

A   B

Fig. 17-11. Patient with psoriasis, 3 hours after topical administration of ALA (A). Excitation with UV light is used, and red fluorescence can be observed in the psoriatic plaques with appropriate filters (B). See Fig. 17-11 on p. 373.

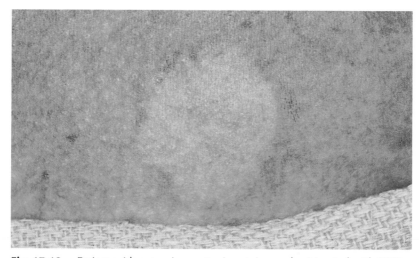

Fig. 17-12. Patient with extensive port-wine stain on chest treated with PDT using Photofrin. This photograph was taken 4 months after PDT. Note the blanching effect. See Fig. 17-12 on p. 374.

Table 12-5.   Disorders for which the
CO$_2$ laser has been used as an ablating tool

I. Epidermal or mucosal disorders:
   A. Actinic cheilitis[a]
   B. Erythroplasia of Queyrat[a]
   C. Oral florid papillomatosis[a]
   D. Sublingual keratosis[a]
   E. Bowenoid papulosis[a]
   F. Balanitis xerotica obliterans[b]
   G. Bowen's disease or squamous cell carcinoma in situ[c]
   H. Superficial basal cell carcinomas[c]
   I. Epidermal nevus[b]
   J. Nail ablation[c]
   K. Lentigines[d]
   L. Lower labial macules[e]
   M. Lichen sclerosus et atrophicus[e]
   N. Zoon's balanitis[e]
   O. Hailey-Hailey disease[e]
   P. Darier's disease[e]
   Q. Porokeratosis[e]
II. Warts:
   A. Verruca vulgaris[c]
   B. Verruca plantaris[c]
   C. Periungual warts[c]
   D. Widespread condyloma acuminatum[b]
   E. Recalcitrant warts[b]
   F. Warts with histologic atypia[b]
III. Dermal processes:
   A. Syringomas[b]
   B. Granuloma faciale[c]
   C. Trichoepitheliomas[c]
   D. Neurofibromas[c]
   E. Xanthelasma[c]
   F. Adenoma sebaceum[c]
   G. Myxoid cysts[e]
   H. Apocrine hydrocystoma[e]
   I. Angiolymphoid hyperplasia[e]
   J. Pearly penile papules[e]
   K. Cowden's disease[e]
   L. Chondrodermatitis nodularis helicis[e]
   M. Debridement of granulation tissue[e]
   N. Cutaneous infections (botryomycosis, leishmaniasis)[e]
   O. Hidradenitis suppurativa[e]
IV. Vascular lesions:
   A. Port-wine stains[d]
   B. Telangiectases[d]
   C. Cherry angiomas[c]
   D. Lymphangioma circumscriptum[e]
   E. Pyogenic granulomas[e]
   F. Angiokeratomas[c]
   G. Angiosarcomas[e]
   H. Venous lakes[c]

Continued

Table 12-5. Continued

V. Miscellaneous:
   A. Tattoos[d]
   B. Red tattoo reactions[b]
   C. Cutaneous resurfacing[e]
   D. Deepithelialization before reconstructive surgical procedure[e]
   E. Aging hands[e]
   F. Sterilization of infected wounds[e]
   G. Debridement of burn wounds[e]

---

[a]Treatment of choice.
[b]Results often better than alternatives.
[c]Results usually same as alternatives; use of the laser may facilitate procedure.
[d]Better results now obtained with newer laser systems.
[e]Results may or may not be acceptable; current information cannot be easily evaluated.
Source: Modified and updated from Olbricht SO. Use of the carbon dioxide laser in dermatologic surgery: a clinically relevant update for 1993. J Dermatol Surg Oncol 1993;19:367.

with the CO_2 laser are now treated using other laser systems that yield better results and minimize adverse effects.

The most important advantage of the CO_2 laser from the standpoint of ablative therapy is its ability to produce limited destruction very rapidly. The continuous-wave beam accomplishes relatively good hemostasis during the procedure. It can heat and seal blood vessels 0.5 mm in diameter and smaller,[42] allowing the procedure to be performed quickly with minimal blood loss.[43,44] Larger vessels can be grasped with a forceps and welded shut without difficulty. The pulse waveform causes minimal adjacent thermal injury but also has a minimal hemostatic effect, so wounds made with a pulsed laser may bleed like those made with a scalpel. The laser also sterilizes as it vaporizes[45,46] and does not interfere with the operation of pacemakers or monitoring devices. Nail and thick hyperkeratotic debris can be melted away, and even bone can be ablated. The surgery is noncontact, thus theoretically limiting the potential transfer of pathogens or malignant cells from the surface of a surgical tool to the wound. The laser has been said to seal nerve endings,[47] but data documenting diminished pain in laser-created wounds are anecdotal. In addition, results from an early histologic study indicated that small lymphatics were sealed,[48] and it had been assumed that the wound would therefore show less postoperative edema. However, two other ultrastructural studies[49,50] showed that lymphatic channels are patent, and in a third study,[51] technetium-labeled colloid was placed in a laser-induced wound and was found to migrate into regional lymph nodes in a fashion similar to the migration noted in scalpel-created wounds. Paired trials evaluating the use of the scalpel and the CO_2 laser in blepharoplasties have yielded mixed findings regarding whether postoperative edema and pain are diminished through the use of the laser.[52–54] However, when compared with electrosurgical techniques for ablation, the CO_2 laser has been found to cause much less adjacent thermal tissue damage[10,42] and the length of the procedure is shorter.[55] Cryosurgery generally produces more edema and pain.[56,57] In addition, blisters cannot form after use of the CO_2 laser, because the epidermis is not intact. One drawback to the use of the CO_2 laser for ablation, however, is that there is no specimen available to be sent for pathologic study. Therefore a biopsy specimen from any questionable process needs to be obtained before the destruction of such a lesion.

EPIDERMAL PROCESSES

The CO_2 laser is the instrument of choice in the treatment of a variety of thin epidermal processes characterized by hyperplasia, atypia, or both. Actinic cheilitis is a disorder in which the pathologic changes, atypical epidermal cells, are confined to the squamatizing mucosa of the lower lip. The mucosa is generally not thickened, and there are no follicles down which the atypia can extend. With the patient under local anesthesia, a thin strip of mucosa can be vaporized rapidly (see Table 12-2). The underlying coagulated tissue and thermal debris separates 3 to 7 days after the procedure, and reepithelialization then occurs within 4 weeks. Morbidity is minimal, results are excellent,[56,58–61] and histologic atypia is absent at 6 months.[40] In addition, scarring is not usually appreciated, and its incidence can be minimized by the selection of treatment parameters that maximize vaporization and minimize charring.[27] Other treatments for actinic cheilitis, such as cryosurgery, electrodesiccation, excision repaired by mucosal advancement flaps, and topical 5-fluorouracil application, are generally associated with greater morbidity, as well as a lower rate of success and greater risk of cosmetic deformity.[56] Lower labial macules and Peutz-Jeghers lentigines[62] may be treated similarly.

Other thin, superficial processes for which the CO_2 laser is the treatment of choice include squamous cell carcinoma (SCC) in situ of the penis (erythroplasia of Queyrat),[63,64] Bowen's disease of the finger,[65] and Bowen's disease of the vulva.[66] Very superficial ablation of clinically apparent lesions surrounded by wide margins of normal tissue can be produced quickly in otherwise difficult surgical sites. The wounds heal without difficulty. Bowenoid papulosis may also be treated by superficial CO_2 laser ablation. It is a disorder that affects genital skin with SCC in situ, like the histologic picture associated with infection by some subtypes of human papillomavirus (HPV). This virus can reside for an indefinite time in clinically normal skin. New lesions may appear, and the patient may require additional treatments over many years. Such a simple procedure that is associated with minimal postoperative morbidity may have the additional benefit of maximizing the likelihood of patient compliance with long-term surveillance. Balanitis xerotica obliterans,[67] lichen sclerosus et atrophicus,[68] Zoon's blanitis,[69] oral leukoplakia,[70] oral florid papillomatosis,[71] and sublingual keratoses[72] may be treated similarly, although the mechanism by which improvement occurs is not clear.

Superficial skin cancers on glabrous skin have also been treated with the CO_2 laser. Fifteen patients with SCC in situ of the nose, upper lip, and cheeks were treated with the Ultrapulse, and results were acceptable.[73] Superficial vaporization in combination with a trichloroacetic acid (TCA) peel may be a useful alternative option in the treatment of a bald scalp with multiple large and recurrent actinic keratoses and SCC in situ.[27] One study of the effectiveness of CO_2 laser vaporization of basal cell carcinomas (BCC) revealed a recurrence rate of 50%,[74] but another large study of 52 patients with 370 carcinomas treated with curettage followed by CO_2 laser vaporization showed no recurrence within 20 months.[75]

The CO_2 laser may be employed to treat other epidermal processes not easily treated using standard physical modalities, which have also not produced uniformly good results. These disorders usually have a superficial dermal component, and to be successful the ablation must extend to that tissue level. Porokeratosis of Mibelli is a single, enlarging hyperkeratotic plaque that is unsightly and may undergo neoplastic transformation to SCC or BCC. CO_2 laser ablation has been successful in its treatment.[76,77] This was shown by a study in which a portion of a single lesion on a hand underwent CO_2 laser vaporization with healing by second intention and another portion was removed by scalpel excision followed by placement of a split-thickness skin graft.[77] The results of CO_2 laser ablation were found to be both cosmetically and functionally superior to the results of scalpel removal, even for lesions over digits and joints. Epidermal nevi may also be ablated, although strict attention to the depth of vaporization is necessary to minimize scarring and the likelihood of recurrence.[27,41,78,79] Symptomatic lesions of Darier's disease and Hailey-Hailey dermatosis unresponsive to standard therapies have also been alleviated by laser ablation, which produces thin, asymptomatic, fully functional scars.[80,81] Large, thick, single or multiple seborrheic keratoses may also be treated easily in a single surgical session.[27]

Experience in the treatment of disorders of medical significance sparked interest in the use of the CO_2 laser for various cosmetic resurfacing procedures, either alone or in conjunction with chemical peeling agents. CO_2 laser ablation with a defocused continuous-wave beam can be used in a fashion similar to dermabrasion to remodel acne scars,[82] full-thickness grafts,[83] or other focal and discrete irregularities.[41,84,85] Because this procedure is performed freehand, experience with the use of the laser is required to ensure excellent, predictable results. The resurfacing of large areas, such as a cheek or an entire face, requires use of the Ultrapulse and an unfocused beam or computerized pattern generator to maintain a uniform high power density and an extremely short duration of power and thereby obtain a uniform and superficial depth of vaporization (see Chap. 13).

The most common current use of the CO_2 laser in cosmetic resurfacing procedures is for the coagulation or vaporization of surface irregularities (thick actinic keratoses, lentigines, sebaceous hyperplasia, rhytides). Dermal filling substances such as Zyderm collagen (Collagen Corporation, Palo Alto, CA) or autologous fat may be injected after wound healing to complete the "rejuvenation" process.[86]

Low-fluence CO_2 laser irradiation has been evaluated for the treatment of epidermal pigmented lesions, such as solar lentigines or lower labial macules. In a study[87] of 121 psoralen-ultraviolet-light–induced lentigines treated by a brief shuttered beam of 3.7 or 4.4 J, complete clearing was seen in 10% and substantial lightening in 66%, with no subsequent depigmentation, hyperpigmentation, or hypertrophic scarring. When low-fluence CO_2 laser radiation was compared with argon laser light delivered by a Dermascan shuttered-delivery system and with cryosurgery using liquid nitrogen in the treatment of 99 solar lentigines, cryosurgery was found to produce a good or excellent result about twice as often as either laser technique, but all therapies appeared to be associated with a low frequency of substantial textural change.[88] This study also underscores the problem with most of the reports of the clinical uses of laser technology: that is, the modality is observed to be effective, but only when it is compared directly with other therapies does it then become clear whether its results are better, similar, or less efficacious than those of the other therapies. Recent advances in technology have led to the more effective treatment of pigmented lesions by the Q-switched ruby laser (see Chap. 9).[89]

WARTS

The CO_2 laser has also been used for the treatment of HPV infection. HPV is a family of at least seventy known subtypes that cause epithelial or mucosal proliferation and sometimes squamous atypia. The epithelial-mucosal proliferation generally is manifested as an excrescence of thickened skin with a rough surface and sometimes thick hyperkeratosis. These papules and plaques may occur on any surface of skin or mucosa but are most common on the hands, feet, and genital skin. Plantar warts are often depressed, because they have been pushed into the dermis or even subcutaneous fat by pressure during ambulation. Because the pathologic process resides on the surface, it appeared that treatment using the CO_2 laser would be effective. Results of early studies were encouraging,[90–92] but more recent data indicate that this procedure is not without its difficulties. In a study of 18 patients with persistent warts on the hands and feet, 56% were found to be cured at follow-up (minimum, 6 months), partial clearance was achieved in 17%, and relapse occurred in 27%.[93] Considerable morbidity, including postoperative pain, temporary loss of function, and scarring, was also associated with the procedure. In a study of 25 patients with warts resistant to other therapies, 32% were cured, 20% showed improvement, and 48% suffered complete relapse.[94] In 17 patients with 24 periungual warts resistant to other therapy, vaporization of the entire wart, with the partial or complete avulsion of the nail, led to a 71% cure rate achieved with one or two treatments with the laser alone and a 94% cure rate with the adjuvant use of other therapies.[95] It took approximately 2 months for complete reepithelialization to occur. Complications reported include significant pain (12%), postoperative numbness (18%), and nail dystrophy (29%). In 46 patients with 300 warts, use of continuous-wave CO_2 and superpulsed CO_2 energy was observed to produce clearing in 68%, whereas the Ultrapulse was observed to produce clearing in 90%.[27] The incidence of scarring depended on the waveform used and was 54%, 33%, and 7%, respectively. All procedures were designed to ablate all appreciable warty tissue.

The reason for the relatively moderate cure rate with its attendant morbidity, despite such vigorous therapy, is not known; however, it probably relates to persistence of the virus in adjacent, but clinically uninvolved, skin. Such persistent subclinical infection has been well studied in women with HPV-related diseases of the genital tract, and it has been found that 50% of the patients studied had a viral genome, shown by Southern blot hybridization, residing in normal-appearing skin 5 to 10 mm away from visible lesions.[96] Detection of persistent viral genome was associated with a 67% incidence of recurrence after laser surgery. Similarly, in a study of 38 men with genitoanal skin lesions, HPV types 16 and 18 were detected in a total of 65% of biopsy specimens obtained before CO_2 laser therapy and in 61% after therapy.[97] In a study of 25 women with recalcitrant and widespread genital disease, the CO_2 laser was used to destroy the entire epithelial-mucosal surface, from the cervix to the anal canal and the entire perineum, regardless of whether there appeared to be condylomatous changes.[98] Thirteen of 19 male consorts also underwent vigorous treatment, which included the entire penile shaft. As expected, the morbidity was high. At 3 months, there was also histologic evidence of persistent wart virus in 88% of the patients and 23 of the 25 women had clinically apparent HPV lesions. In other studies, the success rates for the treatment of condyloma acuminatum in women has ranged from 65% to 100%[99–101] and more than one procedure was required in some patients. Cure rates may be enhanced by treating the male partner simultaneously.[101] Because women generally have warts in more than one perineal location, colposcopy should be carried out to detect vaginal or cervical warts before the external genital or perianal warts are treated.

Results from the treatment of male patients with HPV-induced condylomas are similar. In one study of 119 patients, 82.3% of the lesions were eradicated in one session; however, new areas of involvement appeared in five patients.[102] Two thirds of the patients healed within 3 to 4 weeks, but it took up to 6 weeks in the remainder. Complications such as local infection and cellulitis developed in 13% of the patients. In another study of 43 male patients, acetowhite lesions thought to be characteristic of HPV were treated by the CO$_2$ laser, with or without the intraurethral administration of 5-fluorouracil, and a 50% cure rate was achieved.[103] Other adjuvant therapies, such as the local injection[104] or systemic administration[105] of interferon-alpha-2b, may reduce the risk of recurrence.

The wide difference in the response rates reported may be related to differences in the type of warts treated (recalcitrant or previously untreated, localized or diffuse, small or large), the HPV subtypes, the anatomic sites, and the host immune status, but differences in technique are also apparent. Some authors used low power densities,[93] others used much higher powers,[102] and some debride hyperkeratotic material first.[27] The margin of normal skin treated is often not mentioned but, when reported, has varied from 2 to 10 mm. In a comparative trial in which different waveforms were used, the influence of the treatment parameters used was illustrated.[27] Morbidity also varies, probably for the same reasons. The procedure generally produces a wound that takes 1 to 2 months to heal, causes some pain, and sometimes results in scarring. These anticipated results are complicated by the nearly universal expectation on the part of both patients and referring physicians that laser surgery is easy and painless (without anesthesia!), involves no postoperative care, leaves no scar, and guarantees a cure. Recurrence is further complicated by the fact that some HPV types have an oncogenic potential,[16,18,33–37,41,44,49,53,106] which may be associated with SCC of the skin,[107,108] as well as with bowenoid papulosis, cervical dysplasia, cervical cancer, and anogenital carcinoma.[106] It is also known that the successful laser ablation of the cervical intraepithelial neoplasia associated with HPV infection may not preclude the development of invasive cancer of the cervix.[109]

It is clear at this time that HPV infection cannot truly be eradicated, although CO$_2$ laser treatment may bring about complete clearing of the clinical lesions. Laser therapy may therefore be best reserved for those warts that are recalcitrant to treatments associated with less morbidity and to those that are bulky, painful, or histologically atypical. In addition, the treatment of warts in sites difficult to treat using other modalities may be facilitated by use of the CO$_2$ laser. Thick plantar warts can be treated faster by lasers than by electrosurgical devices. Periungual warts can be ablated easily without avulsing the nailplate. Laser treatment does not, however, preclude the use of other adjuvant therapies or treatments causing less morbidity for the management of small recurrences, but rigorous and long-term follow-up must be carried out in any patient with a lesion so treated that has a potential for malignant degeneration. Follow-up of the female partners of male patients with genital lesions associated with HPV infection must include yearly surveillance for cervical disease, regardless of whether the therapy causes the visible lesions to clear in either partner.

DERMAL PROCESSES

Use of the CO_2 laser facilitates the removal of a variety of dermal processes producing tumors or nodules. When laser treatment has been compared with standard surgical excision and closure or with electrosurgery, it has been found that the laser allows the removal of many more lesions much more quickly.[55] In patients with multiple or confluent tumors, the atrophic scarring produced by laser ablation can be a marked cosmetic improvement.[55] In some situations, scarring has been reported to be minimized by utilizing a pulsed waveform.[27] Vaporization with the CO_2 laser has been reported to facilitate removal and produce good results in the treatment of multiple trichoepitheliomas,[110,111] neurofibromas,[55,112] apocrine hidrocystomas,[113] cylindromas,[114] trichilemmomas of Cowden's disease,[27] adenoma sebaceum in tuberous sclerosis,[41,115,116] and pearly penile papules.[117] The treatment of syringomas with the CO_2 laser has proved especially satisfying, because the procedure is fast and precise, results are excellent, and recurrence has not been observed.[39,40,118] The palliative treatment of multiple cutaneous metastatic lesions may also be similarly accomplished.[119] Some inflammatory conditions that produce nodules or plaques, most of unknown etiology, may also be alleviated by ablation with the CO_2 laser, even though the mechanism by which the laser works may be unclear. These processes include xanthelasma palpebrarum,[120] chondrodermatitis nodularis chronica helicis,[121] granuloma faciale,[122] lichen myxedematosus,[123] angiolymphoid hyperplasia,[124] nodular amyloidosis,[125] and digital mucous cysts.[126] Excessive granulation tissue in difficult sites, such as posttracheostomy wounds,[127] may also be managed by ablation with the CO_2 laser.

Because of data indicating that the CO_2 laser can sterilize wounds[45,46] and because of the ease with which it can be used for ablation, it has been used to treat some infectious processes for which medical therapy is either not readily available or routinely effective. The cutaneous lesions of blastomycosis,[128] chromomycosis,[129] and leishmaniasis[130] have cleared after vaporization with the laser. Cutaneous botryomycosis, a chronic skin infection caused by *Staphylococcus aureus,* can be poorly responsive to antibiotic therapy but may respond to laser ablation.[131] Isolated cases of inflammatory disorders of the epidermal appendages complicated by infection, such as perifolliculitis capitis abscedens et suffodiens[132] and hidradenitis suppurativa,[133–135] have been treated with good results. Ablation of nails affected by chronic recalcitrant dermatophyte infection and matrixectomy to prevent regrowth may be performed easily, with minimal postoperative morbidity.[136]

In the first decade of cutaneous laser surgery, the CO_2 laser was an important option in the treatment of vascular lesions such as port-wine stains[137] and telangiectases.[138] Good to excellent results were noted in 50% to 60% of patients with port-wine stains treated with the CO$_2$ laser, with hypertrophic scarring in less than 10% of the treated areas. These results were not dissimilar from those reported in the same period for argon laser treatment,[139-141] with both lasers producing nonspecific superficial thermal damage. A recent report[142] summarized the results of CO$_2$ laser treatment in 29 adult patients with mature port-wine stains that had not responded to treatment with the argon laser and the continuous-wave dye laser. Excellent to good results were seen in 74%, and no hypertrophic scars were seen. Seventeen children with pink port-wine stains were also treated; excellent or good results were seen in 53%, with hypertrophic scars developing in two children (12%). Today, improvements in technique and new technology (robotized scanning devices, the pulsed dye laser) have led to the development of a variety of visible light lasers that produce better results with a negligible risk of scarring (see Chaps. 5, 6, and 8). With the better treatments now available, the CO$_2$ laser no longer has a large role in the therapy of port-wine stains and telangiectases. The laser treatment of thick vascular tumors, however, entails nonspecific thermal damage, regardless of the wavelength, fluences, and pulse durations used. The CO$_2$ laser may therefore continue to be used in that setting because it can produce results equivalent to treatments with other laser treatments. For example, good results have been reported for the CO$_2$ laser treatment of cherry angiomas,[143] pyogenic granulomas,[41] and digital angiosarcomas.[144] The CO$_2$ laser may also successfully ablate lymphangioma circumscriptum,[41,145,146] probably because the fibrosis that develops during normal wound healing when ablation extends to the deep dermis prevents the blood and lymphatic vessels from becoming ectatic again. Successful treatment requires the vaporization of the entire lesion, however, including the deep communicating cistern.

Ten years ago, tattoos were commonly treated by CO$_2$ laser vaporization. The procedure was similar to dermabrasion but offered the advantages of providing a relatively bloodless field, being versatile in its ability to work over angular surfaces, and requiring a short operating time. The surgeon could visualize the pigment and remove it in toto, even that in large or wide tattoos. The complete removal of tattoo pigment generally required vaporization to at least the depth of the pigment, and therefore the wound healed with a scar, which was usually atrophic but sometimes hypertrophic. Regardless, many patients were willing to exchange their tattoo for a scar. Traumatic tattoos[147] and other pigmented disorders[41] were treated similarly. In one variation of the treatment, urea paste was applied after the epidermis has been ablated.[148] Today, tattoos and other pigmented disorders may be treated with good results and with minimal risk of scarring using the Q-switched ruby, Q-switched Nd:YAG, and Q-switched alexandrite lasers (see Chap. 9). However, multiple treatments are required for excellent results to be achieved using these lasers.[149] For this reason, the CO$_2$ laser is still used in a few situations. For instance, some patients desire treatment to be accomplished in a single treatment session and are willing to accept healing with a scar.

In addition, red tattoo reactions may be best treated by the CO_2 laser,[150] because all the cinnabar dye is removed completely in one session. The ablation can be done precisely so that the rest of the tattoo is preserved. Unwanted eyeliner tattoo pigment may also be removed in one treatment with the CO_2 laser, with good results.[27]

Investigators at several centers have studied the use of the CO_2 laser for the vaporization of necrotic or infected tissue, such as the debridement of burns. In early studies,[151–153] the laser was used as an excising tool. The primary benefit to use of this modality was the hemostasis and preservation of blood volume it afforded; however, the procedure was little used because arguments abounded regarding wound healing and graft survival.[20,154,155] In addition, the procedure was cumbersome and slow to perform over a large area. Recent experimental work with a superpulsed CO_2 laser coupled to a mechanical scanner has indicated that ablation may be easily performed using this equipment and that the wounds produced may take grafts.[26,156] The development of an accompanying intelligent scanning mechanism that could differentiate necrotic skin from viable tissue through the use of a dye[157] would allow the procedure to be fully automatic and rapid, with the result that there would be little residual thermal damage. Unwanted normal tissue can also be removed by ablation. For example, this laser could be used to deepithelialize skin before flap transposition and grafting. There would also be an advantage to utilizing the laser in situations in which rigid skin immobilization is impossible, such as the breast,[158] or in which a more conventional approach might pose a risk to an underlying structure.

Complications

In a survey of more than a hundred cutaneous laser surgeons reported on in 1986,[159] it was found that 1% to 4% of procedures done using the CO_2 laser were associated with complications. A slowly healing wound, pain necessitating narcotic use for up to 1 week, the formation of a thin, pliable, burnlike scar, and regrowth of excised keloid tissue were considered normal sequelae and not treatment complications.

The most frequently noted complication was hypertrophic scarring. It was the only complication noted by more than a fourth of the respondents and was encountered in 64% of their patients. In particular, the treatment of tattoos seemed to be commonly followed by this type of wound healing, with the incidence ranging from 10% to 100% and the median incidence ranging from 20% to 35%. Scarring following tattoo removal with the CO_2 laser had been noted before this report[160,161] and since[162] and was the primary impetus to the development of new laser technology for their treatment. Although the occurrence of hypertrophic scarring is related in part to the degree of thermal damage and the wound depth, it also depends on the anatomic location of the wound. Hypertrophic scars are particularly likely to form at the sites of tattoos removed from the upper arm and shoulder. In the survey, hypertrophic scarring was also noted to occur after the laser surgery treatment of warts, nevus of Ota, rhinophyma, port-wine stain, and an epidermal nevus. The arm, chest, and lip were reported as being at high risk, but sites such as the periungual area and feet also developed hypertrophic scars. In addition, six physicians reported the de novo development of keloids in sites treated by the CO$_2$ laser. Keloids have also been reported to form after the CO$_2$ laser treatment of molluscum contagiosum.[163]

Attention to good surgical technique, optimal treatment parameters, and appropriate wound care all speed wound healing and minimize scarring. Appropriate wound care is especially important for the wounds created by CO$_2$ laser ablation, because healing by second intention is intended and may take weeks to occur if the defect is large or deep. Wound care should be simple for the patient to perform and repeat and also supply comfort and protection. Early wound care involves cleansing the wound twice a day with diluted hydrogen peroxide or mild soap and water, followed by the application of bacitracin or Neosporin ointment in a thin layer. A moist wound heals faster than a dry wound,[22] and bacitracin or Neosporin ointment is known to promote reepithelialization, as opposed to petrolatum[164] or povidone-iodine.[165] The wound is then protected by a Telfa dressing and gauze. Alternatively, semipermeable occlusive dressings such as Vigilon, Duoderm, or OpSite can be used. The effectiveness of some of these dressings was documented in a study comparing them with no treatment at all.[164] Wound care is continued until complete reepithelialization has occurred. Complete healing may take 2 to 8 weeks, depending on the site of the wound and the extent of surgery. Wound care is continued after complete reepithelialization to decrease or prevent hypertrophic scarring.[167] Moisturing and massaging healed wounds for 2 to 6 months is also standard advice. Constant-pressure measures (e.g., tailor-made pressure garments, surgical compression earrings) and splints are effective deterrents to hypertrophic scarring. Intralesional corticosteroid injections (10 to 40 mg/ml of triamcinolone diacetate or acetonide) administered at monthly intervals may be required if thick areas of scar develop.

The survey mentioned earlier also showed other complications of CO$_2$ laser procedures to be less frequent or rare. Twenty to thirty percent of the users of CO$_2$ lasers had one or more patients who experienced hemorrhage, unexpected pain, unexpected prolonged healing, or infection, with estimated incidences ranging from 0.2% to 0.6%. The formation of reactive benign growths after surgery were also reported. These included lip mucocoele, excess granulation tissue, and pyogenic granuloma.

Attention to safety issues affecting the patient, physician, and assistants is essential in the practice of laser surgery (see Chap. 19). In the survey, 10% of the physicians reported the occurrence of either unintentional burns to the patient or operating room personnel (usually to the finger of the operator or an assistant providing exposure) or fire. One such incident was attributed to reflection of the laser beam off a metal instrument. This type of accident was also noted to occur in 9% of gynecologic procedures and was not always prevented by the use of wet drapes.[168] In addition, laryngitis developed in a physician and his assistant that was attributed to the aspiration of laser plume when the smoke evacuation system failed.[159] Certainly, viable infectious agents[169–171] and lung-damaging dust[172] may be present in the plume, and for this reason, adequate plume evacuation systems must be used intraoperatively. The risk of acquiring HPV from the plume is debated but may be increased in the treatment of genital warts, which seem to have a predilection for infecting the upper airway mucosa.[173]

Two potentially life-threatening complications of CO_2 laser procedures have been reported, both by respondents to the survey. One occurred in a middle-aged woman who underwent extensive CO_2 laser surgery for the removal of plantar warts, which produced an open wound that persisted for several months. A popliteal artery bypass was finally necessary to accomplish healing. The other occurred in a 16-year-old pregnant girl, in whom a systemic bacterial infection developed after the treatment of a massive condyloma. Regardless of her experience, the treatment of genital condyloma during pregnancy is generally safe.[174] To date, no deaths and no serious chronic functional morbidity, ocular damage, or secondary malignant neoplasms have been reported to result from the use of the CO_2 laser during an operative procedure.

Conclusion

The CO_2 laser is certainly now far beyond the experimental stage. It simplifies many procedures, is usually safe, is effective for its intended uses, and is now the preferred treatment for several cutaneous disorders. At one time it was thought that every dermatology office would have a CO_2 laser. However, the realistic appreciation of its limitations and the expense of the technology have probably been responsible for precluding its routine clinical use. Nevertheless, the unique properties of the CO_2 laser have definitely created a vast potential for its use in various clinical settings and as a research tool for increasing our understanding of laser-tissue interactions and wound healing. As more experience is gained and rigorous studies performed, the future is bound to yield further innovative advances in biomedical laser instrumentation as well as modifications in current laser techniques.

References

1. Hobbs ER, Bailin PL, Wheeland RG, Ratz JL. Superpulsed lasers: minimizing thermal damage with short duration, high irradiance pulses. J Dermatol Surg Oncol 1987;13:955–964.

2. McKenzie AL. A three-zone model of soft-tissue damage by a CO$_2$ laser. Phys Med Biol 1986;31:967–983.
3. Schomacker KT, Walsh JT, Flotte TJ, Deutsch TF. Thermal damage produced by high-irradiance continuous wave CO$_2$ laser cutting of tissue. Lasers Surg Med 1990;10:74–84.
4. Bailin PL. Treatment of port wine stains with the CO$_2$ laser: early results. In: Arndt KA, Noe JM, Rosen S, eds. Cutaneous laser therapy: principles and methods. New York: Wiley, 1983:129–136.
5. Polanyi TG. Laser physics: medical applications. Otolaryngol Clin North Am 1983;16:753–774.
6. Kamat BR, Tang SV, Arndt KA et al. Low fluence CO$_2$ laser irradiation: selective epidermal damage to human skin. J Invest Dermatol 1985;85:274–278.
7. Anderson RR, Parrish JA. Selective photothermolysis: precise microsurgery by selective absorption of pulsed radiation. Science 1983;220:524–527.
8. Mihaslin S, Jako GJ, Incze J et al. Laser surgery in otolaryngology: interaction of CO$_2$ laser and soft tissue. Ann NY Acad Sci 1976;267:264–294.
9. Walsh JT, Flotte TJ, Anderson RR, Deutsch TF. Pulsed CO$_2$ laser tissue ablation: effect of tissue type and pulse duration on thermal damage. Lasers Surg Med 1988;8:108–118.
10. Montgomery TC, Sharp JB, Bellina JH et al. Comparative gross and histological study of the effects of scalpel, electric knife, and carbon dioxide laser on skin and uterine incisions in dogs. Lasers Surg Med 1983;3:9–15.
11. Hall RR, Hill DW, Beach AD. A carbon dioxide surgical laser. Ann R Coll Surg Engl 1971;48:181–187.
12. Kanzler MH, Gorsulowsky DC, Swanson NA. Basic mechanisms in the healing cutaneous wound. J Dermatol Surg Oncol 1986;12:1156–1164.
13. Levensen SM, Geever EG, Crowley LV et al. The healing of rat skin wounds. Ann Surg 1965;161:293–308.
14. Weigel J, Dolmaniecki J, Orlowski I et al. Healing of liver wounds inflicted with CO$_2$ lasers. Acta Med Pol 1981;22:105–118.
15. Carney JM, Kamat BR, Stern RS et al. Cutaneous tissue repair after focused CO$_2$ laser irradiation. Lasers Surg Med 1985;5:180–181.
16. Hall RR. The healing of tissues incised by a carbon dioxide laser. Br J Surg 1971;58:222–227.
17. Hishimoto K, Rockwell JR, Epstein RA et al. Laser wound healing compared with other surgical modalities. Burns 1973;1:13–21.
18. Moreno RA, Hebda PA, Zitelli JA et al. Epidermal cell outgrowth from CO$_2$ laser- and scalpel-cut explants: implications for wound healing. J Dermatol Surg Oncol 1984;10:863–869.
19. Rainoldi R, Candiani P, Virgilis G et al. Connective tissue regeneration after CO$_2$ laser therapy. Int Surg 1983;68:167–171.
20. Fry TB, Gerba RW, Bostros SB et al. Effects of laser, scalpel and electrosurgical excision on wound contracture and graft "take." Plast Reconstr Surg 1980;65:729–731.
21. Bueh BR, Schuller DE. Comparison of tensile strength in CO$_2$ laser and scalpel skin incisions. Arch Otolaryngol 1983;109:465–471.
22. Winter GD. Formation of the scab and the rate of epithelialization of superficial wounds in the skin of the young domestic pig. Nature 1962;4812:292–294.

23. Cochrane JPS, Beacon JP, Creasy GH et al. Wound healing after laser surgery: an experimental study. Br J Surg 1980;67:740–743.

24. Badawy SZA, Mohammed EM, Baggish MS. Comparative study of continuous and pulsed CO_2 laser on tissue healing and fertility outcome in tubal anastomosis. Fertil Steril 1987;47:843–847.

25. Baggish MS, Mohamed ME. Comparison of electronically superpulsed and continuous wave CO_2 laser on the rate of uterine horn. Fertil Steril 1986;45:120–125.

26. Green HA, Burd E, Nishioka NS et al. Middermal wound healing: a comparison between dermatomal excision and pulsed carbon dioxide laser ablation. Arch Dermatol 1992:639–642.

27. Fitzpatrick RE, Goldman MP. CO_2 laser surgery. In: Goldman MP, Fitzpatrick RE, eds. Cutaneous laser surgery: the art and science of selective photothermolysis. St. Louis: Mosby, 1994:198–258.

28. Reid R. Physical and surgical principles governing carbon dioxide laser surgery on the skin. Dermatol Clin 1991;9:297–304.

29. Fleming MG, Brody N. A new technique for laser treatment of cutaneous tumors. J Dermatol Surg Oncol 1986;12:1170–1175.

30. Dobry MM, Padilla RS, Pennino RP. Carbon dioxide laser vaporization: relationship of scar formation to power density. J Invest Dermatol 1989;93:75–77.

31. Kamat BR, Tang SV, Arndt KA et al. Low-fluence CO_2 laser irradiation: selective epidermal damage to human skin. J Invest Dermatol 1985; 85:274–278.

32. Herbich G. Epidermal changes limited to the epidermis of guinea pig skin by low-power carbon dioxide laser irradiation. Arch Dermatol 1986;122:132–135.

33. Moritz AR, Henriques FC. Studies of thermal injury. II. The relative importance of time and surface temperatures in the causation of cutaneous burns. Am J Pathol 1947;23:695–703.

34. Moritz AR. Studies of thermal injury. III. The pathology and pathogenesis of cutaneous burns: an experimental study. Am J Pathol 1947; 23:915–921.

35. Brugmans MJP, Kemper J, Gijsberg GHM et al. Temperature response of biological materials to pulsed non-ablative CO_2 laser irradiation. Lasers Surg Med 1989;9:405–406.

36. Van Gemert MJC, Welch AJ. Time constants in thermal laser medicine. Lasers Surg Med 1989;9:405–421.

37. Rattner NH, Rosenberg SK, Fuller T. Difference between continuous wave and superpulse CO_2 laser in bladder surgery. Urology 1979;13: 264–269.

38. Wheeland RG, McGillis ST. Cowden's disease—treatment of cutaneous lesions using carbon dioxide laser vaporization: a comparison of conventional and superpulsed techniques. J Dermatol Surg Oncol 1989; 1055–1059.

39. Apfelberg DB, Maser MR, Lash H et al. Superpulse CO_2 laser treatment of facial syringomata. Lasers Surg Med 1987;7:533–535.

40. Whitaker DC. Microscopically proven cure of actinic cheilitis by CO_2 laser. Lasers Surg Med 1987;7:520–523.

41. Dover JS, Arndt KA, Geronemus RG. Illustrated cutaneous laser surgery. A practitioner's guide. East Norwalk, CT: Appleton & Lange, 1990:21–73.

42. Hall RR. Haemostatic incisions of the liver. CO$_2$ laser compared with surgical diathermy. Br J Surg 1971;58:538–541.

43. Slutzki S, Shafir R, Bornstein LA. Use of the carbon dioxide laser for large excisions with minimal blood loss. Plast Reconstr Surg 1977;60:250–257.

44. Kaplan I, Sarig A, Taube E et al. The CO$_2$ laser in pediatric surgery. J Pediatr Surg 1984;19:248–257.

45. Reid AB, Stranc MF. Healing of infected wounds following iodine scrub or CO$_2$ laser treatment. Lasers Surg Med 1991;11:475–480.

46. Mullarky MB, Norris CW, Goldberg ID. The efficacy of the CO$_2$ laser in the sterilization of skin seeded with bacteria: survival at the skin surface and in the plume emissions. Laryngoscope 1985;95:186–187.

47. Aschler P, Ingolitsch E, Walter G et al. Ultrastructural findings in CNS tissue with CO$_2$ laser. In: Kaplan I, ed. Laser surgery. Jerusalem: Academic Press, 1976.

48. Ben-Bassat M, Ben Bassat J, Kaplan I. An ultrastructural study of the cut edges of skin and mucous membrane specimens excised by carbon dioxide laser. In: Kaplan I, ed. Laser surgery. Jerusalem: Academic Press, 1976.

49. Ehrenberger K, Inniton J. The effect of carbon dioxide laser on skin lymphatics. Wien Klin Wochenschr 1978;90:307–309.

50. Schenk P. Ultrastructure of skin and mucous membranes after incision with a CO$_2$ laser. Laryngol Rhinol Otol (Stuttg) 1979;58:770–777.

51. Fruhling J, Lejoune E, Van Hoof G, Gerard A. Lymphatic migration after laser surgery. Lancet 1977;2:973–974.

52. Morris DM, Morrow LB. CO$_2$ laser blepharoplasty. A comparison with cold-steel surgery. J Dermatol Surg Oncol 1992;18:307–313.

53. David LM, Sanders G. CO$_2$ laser blepharoplasty: a comparison to cold steel and electrocautery. J Dermatol Surg Oncol 1987;13:110–114.

54. Mittelman H, Apfelberg DB. Carbon dioxide laser blepharoplasty—advantages and disadvantages. Ann Plast Surg 1990;24:1–6.

55. Becker DW. Use of the carbon dioxide laser in treating multiple cutaneous neurofibromas. Ann Plast Surg 1991;26:582–586.

56. Stanley TH, Roenigk RK. The carbon dioxide laser treatment of actinic cheilitis. Mayo Clin Proc 1988;63:230–235.

57. Kardos TB, Ferguson MM. Comparison of cryosurgery and the carbon dioxide laser in mucosal healing. Int J Oral Maxillofac Surg 1991;20:108–111.

58. Zelickson BD, Roenigk RK. Actinic cheilitis. Treatment with the carbon dioxide laser. Cancer 1990;65:1307–1311.

59. Dufresne RG, Garett AB, Bailin PL et al. Carbon dioxide laser treatment of chronic actinic cheilitis. J Am Acad Dermatol 1988;19:876–878.

60. David LM. Laser vermilion ablation for actinic cheilitis. J Dermatol Surg Oncol 1985;11:605–609.

61. Johnson TM, Sebastien TS, Lowe L et al. Carbon dioxide laser treatment of actinic cheilitis: clinicohistopathologic correlation to determine the optimal depth of destruction. J Am Acad Dermatol 1992;27:737–745.

62. Benedict LM, Cohen B. Treatment of Peutz-Jeghers lentigines with the carbon dioxide laser. J Dermatol Surg Oncol 1991;17:954–955.

63. Greenbaum SS, Glogau R, Stegman SJ et al. Carbon dioxide laser treatment of erythroplasia of Queyrat. J Dermatol Surg Oncol 1989;15:747–750.

64. Malek RS. Laser treatment of squamous cell lesions of the penis. Lasers Surg Med 1992;12:246–249.

65. Gordon KB, Robinson J. Carbon dioxide laser vaporization for Bowen's disease of the finger. Arch Dermatol 1994;130:1250–1252.

66. Eliezri YD. The toluidine blue test: an aid to the diagnosis and treatment of early squamous cell carcinoma of mucous membranes. J Am Acad Dermatol 1988;18:1339–1349.

67. Ratz JL. Carbon dioxide laser treatment of balanitis xerotica obliterans. J Am Acad Dermatol 1984;10:925–928.

68. Windahl T, Hellstens. CO_2 laser treatment of lichen sclerosus et atrophicus. J Urol 1993;150:868–870.

69. Baldwin HE, Geronemus RG. The treatment of Zoon's balanitis with the carbon dioxide laser. J Dermatol Surg Oncol 1989;15:491–494.

70. Roodenburg JLN, Panders AK, Vermey A. Carbon dioxide laser surgery of oral leukoplakia. Oral Surg Oral Med Oral Pathol 1991;71:670–674.

71. Persley MS. Carbon dioxide laser treatment of oral florid papillomatosis. J Dermatol Surg Oncol 1984;10:64–66.

72. Frame JW. Treatment of sublingual keratosis with the carbon dioxide laser. Br Dent J 1984;156:243–246.

73. Fitzpatrick RE. The Ultrapulse CO_2 laser: selective photothermolysis of epidermal tumors. Lasers Surg Med 1993;5(suppl):803–804.

74. Adams EL, Prince NM. Treatment of basal cell carcinomas with a carbon dioxide laser. J Dermatol Surg Oncol 1979;5:803–806.

75. Wheeland RG, Bailin PL, Ratz JL et al. Carbon dioxide laser vaporization and curettage in the treatment of large or multiple superficial basal cell carcinomas. J Dermatol Surg Oncol 1987;13:119–124.

76. Groot DW, Johnston PA. Carbon dioxide laser treatment of porokeratosis of Mibelli. Lasers Surg Med 1985;5:603–606.

77. Rabbin PE, Baldwin HE. Treatment of porokeratosis of Mibelli with CO_2 laser vaporization versus surgical excision with split-thickness skin graft. A comparison. J Dermatol Surg Oncol 1993;19:199–202.

78. Ratz JL, Bailin PL, Lakeland RF. Carbon dioxide laser treatment of epidermal nevi. J Dermatol Surg Oncol 1986;12:567–571.

79. Hohenleutner U, Wlotzke U, Konz B et al. Carbon dioxide laser therapy of a widespread epidermal nevus. Lasers Surg Med 1995;16:288–291.

80. McElroy JA, Mehregan DA, Roenigk RK. Carbon dioxide laser vaporization of recalcitrant symptomatic plaques of Hailey-Hailey disease and Darier's disease. J Am Acad Dermatol 1990;23:893–897.

81. Kartamaa IM, Reitamo S. Familial benign chronic pemphigus (Hailey-Hailey disease): treatment with carbon dioxide laser vaporization. Arch Dermatol 1992;128:646–648.

82. Garrett AB, Dufresne RG, Ratz JL et al. Carbon dioxide laser treatment of pitted acne scarring. J Dermatol Surg Oncol 1990;16:737–740.

83. Wheeland RG. Revision of full-thickness skin grafts using the carbon dioxide laser. J Dermatol Surg Oncol 1988;14:130–132.

84. Spandoni D, Cain CL. Facial resurfacing using the carbon dioxide laser. AORN J 1989;50:1007–1013.

85. Solotoff S. Treatment for pitted acne scarring—postauricular punch grafts followed by dermabrasion. J Dermatol Surg Oncol 1986;12:10–15.

86. Abergel RP, David LM. Aging hands: a technique of hand rejuvenation by laser resurfacing and autologous fat transfer. J Dermatol Surg Oncol 1989;15:725–729.

87. Dover JS, Smoller BR, Stern RS et al. Low-fluence carbon dioxide laser irradiation of lentigenes. Arch Dermatol 1988;124:1219–1224.

88. Stern RS, Dover JS, Levin J et al. Laser therapy versus cryotherapy of lentigenes: a comparative trial. J Am Acad Dermatol 1994;30:985–987.

89. Goldberg DJ. Benign pigmented lesions of the skin. Treatment with the Q-switched ruby laser. J Dermatol Surg Oncol 1993;19:376–379.

90. Bailin PL. CO_2 laser therapy for non-PWS lesions. In: Arndt KA, Noe JM, Rosen S, eds. Cutaneous laser therapy: principles and methods. New York: Wiley, 1983:195–196.

91. Mueller TF, Carlson BA, Lundy MP. The use of the carbon dioxide surgical laser for treatment of verrucae. J Am Pediatr Assoc 1980;70:136–141.

92. McBurney EI, Rosen DA. Carbon dioxide laser treatment of verrucae vulgares. J Dermatol Surg Oncol 1984;10:45–48.

93. Logan RA, Zachary CB. Outcome of carbon dioxide laser therapy for persistent cutaneous viral warts. Br J Dermatol 1989;121:99–105.

94. Apfelberg DB, Druber D, Maser MR et al. Benefits of the CO_2 laser for verruca resistant to other modalities of treatment. J Dermatol Surg Oncol 1989;15:371–375.

95. Street ML, Roenigk RK. Recalcitrant periungual verrucae: the role of carbon dioxide laser vaporization. J Am Acad Dermatol 1990;23:115–120.

96. Ferenczy A, Mitao M, Nagai N et al. Latent papilloma virus and recurring genital warts. N Engl J Med 1985;313:784–788.

97. Lessus J, Happonen HP, Niemi KM et al. Carbon dioxide laser therapy cures macroscopic lesions, but viral genome is not eradicated in men with therapy-resistant HPV infection. Sex Transm Dis 1994;21:297–302.

98. Riva JM, Sedlacek TW, Cunnane MF et al. Extended carbon dioxide laser vaporization in the treatment of subclinical papilloma virus infection of the lower genital tract. Obstet Gynecol 1989;73:25–30.

99. Calkins JW, Masterson BJ, Magrina JE et al. Management of condyloma acuminata with the carbon dioxide laser. Obstet Gynecol 1982;59:105–108.

100. Baggish MS. CO_2 laser surgery for condyloma acuminata venereal infection. Obstet Gynecol 1980;55:711–715.

101. Bellina JH. The use of the CO_2 laser in management of condyloma acuminata with eight year follow-up. Am J Obstet Gyncol 1983;147:375–378.

102. Bar-Am A, Shilon M, Peyser MR et al. Treatment of male genital condylomatous lesions by carbon dioxide laser after failure of previous non-laser methods. J Am Acad Dermatol 1991;24:87–89.

103. Carpiniello VL, Schoenberg M, Malloy TR. Longterm follow-up of subclinical human papillomavirus infection treated with the carbon dioxide laser and intrauretheral 5-fluorouracil: a treatment protocol. J Urol 1990;143:726–728.

104. Vance JC, Davis D. Interferon alpha-2b infections used as an adjuvant therapy to carbon dioxide laser vaporization of recalcitrant ano-genital condylomata acuminata. J Invest Dermatol 1990;95:146S–148S.

105. Reid R, Greenberg MD, Pizzuti DJ et al. Superficial laser vulvectomy. V. Surgical debulking is enhanced by adjuvant systemic interferon. Am J Obstet Gynecol 1992;166:815–820.

106. Cobb MW. Human papillomavirus infection. J Am Acad Dermatol 1990;22:547–566.

107. Moy RL, Eliezri YD, Nuovo GJ et al. Human papillomavirus type 16 DNA in periungual squamous cell carcinomas. JAMA 1989;261:2669–2673.

108. Kawashima M, Jablonska S, Favre M et al. Characterization of a new type of human papillomavirus found in a lesion of Bowen's disease of the skin. J Virol 1986;57:688–692.

109. Pearson SE, Whittaker J, Ireland D et al. Invasive cancer of the cervix after laser treatment. Br J Obstet Gynecol 1989;96:486–488.

110. Wheeland RG, Bailin PL, Kronberg E. Carbon dioxide laser vaporization for treatment of multiple tricho-epithelioma. J Dermatol Surg Oncol 1984;10:470–475.

111. Sawchuk WS, Heald PW. CO_2 laser treatment of trichoepithelioma with focused and defocused beam. J Dermatol Surg Oncol 1984;10:905–907.

112. Roenigk RK, Ratz JL. CO_2 laser treatment of cutaneous neurofibromas. J Dermatol Surg Oncol 1987;13:187–189.

113. Bickley LK, Goldberg DJ, Imaeda S et al. Treatment of multiple apocrine hidrocystomas with the carbon dioxide laser. J Dermatol Surg Oncol 1989;15:599–602.

114. Stoner MF, Hobbs ER. Treatment of multiple dermal cylindromas with the carbon dioxide laser. J Dermatol Surg Oncol 1988;14:1263–1267.

115. Janniger CK, Goldberg DJ. Angiofibromas in tuberous sclerosis: comparison of treatment by carbon dioxide and argon laser. J Dermatol Surg Oncol 1990;16:317–320.

116. Boixeda P, Sanchez-Miralles E, Azana JM et al. CO_2, argon, and pulsed dye laser treatment of angiofibromas. J Dermatol Surg Oncol 1994;20:808–812.

117. Magid M, Garden JM. Pearly penile papules: treatment with the carbon dioxide laser. J Dermatol Surg Oncol 1989;15:552–554.

118. Wheeland RG, Bailin PL, Reynolds OD et al. Carbon dioxide laser vaporization of multiple facial syringomas. J Dermatol Surg Oncol 1986;12:225–228.

119. Waters RA, Clement RM, Thomas JM. Carbon dioxide laser ablation of cutaneous metastases from malignant melanoma. Br J Surg 1991;78:493–494.

120. Apfelberg DB, Maser MR, Lash H et al. Treatment of xanthelasma palpebrarum with the carbon dioxide laser. J Dermatol Surg Oncol 1987;13:149–151.

121. Taylor MB. Chrondrodermatitis nodularis chronical helicis. Successful treatment with the carbon dioxide laser. J Dermatol Surg Oncol 1991;17:862–864.

122. Wheeland RG, Ashley JR, Snick DA et al. CO_2 laser treatment of granuloma faciale. J Dermatol Surg Oncol 1984;10:730–733.

123. Kaymen AH, Nasr A, Grekin RC. The use of carbon dioxide laser in lichen myxedematous. J Dermatol Surg Oncol 1989;15:862–865.

124. Hobbs ER, Bailin PL, Ratz JF et al. Treatment of angiolymphoid hyperplasia of the external ear with carbon dioxide laser. J Am Acad Dermatol 1988;19:345–349.

125. Truhan AP, Garden JM, Roenigk HH. Nodular primary localized cutaneous amyloidosis: immunohistochemical evaluation and treatment with the carbon dioxide laser. J Am Acad Dermatol 1986;14:1058–1062.

126. Huerter CJ, Wheeland RG, Bailin PL et al. Treatment of myxoid cysts with carbon dioxide laser vaporization. J Dermatol Surg Oncol 1987;13:723–727.

127. Werkhaven J, Maddern BR, Stool SE. Post-tracheostomy granulation tissue managed by carbon dioxide laser excision. Ann Otol Rhinol Laryngol 1989;98:828–830.

128. Kantor GR, Roenigk RK, Bailin PL et al. Cutaneous blastomycosis: report of a case presumably acquired by direct inoculation and treated with carbon dioxide laser vaporization. Cleve Clin J Med 1987;54:121–124.

129. Kuttner BJ, Siegle RJ. Treatment of chromomycosis with a CO_2 laser. J Dermatol Surg Oncol 1986;12:965–968.

130. Babejev KB, Babajev OG, Korepanov VI. Treatment of cutaneous leishmaniasis using a carbon dioxide laser. Bull WHO 1991;69:103–106.

131. Lefell DJ, Brown MD, Swanson NA. Laser vaporization: a novel treatment of botryomycosis. J Dermatol Surg Oncol 1989;15:703–705.

132. Glass LF, Berman B, Laub D. Treatment of perifolliculitis capitis abscedens et suffodiens with the carbon dioxide laser. J Dermatol Surg Oncol 1989;15:673–676.

133. Dalrymple JC, Monaghan JM. Treatment of hidradenitis suppurativa with the carbon dioxide laser. Br J Surg 1987;74:420–424.

134. Sherman AI, Reid R. CO_2 laser for suppurativa hidradenitis of the vulva. J Reprod Med 1991;36:113–117.

135. Lapins J, Marcusson JA, Emtestam LB. Surgical treatment of chronic hidradenitis suppurativa: CO_2 laser stripping—secondary intention technique. Br J Dermatol 1994;131:551–556.

136. Leshin B, Whitaker DC. Carbon dioxide laser matrixectomy. J Dermatol Surg Oncol 1988;14:608–611.

137. Ratz JL, Bailin PL, Levine HL. CO_2 laser treatment of portwine stains: a preliminary report. J Dermatol Surg Oncol 1982;8:1039–1043.

138. Kaplan I, Peled I. The CO_2 laser in the treatment of superficial telangiectases. Br J Plast Surg 1975;28:214–215.

139. Apfelberg DB, Maser MR, Lash H. Argon laser treatment of cutaneous vascular abnormalities. Ann Plast Surg 1978;1:14–18.

140. Cosman B. Experience in the argon laser therapy of portwine stains. Plast Reconstr Surg 1980;65:119–127.

141. Noe JM, Barsky S, Gerr D et al. Portwine stains and the response to argon laser therapy: successful treatment and the predictive role of color, age, and biopsy. Plast Reconstr Surg 1980;65:130–137.

142. Lanigan SW, Cotterill JA. The treatment of portwine stains with the carbon dioxide laser. Br J Dermatol 1990;123:229–235.

143. Bailin PL. Use of the CO_2 laser for non-PWS cutaneous lesions. In: Arndt KA, Noe JM, Rosen S, eds. Cutaneous laser therapy: principles and methods. New York: Wiley, 1983:187–200.

144. Goldman L, Naprstek Z, Johnson J. Laser surgery of a digital angiosarcoma: report of a case and 6 year follow-up study. Cancer 1977;39:1738–1742.

145. Bailin PL, Kantor GR, Wheeland RG. Carbon dioxide laser vaporization of lymphangioma circumscriptum. J Am Acad Dermatol 1986;14:257–262.

146. Kaplan I. The Sharplan CO_2 laser in neonatal surgery. Ann Plast Surg 1982;8:426–428.

147. Dufresne RG Jr, Garrett AB, Bailin PL et al. CO_2 laser treatment of traumatic tattoos. J Am Acad Dermatol 1989;20:137–138.

148. Ruiz-Esparza J, Fitzpatrick RE, Goldman MP. Tattoo removal with

minimal scarring: the chemo-laser technique. J Dermatol Surg Oncol 1989;14:1372–1376.

149. Kilmer SL, Lee MS, Grevelink JM et al. The Q-switched Nd:YAG laser effectively treats tattoos. A controlled, dose-response study. Arch Dermatol 1993;129:971–978.

150. Kyanko ME, Pontasch MJ, Brodell RT. Red tattoo reactions: treatment with the carbon dioxide laser. J Dermatol Surg Oncol 1989;15:652–656.

151. Levin NS, Salisbury RE, Paterson HD et al. Clinical evaluations of the carbon dioxide laser for burn wound excisions: a comparison of the laser, scalpel, and electrocautery. J Trauma 1975;15:800–805.

152. Fidler JP, Law E, MacMillan BG et al. Comparison of carbon dioxide laser excision of burns with other thermal knives. Ann NY Acad Sci 1976;267:254–256.

153. Stellar S, Levine N, Ger R et al. Laser excision of acute third-degree burns followed by immediate autograft replacement: an experimental study in the pig. J Trauma 1973;13:45–48.

154. Lejeuene EJ, Van Hook G, Gerard A. Impairment of graft take after CO_2 laser surgery in melanoma patients. Br J Surg 1980;67:318–320.

155. Cochrane TP, Beacon JP, Creasey Gal et al. Wound healing after laser surgery: an experimental study. Br J Surg 1980;67:740–743.

156. Green HA, Domankevitz Y, Nishioba NS. Pulsed carbon dioxide laser ablation of burned skin: in vitro and in vivo analysis. Lasers Surg Med 1980;10:476–484.

157. Green HA, Bua D, Anderson RR et al. Burn depth estimation using indocyanine green fluorescence. Arch Dermatol 1992;128:43–49.

158. Hallock GG. Extended applications of the carbon dioxide laser for skin deepithelialization. Plast Reconstr Surg 1989;83:717–721.

159. Olbricht SM, Stern RS, Tang SV et al. Complications of cutaneous laser surgery. A survey. Arch Dermatol 1987;123:345–349.

160. Reid R, Muller S. Tattoo removal by carbon dioxide laser dermabrasion. Plast Reconstr Surg 1980;65:717–728.

161. Zimmerman MC. Tattoo removal. J Dermatol Surg Oncol 1984;10:911–918.

162. Ruiz-Esparza J, Fitzpatrick RE, Goldman MP. Tattoo removal: selecting the right alternative. Am J Cosmetic Surg 1992;9:171–179.

163. Friedman M, Gal D. Keloid scars as a result of CO_2 laser for molluscum contagiosum. Obstet Gynecol 1987;70:394–396.

164. Eaglstein WH, Mertz PM. "Inert" vehicles do affect wound healing. J Invest Dermatol 1980;74:90–91.

165. Geronemus RG, Mertz PM, Eaglstein WH. Wound healing. The effects of topical antimicrobial agents. Arch Dermatol 1979;115:1311–1314.

166. Chan P, Vincent JW, Wangemann RT. Accelerated healing of carbon dioxide laser burns in rats treated with composite polyurethane dressing. Arch Dermatol 1987;123:1042–1045.

167. Larson DL, Abston S, Evans EB et al. Techniques for decreasing scar formation and contractions in the burned patient. J Trauma 1971;11:807–823.

168. Brodman M, Port M, Friedman F Jr et al. Operating room personnel morbidity from carbon dioxide laser use during precepted surgery. Obstet Gynecol 1993;81:607–609.

169. Kashima HK, Kessis T, Mounts P et al. Polymerase chain reaction identification of human papillomavirus DNA in CO_2 laser plume from re-

current respiratory papillomatosis. Otolaryngol Head Neck Surg 1991; 104:191–195.

170. Ferenczy A, Bergeron C, Richart RM. Carbon dioxide laser energy disperses human papillomavirus deoxyribonucleic acid onto treatment fields. Am J Obstet Gynecol 1990;163:1271–1274.

171. Matchette LS, Faaland RW, Royston DD et al. In vitro production of viable bacteriophage in carbon dioxide laser. Am J Obstet Gynecol 1984; 148:9–12.

172. Nezhat C, Winer WK, Nezhat F et al. Smoke from laser surgery: is there a health hazard? Lasers Surg Med 1987;7:376–382.

173. Gloster HM Jr, Roenigk RK. Risk of acquiring human papillomavirus from the plume produced by the carbon dioxide laser in the treatment of warts. J Am Acad Dermatol 1995;32:432–441.

174. Ferenczy A. Treating genital condyloma during pregnancy with carbon dioxide laser. Am J Obstet Gynecol 1984;148:9–12.

13 ___ Laser Skin Resurfacing

George J. Hruza
Richard E. Fitzpatrick
Jeffrey S. Dover

There has always been great interest in facial rejuvenation. As proof of this, for thousands of years, topical agents, such as sour milk, vegetable extracts, and mud packs, have been used with this object in mind, but with only limited success. More recently, prepared concentrations of topical agents have been used; these include vitamin A derivatives, such as retinoic acid, and a group of hydroxy acids, most notably alpha-hydroxy acid. However, although public interest has been great, the clinical effects have been only minimal.

In an effort to more effectively rejuvenate very photodamaged skin, a variety of chemical agents have been used to strip off a variable thickness of skin, in the expectation that reepithelialization will occur, resulting in a more youthful skin appearance. Mechanically removing varying layers of dermis with dermabrasion can also alleviate wrinkles.

In the 1980s and early 1990s continuous-wave CO_2 lasers were used in an effort to resurface photoaged skin.[1] Although the results of this procedure in the hands of a few practitioners were quite impressive, the risk-benefit ratio associated with the procedure was very high. This was due to the fact that dwelling too long on a specific area led to significant thermal diffusion, thermal damage, and, ultimately, scarring. For this reason the technique was never widely used. However, with the development of short-pulsed, high peak power, rapidly scanned, focused-beam CO_2 lasers, it became possible to remove photodamaged skin layer by layer in a precisely controlled manner while leaving behind a very narrow zone of thermal damage.[2-8] Because of its effectiveness there has been an explosion of interest in this new technology for the resurfacing of photoaged skin, as well as for the treatment of scars.

Laser-Tissue Interactions for CO_2 Lasers

In general, lasers are used in dermatology for their laser-induced heating. When they are used in this way, with close attention to the principles of selective photothermolysis, then very precise tissue effects can be achieved. The basic principles of this theory are that selective heating is achieved by means of preferential laser light absorption and heat production in the target chromophore, with the heat being localized to the target by using a pulse duration shorter than the tissue's thermal relaxation time (or cooling time).[9]

The tissue chromophore that absorbs the 10,600-nm wavelength of the CO_2 laser is water. The depth of penetration of this wavelength into tissue depends only on the tissue water content, with the degree of pigmentation and vascularity being irrelevant. The extinction length, or thickness of tissue that absorbs 90% of the radiant energy of the incident beam of the CO_2 laser, is approximately 30 μm.[10–12]

The vaporization or boiling temperature of water at 1 atmosphere pressure is 100°C. When the CO_2 laser is used for vaporization in the continuous mode at modest powers, the skin surface temperature fluctuates in cycles between about 120° and 200°C during ablation. Charring occurs when desiccated tissue becomes extremely hot and then carbonizes. The immediate tissue effects depend on the spot size and power as well as on the speed with which the laser beam is moved across the tissue surface. When a very small beam diameter of 100 to 300 μm is used, very high irradiances can be achieved, resulting in rapid tissue vaporization. However, unless the beam is moved rapidly across the tissue surface, desiccation, charring, and heat diffusion occur. When a large beam size of greater than 2 mm is used, nonvaporization heating occurs and the potential for deep thermal damage increases because of the need to apply the low irradiances for long tissue dwell times to achieve vaporization or visible thermal effects. In all of these situations, the duration of the laser-tissue interaction is the critical factor in determining the depth of residual thermal damage.[2]

Though the laser energy penetrates only 30 μm or so and is absorbed within that layer, thermal coagulation occurs to a depth of about 1 mm because of heat diffusion. Temperatures reach an excess of 300°C when visible tissue charring occurs, and temperatures in excess of 600°C may be achieved when the laser is held stationary on this carbonized tissue until it glows red, as occurs with burning coals. This results in widespread thermal necrosis that interferes with wound healing and results in scarring.

The ability of the CO_2 laser to photocoagulate blood vessels less than 0.5 mm in diameter, as well as to seal small lymphatics and nerve endings, has made it possible to achieve relatively bloodless surgical procedures, accompanied by less postoperative edema and pain.[13,14] However, the risk of scarring and the unpredictable levels of thermal damage with delayed healing that often occur have been responsible for limiting the clinical applications of the continuous-wave CO_2 laser. It has remained difficult to achieve excellent clinical results using this laser.

To control the depth of thermal damage that occurs in tissue, the continuous-wave CO_2 laser beam needs to be scanned at a rate that results in a tissue dwell time of less than the thermal relaxation time, or the energy must be delivered in a pulse shorter than this time. The thermal relaxation time of the 30-μm tissue layer heated by the CO_2 laser has been calculated to be less than 1 msec.[15]

Superpulsed CO_2 lasers were developed to deliver peak powers two to ten times higher and pulse durations ten to a hundred times shorter than those of conventional CO_2 lasers with shuttered pulses. The basic principle of superpulsed CO_2 lasers is to use high peak powers with a short pulse duration to vaporize tissue with minimal thermal injury.[16-18]

Further calculations as well as experimental data revealed that the pulse fluence needed to ablate skin tissue using a pulsed laser is approximately 5 J/cm^2.[10-12] The pulse energy of a single pulse from a superpulsed laser is in the 30- to 50-mJ range, so for single pulse vaporization to occur, the beam diameter must be less than 1 mm. Such a narrow beam cannot be used efficiently for resurfacing vaporization, because this grooves the tissue and also causes the procedure to be slow and tedious. In general, a beam diameter of at least 2.5 mm is desirable for these applications. In this situation, six to ten pulses of 30 to 50 mJ are necessary to reach the tissue vaporization threshold. This can be accomplished by manually shuttering the beam, and this has the effect of minimizing residual thermal damage. However, if the superpulsed laser pulses are delivered in an uninterrupted stream, often at a rate of 200 Hz or more, this semicontinuous beam reacts no differently with tissue than a continuous beam. To prevent heat from accumulating between pulse delivery, if the only mechanism for heat removal is conduction, with no vaporization occurring, a rate of 5 Hz is considered optimal when the spot is not moved.[19] It is clear that the effect of multiple laser pulses striking the same tissue points is deeper thermal damage.

HIGH PEAK POWER LASER

To achieve maximal vaporization with minimal thermal damage, tissue needs to be vaporized in a single pulse. If a beam diameter of 2.5 mm or greater is used, a pulse energy greater than 250 mJ is necessary, which delivers the required 5 or more J/cm^2. This laser energy vaporizes tissue to the 20- to 30-μm optical penetration depth of the laser and leaves 40 to 120 μm of residual thermal damage, which is two to four times the optical penetration depth.[4,5] This high-energy pulsed laser has been developed by Coherent, Inc., and has been named the *UltraPulse laser.*

If this laser is used for single-pulse vaporization of the epidermis, intracellular water is vaporized, leaving behind cellular proteinaceous debris. The depth of vaporization is directly proportional to the pulse energy. However, there is a large amount of extracellular matrix in the dermis, dominated by structural proteins, collagen, and elastin. Elastin is very stable and may survive very high temperatures intact. Type I collagen undergoes a sharp melting transition between 60° and 70°C. However, energy fluences much higher than 5 J/cm^2 are necessary to vaporize the proteinaceous matrix. Nonvaporization heating of the dermis has little additive effect if the pulse duration is less than 1 msec and the pulses are delivered at a rate of 5 Hz or less.[19] If the delivery rate is greater than this, heat accumulates in tissue, leading to possible thermal damage by diffusion, and hence poor wound healing or scarring.

In a study conducted on pig skin, the resurfacing depth produced by 150 to 450 mJ per pulse delivered in one to three passes was compared with the depth achieved with 30% trichloroacetic acid (TCA) medium-depth chemical peel, dermabrasion, and Baker's phenol deep peel.[4] Reepithelialization of all sites treated with the different methods was complete at 7 days, with the exception of the phenol-treated skin, which took approximately 3 weeks to heal completely with a normally configured epidermis. Healing of the TCA-treated site was comparable clinically and histologically to the healing of laser-treated sites receiving 150 mJ per pulse (three passes) and 250 mJ per pulse (one or two passes). Healing of the dermabrasion-treated site was comparable clinically and histologically to that of the laser-treated sites receiving 250 to 450 mJ per pulse and two or three passes. The phenol-treated site had not returned histologically to normal at the end of the study (6 weeks) and showed a deeper and slower-healing wound than that produced by any combination of laser pulse energy and numbers of passes studied. Overall, the severity of the clinical wound and time to completion of healing correlated with the depth of tissue removal. Scarring was not observed in any of the treatment sites at the end of the study period.

The precise depth of vaporization was difficult to measure, because once the epidermis is removed, the heat generated in the tissue causes the collagen to contract, and this alters the visible dermal thickness. Instead, the total zone of vaporization–tissue contraction plus residual thermal damage was measured to determine the laser resurfacing depth. This was also more appropriate, because the thermally coagulated tissue sloughs within days and it is this combination of tissue effects that is relevant clinically. A single pass was found to result in partial or complete epidermal loss with minimal dermal effects, regardless of the pulse energy, though higher energy fluences resulted in more complete epidermal vaporization. Subsequent passes resulted in progressive tissue loss into the dermis. The dermal vaporization plus necrosis depth was directly proportional to the pulse energy and the number of passes utilized. The depth of residual thermal necrosis in the dermis after single laser passes of various energies was minimal (<4 μm); however, the residual thermal damage after two and three passes ranged from 53 to 106 μm in depth and increased with increasing pulse energies as well as increasing numbers of passes.

In rabbit skin, with its very thin epidermis, one laser pass delivering 250 mJ of energy to a 3-mm collimated spot size was found to vaporize the epidermis and portions of the papillary dermis and leave behind residual thermal damage to a depth of approximately 70 μm.[5] In human skin, one pass with the UltraPulse laser was found to leave behind a 20-μm-deep zone of thermal damage, a second pass a 40-μm-deep zone, and a third pass a 70-μm-deep zone.[20]

FLASHSCANNER

A focused CO_2 laser beam with a spot size of 0.1 to 0.25 mm can completely vaporize tissue water by delivering more than 5 J/cm^2 to the target tissue in less than 1 msec. However, a focused laser beam delivering such a high energy fluence would be very difficult to control freehand. For this reason, a flashscanner (Sharplan SilkTouch) was developed that, with the help of rapidly oscillating mirrors in the handpiece, scans the focused laser beam in a spiral pattern across the tissue. This device is able to keep the laser beam at any given spot for less than 1 msec, which for the tissue is equivalent to a 1-msec laser pulse. This dwell time allows for complete vaporization of well-hydrated target tissue and is also short enough so that peripheral thermal damage is confined to a 40- to 50-μm-wide zone around the impact site.[6,7] The scanner is microprocessor controlled and can be programmed to scan areas of various sizes ranging from 1 to 16 mm in diameter, depending on the focal length of the handpiece lens. Scan shapes can be circular, elliptical, or even square. A complete scan for skin resurfacing takes 0.2 to 0.45 second, depending on the scan size.

One pass with the flashscanner vaporizes the epidermis, leaving behind a 30-μm-deep zone of thermally coagulated dermis. A second pass deepens the zone of thermal damage to 80 μm and a third pass to 150 μm.[20] The additive depth of thermal damage observed is probably due to the desiccated thermally denatured collagen left behind after each pass. This material contains very little water, thus preventing significant additional vaporization after the initial pass. When vaporization is less complete, there is more energy left in the tissue to cause thermal coagulation.

HIGH PEAK POWER LASER VERSUS FLASHSCANNER

As tissue is vaporized using either laser system, the remaining dermis noticeably shrinks. As noted earlier, collagen contracts significantly as it is heated. It is unclear, at this time, however, whether this collagen shrinkage adds to the final clinical improvement or whether the collagen that has contracted is sloughed off with all the other necrotic material. The different laser systems appear to achieve equivalent clinical results in properly trained hands. In clinical use, two passes with the flashscanner are equivalent to three passes with the UltraPulse laser in terms of the amount of tissue removed and the depth of residual thermal damage. The main differences between the two laser systems are in the specific parameters used with each (Table 13-1).

Table 13-1. High peak power CO_2 lasers versus flashscanner

	Coherent UltraPulse	Tissue Technology TruPulse	Sharplan SilkTouch
Laser type	100-W CO_2	6-W CO_2	40 or more W CO_2
Delivery method	Individual gaussian pulses	Individual square pulses	Spiral scan, focused beam
Power	500-W peak power, pulsed	10,000-W peak power, pulsed	6- to 18-W average power, continuous-wave beam
Pulse duration	950 μsec	60–100 μsec	0.2–0.45 sec scan duration; <1-msec tissue dwell time
Energy	50–500 mJ/pulse, adjustable by changing pulsewidth	10–500 mJ/pulse, adjustable by changing peak power	—
Energy fluence (J/cm^2)	5–7	5–7	5–15 or more
Spot size	3-mm collimated, computer pattern generator	1 and 3 mm; 5 mm in development	1- to 16-mm scan size with 0.1- to 0.25-mm focused beam
Spot shape	Round spot, varies with computer pattern generator	Square spot	Round, square, or elliptical scan
Effect of increasing power setting	Increases rate of pulsing	Increases rate of pulsing	Increases thickness of tissue removed with each scan

Preoperative Considerations

PATIENT SELECTION

In evaluating the prospective patient and assessing his or her potential response to laser resurfacing, the two primary areas of focus are the perioral (Fig. 13-1) and periorbital (Fig. 13-2) regions. Wrinkling in these areas has been traditionally unresponsive to face-lifting procedures, because the laxity of the skin removed and tightened by these techniques does not include these areas. Chemical peeling and dermabrasion in these locations, though helpful, have often produced disappointing results. However, we have found laser resurfacing to achieve excellent results in these locations. Though any facial wrinkles may respond excellently to laser therapy, it is the results seen in these locations that have established the success of laser resurfacing, primarily because historically they have been difficult to treat.[3,7,8,21,22]

In general, both wrinkling and photodamage to the epidermis and dermis respond to treatment. With regard to the epidermal abnormalities associated with aging, actinic keratoses, squamous cell carcinoma in situ, lentigines, and seborrheic keratoses can all be removed by stripping of the epidermal layer. Photodamage of the dermis results in fragmentation of the elastin and collagen fibrils, most profoundly in the papillary dermis. This is seen clinically in the form of an altered surface texture and pallor, with crepelike changes progressing to those typical of cutis rhomboidalis nuchae. These layers of altered dermal tissue may be removed by vaporization and thermal necrosis and replaced with new, healthy collagen that develops over a tightened matrix of shrunken collagen. The ability to change these tissues dramatically depends on the depth of damage, with the more superficial damage being more responsive. These altered dermal changes result in loose, sagging, or folded skin. The folds may be particularly visible under the eyes, on the medial lower cheeks, on the lateral cheeks anterior to the ears, and to a certain extent at the nasolabial folds. These areas tend to be very responsive to the tightening effects achieved with laser resurfacing.[3,7,8,21,22]

Lines of expression, such as forehead creases, glabellar furrows, "crow's feet," and nasolabial folds, may respond if they are superficial, but deep folds and palpable deep creases may only be softened. Even if these lines completely disappear after treatment, they recur much sooner than sun-induced wrinkles because of the unavoidable effects of muscular contractions compressing and folding the skin during facial expressions. This is true of certain perioral lines as well.

As with any cosmetic procedure, patient expectations are the most important determinant of patient satisfaction. A patient must have realistic expectations as to the improvement that can be achieved. He or she must understand that laser resurfacing cannot eliminate all or even most wrinkles. Showing patients before-and-after photographs may be helpful, but photographs of patients with rhytides before and after treatment can often be misleading, because of changing light

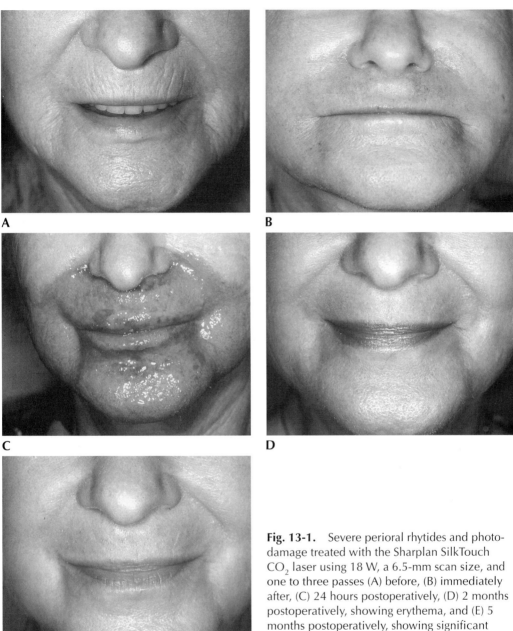

Fig. 13-1. Severe perioral rhytides and photo-damage treated with the Sharplan SilkTouch CO_2 laser using 18 W, a 6.5-mm scan size, and one to three passes (A) before, (B) immediately after, (C) 24 hours postoperatively, (D) 2 months postoperatively, showing erythema, and (E) 5 months postoperatively, showing significant rhytid effacement without skin texture or pigment changes. See Fig. 13-1 in color section.

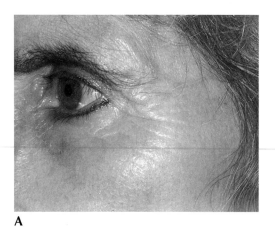
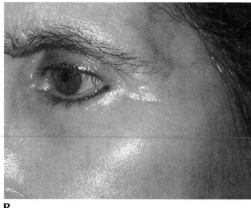

A   B

Fig. 13-2.   Periorbital rhytides treated with the Coherent UltraPulse computerized-pattern generator using 300 mJ, 100 W, a 2.25-mm spot size, and two full passes overall, then one pass in select areas, followed by two to three passes in select areas using 500 mJ and 4 W with a freehand 3-mm spot size. (A) Before and (B) 6 weeks after the procedure.

conditions, camera angles, and patients' facial expressions. If photographs are used, both good and less-than-ideal results should be shown to the patient. A detailed discussion as to the potential complications and expected postoperative course is imperative to reduce patient anxiety. Having patients call frequently in the immediate postlaser period to discuss the status of healing is also important to reducing anxiety.

Patients of any age who are in reasonably good health can undergo laser resurfacing. Screening laboratory tests are generally not necessary, because the procedure is most often done with the patient under local anesthesia. Contraindications to the procedure are similar to those of dermabrasion. Patients who are keloid formers should not undergo laser resurfacing. Laser resurfacing should also not be done in patients with a reduced number of adnexal structures, such as those whose skin has been exposed to x-ray treatment or those with scleroderma, because a successful result relies on reepithelialization from normal and intact adnexal structures remaining after laser resurfacing.

Patients who have undergone isotretinoin treatment sometimes show atypical scarring after dermabrasion or chemical peel, even if the procedure is performed more than 1 year after the isotretinoin treatment.[23] The frequency with which this complication occurs is unknown. Therefore patients who have taken isotretinoin should be given additional warnings about the risk of scarring from laser resurfacing treatment, and the procedure should probably be done more conservatively. We recommend that a patient wait at least 1 to 2 years after isotretinoin treatment before undergoing laser resurfacing.

Blood circulation in skin that has recently been undermined, as is done in a face-lift or blepharoplasty, is altered for several months. The risk of skin necrosis with associated scarring is therefore greater in patients who undergo resurfacing procedures at the same time as or soon after skin undermining.[24,25] We recommend that laser resurfacing of undermined skin be deferred for 6 months after the original surgical procedure. Conversely, it is unknown how long after laser resurfacing a patient can safely undergo a procedure that undermines the resurfaced skin, but a wait of 3 to 6 months seems prudent.

MEDICATIONS

Numerous medications are used in making the procedure safer and more comfortable for the patient. Retin-A (tretinoin) used before dermabrasion has been shown to speed reepithelialization after dermabrasion,[26] and it appears to work similarly after laser resurfacing. Therefore patients are encouraged to use Retin-A daily for at least 6 weeks before the procedure.[27]

Postinflammatory hyperpigmentation is a frequent occurrence after laser resurfacing. It develops in most patients with Fitzpatrick type IV skin and in almost all darker-skinned patients.[3] To reduce its incidence, all patients are encouraged to avoid having a suntan at the time of the procedure and patients with type III to VI skin are given hydroquinone, kojic acid, or azelaic acid, which is used for several weeks before the procedure.[27] The ideal time for laser resurfacing is late fall and winter.

In patients with a history of herpes labialis, laser resurfacing can trigger an outbreak that can spread to involve the entire denuded skin surface, with resulting increased pain, prolonged healing, and an increased risk of scarring. Therefore all patients with any history of cold sores or fever blisters are given prophylactic acyclovir (200 mg orally five times per day or 400 mg three times per day), starting the day before or the day of the procedure and continued for at least 10 days. We have encountered several patients who denied any history of herpes labialis and suffered severe herpes outbreaks after laser resurfacing. Therefore we now give all patients scheduled to undergo resurfacing in the perioral area acyclovir prophylactically.

After laser resurfacing, there is a layer of necrotic, thermally coagulated dermis that sloughs over several days (see Fig. 13-1C). This material serves as an ideal bacterial culture medium. Therefore patients are usually given prophylactic antibiotics, such as dicloxacillin, with penicillin-allergic patients receiving erythromycin, starting on the morning of surgery and continuing for 1 week.[27] Since the introduction of prophylactic treatment with oral antibiotics, impetiginization of the treated areas has been almost totally eliminated.

A short, 3- to 4-day, course of oral corticosteroids can be given to the patient perioperatively to reduce the substantial edema that usually occurs during the first 72 hours after the procedure.

Anesthesia

Facial resurfacing with a laser requires the use of an anesthetic that will effectively block the pain that results from the vaporization of epidermal and dermal tissue. Though many physicians have attempted to perform the procedure using topical anesthetic agents, such as EMLA, the success of this has been very limited, in that either only superficial anesthesia is developed or the occlusion necessary to induce deeper anesthesia results in significant tissue maceration that alters the desired laser-tissue interaction. Because this topical anesthesia approach has proved too impractical to be useful, either local infiltration or regional nerve blocks have come to be preferred for localized areas. Supraorbital, infraorbital, and mental nerves are easily blocked, providing complete anesthesia of the central face but excluding the upper and lower eyelids and the corners of the mouth. These areas, as well as any locations on the lateral and inferior cheeks, temples, and along the jawline, must be anesthetized using local infiltration. The local anesthetic should be injected into the subcutaneous plane to minimize distortion of the surface rhytides. It is often helpful to mark out the rhytides with gentian violet before injecting the anesthetic.

Sedatives and analgesics are commonly administered before these nerves are blocked. Diazepam, midazolam, meperidine, promethazine, triazolam, and lorazepam have been used in various combinations for this purpose. When full-face resurfacing is to be done, it is advisable to use intravenous sedation administered by an anesthesiologist, using appropriate monitoring. Midazolam and propofol are commonly used, and intubation is not required. Performance of nerve blocks in combination with intravenous sedation allows the anesthesiologist to keep the patient in a lighter plane of induced sleep with better control over respiration and oxygen saturation.

Technique for Removal of Rhytides

The technique for the removal of rhytides is as follows.[3,7,8,21,22] The skin is prepared with an antiseptic such as Betadine (povidone-iodine). If alcohol antiseptics are used, they should be allowed to dry completely before the procedure is started. Chlorhexidine should not be used because of its ocular toxicity, which might be aggravated if it is vaporized by the laser. Extensive preparation of the skin is usually not necessary before laser resurfacing, because the laser sterilizes the surface as it vaporizes.[28]

Free-flowing oxygen should be kept away from the surgical field to reduce the risk of fire. The treatment area is wrapped with wet towels. Depending on the area being treated, the patient's eyes are covered with laser safety glasses, small opaque goggles, or wet eyepads. Stainless steel eyeshields are placed under eyelids being resurfaced.

The most commonly requested areas for laser resurfacing are the perioral, periorbital, and glabellar-forehead regions, done as isolated units. When treating any of these areas, it is important to follow the treated wrinkles out to their end. That means that, for instance, when treating the periorbital area, the crow's feet of the lateral canthus area must be followed out to the temporal area as well as to their points over the superior lateral cheeks and the medial lines followed out over the nasal bridge (see Fig. 13-2).

When treating the perioral area alone, the wrinkle lines that often flare laterally off the lower nasolabial fold and the crescent lines of the medial lower cheek just lateral to the mouth should be treated as well. The treatment should be carried over the jawline to the level of the submental crease. The vermilion border should be treated to remove the fine vertical wrinkles that cross it and cause lipstick to "bleed" into them (see Fig. 13-1).

If these areas are treated in this manner, for cosmetic purposes the treatment zone should be extended beyond what is commonly accepted as the anatomic unit of each area. Because of this extension beyond the most visible anatomic markers, such as the nasolabial fold and the orbital rim, it is important to use a feathering technique to blend the laser-treated area into the untreated skin.

If both the perioral and periorbital regions are to be treated, it is far preferable to treat the entire face or at least the full face from the eyebrows down (Fig. 13-3). The treatment of the cheeks then secondarily improves the other two areas. In addition, the erythema or transient pigmentary changes are less visible because they are more uniformly distributed.

Patients sometimes request treatment of only the glabellar lines. Though this may be done, it results in very visible erythema of only this location, which is difficult to conceal with makeup or other camouflage. It is therefore preferable to resurface the entire forehead.

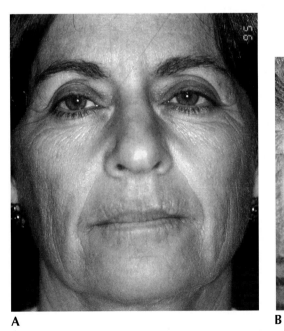
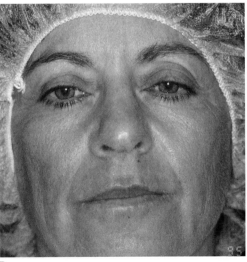

A   **B**

Fig. 13-3. Full-face rhytides treated with the Coherent UltraPulse computerized-pattern generator using 300 mJ, 100 W, a 2.25-mm spot size, and two full passes overall, then one pass in select areas, followed by two to three passes in select areas using 500 mJ and 4 W with a freehand 3-mm spot size. (A) Before and (B) 4 months after the procedure.

The epidermis of the area to be treated is first removed using a confluent application of single vaporizing laser pulses. The desiccated proteinaceous debris that remains represents keratinous cellular remnants resulting from the effects of intracellular vaporization. This debris must be wiped clear because it no longer contains water as a target for the laser energy and it will prevent the energy from reaching its target of dermal tissue underlying this layer. Wiping this layer away with saline not only removes this obstacle but also serves to rehydrate the underlying tissue. Once this debris has been wiped away, a dry gauze must be used to remove any water remaining on the skin surface, because this will absorb the laser energy and block its reaction with dermal tissue. A second laser pass is then performed over the entire area of photodamaged dermis. This is most easily performed in an even, confluent application. However, the area treated with each pass generally becomes smaller as multiple passes are performed and more superficially damaged areas are normalized with tissue vaporization. With each additional pass, there is further wrinkle smoothing, but along with this there is an increased risk of complications because of the greater depth of tissue injury. The endpoint of treatment is the smoothing away of tissue irregularities and visible wrinkle lines so that a smooth and even surface results (see Fig. 13-1B). This is sometimes accomplished more efficiently by concentrating the laser beam on the high points of tissue—on the shoulders of wrinkle lines. This causes them to flatten, both through the process of vaporization and collagen contraction. Bleeding is rarely encountered.

The tissue changes color as resurfacing proceeds deeper into the dermis. Entry into the papillary dermis is evidenced by the pink color of the surface, which changes to gray with deeper papillary dermal ablation. With further ablation the tissue acquires a yellowish hue, which indicates ablation into the upper reticular dermis and is usually the end-point of treatment (see Fig. 13-1B). Additional passes cause the yellow to darken and become brown. The color changes are probably related to the buildup of thermally denatured collagen rather than to some intrinsic property of different dermal layers.

COHERENT ULTRAPULSE

When using the UltraPulse 5000, it is preferable to use the computer pattern generator because it ensures faster, more uniform, and safer treatment, as the computer precisely and rapidly places each laser spot within the pattern.[29] However, all areas of the face may be treated using the 3-mm collimated-beam handpiece and confluent single-pulse vaporization with 10% or less overlap. Because of the lateral heat spread that occurs at the dermal-epidermal juncture, small areas that have been skipped can be removed when the epidermal debris is wiped away. These areas serve as a protective zone that helps to prevent the heat accumulation that may occur if pulses are placed rapidly on top of each other. For this reason, it is far preferable to leave small skip spaces during treatment rather than to overlap pulses too much.[30]

Feathering with the laser is accomplished by decreasing the pulse energy and the density of the pulses. To do this, it is advisable to create two concentric peripheral zones of about 10 to 15 mm in diameter. To create the first zone, the operator should start with a confluent application of pulse energy of 100 to 200 mJ less than that used for treatment and gradually decrease the density so that, at the end of this zone, pulses have 2 to 4 mm of untreated skin between them. To create the second zone of feathering, the pulse energy should be decreased another 100 to 150 mJ and the pulses gradually spread in an irregular, uneven manner so that they are 5 to 6 mm apart.

SHARPLAN SILKTOUCH

The settings used for the Sharplan SilkTouch laser vary depending on the patient's skin type, sex, degree of sun damage, and deepness of the rhytides. In general, the power is set to 6 to 8 W continuous with the 3.7-mm spot size (125-mm handpiece; scanner "+" setting) and 15 to 20 W continuous with the 6.5-mm spot size (200-mm handpiece; scanner "+" setting). The scan duration is 0.2 second on and 0.3 to 0.4 second off in the repetitive mode. For larger or square scans, the laser settings have to be adjusted accordingly.[31]

It is often helpful after the first pass to switch from a 6.5- to 3.7-mm spot size for going down the shoulder of each remaining rhytid. One pass with the laser achieves approximately the same depth of ablation as a medium-depth Jessner's solution plus 35% TCA chemical peel. Two to three passes accomplish approximately the same depth of ablation as dermabrasion and four or more passes approach the depth of a Baker's phenol deep peel. Only one pass is used at the edges of the treatment field to allow for feathering of the edges. Further feathering can be achieved by angling the handpiece so that the laser beam is not exactly perpendicular to the skin surface. This spaces the individual laser passes in the spiral scan farther apart at the edge of the treatment field.

Rhytides in the perioral area require two to three laser passes for adequate effacement. The vermilion region should be treated with a single laser pass. Cheek, forehead, and glabellar rhytides usually respond to two laser passes, and only occasionally are three passes necessary. The temples, with their relatively thin skin, should receive only one to two laser passes. Because of their extremely thin skin, lower eyelids require special care. One laser pass is usually sufficient, and the treatment is extended almost to the lash line. Great care should be taken not to singe the upper and lower eyelashes with the laser beam.

Other Indications

Other skin lesions that can be treated with the CO_2 laser are listed in Table 13-2. Acne scars have traditionally been treated with dermabrasion.[32,33] Although moderate improvement can be achieved using this method, the procedure is quite bloody and the blood microdroplets can hang suspended in the air for several hours, posing a threat to the physician, staff, and other patients.[34] Laser resurfacing can partially efface acne scars with much less risk to the surgical team. In addition, the procedure can be done very precisely, in that the edges of the scars can be sculpted and more tissue vaporized only in the areas of scar tissue, while only superficial resurfacing is done in the rest of the cosmetic unit being treated. The procedure is most suited for the treatment of distensible depressed or elevated acne scars (Fig. 13-4). Ice-pick and bound-down scars should first be removed with punch excision, punch elevation, or punch grafting, with laser resurfacing performed 6 to 8 weeks later.[35]

Crateriform varicella scars can be lessened with spot laser resurfacing. To do this, the area around and over the scar is first vaporized with one pass of the laser, with additional passes concentrated along the edge of the scar crater until it has been completely effaced. The scar can be almost totally effaced if laser treatment is done 6 to 10 weeks after resolution of the infection. Older scars do respond, but less completely. Postoperative and traumatic scars can be dramatically lessened (Fig. 13-5), especially if resurfacing is done 6 to 10 weeks after the surgery or injury.[21,36]

Table 13-2. Indications for resurfacing CO_2 lasers

Actinic cheilitis

Actinic keratoses

Adenoma sebaceum

Dermatosis papulosa nigra

Epidermal nevi

Erythroplasia of Quyerat

Rhinophyma

Rhytides (facial)

Scars (facial)

  Acne

  Surgical

  Traumatic

  Varicella

Sebaceous hyperplasia

Solar lentigines (facial)

Syringoma

Trichoepithelioma

Xanthelasma

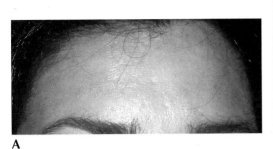
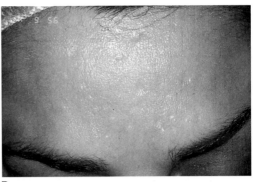

A   B

Fig. 13-4.   Acne scars treated with the Coherent UltraPulse computerized-pattern generator using 300 mJ, 100 W, a 2.25-mm spot size, and two full passes overall, then one pass in select areas, followed by two to three passes in select areas using 500 mJ and 4 W with a freehand 3-mm spot size. (A) Before and (B) 6 months after the procedure.

Actinic cheilitis can be treated successfully by performing a vermilionectomy using one of the resurfacing lasers (Fig. 13-6).[21] Usually only one pass of the laser beam over the vermilion region, including the vermilion border, is needed, and it takes approximately 10 days for the treated area to heal. This is in contrast to the 4 weeks it took for such areas treated with the conventional CO_2 laser to heal.[37–47] The risk of scarring would also be expected to be greatly reduced, because there is much less thermal damage. Actinic keratoses unresponsive to conventional treatment with liquid nitrogen and topical 5-fluorouracil can be removed by removing the epidermis with one pass using one of the resurfacing lasers. This is especially useful for the removal of lesions on the dorsal hands and scalp.

Pigmentation irregularities, such as postinflammatory hyperpigmentation, can sometimes be lessened with laser resurfacing. However, it is very important to use Retin-A and hydroquinone for an

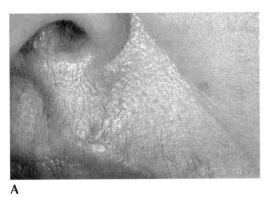
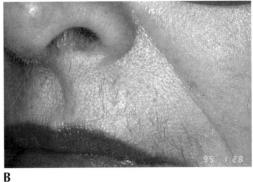

A   B

Fig. 13-5.   Two-month-old excisional scar treated with the Coherent UltraPulse CO_2 laser using 4 W, a 3-mm spot size, 500 mJ/pulse, and three passes. (A) Before and (B) 9 months after laser resurfacing.

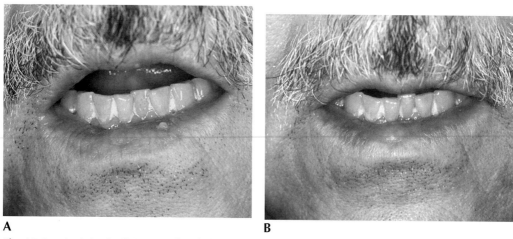

A   **B**

Fig. 13-6. Actinic cheilitis treated with the Sharplan SilkTouch CO_2 laser using 18 W, a 6.5-mm scan size, and one to two passes. (A) Before and (B) 3 months after the procedure.

extended period of time before and after the procedure. Treatment with lasers emitting wavelengths more specific for melanin or with medium-depth chemical peels is often preferable, because these methods do not require anesthesia and the recovery time is much shorter.[48–52] Melasma responds variably, similar to the way in which it responds to other treatments.[53]

Rhinophyma (Fig. 13-7),[54,55] epidermal nevi (Fig. 13-8),[56,57] and various small benign growths, such as syringoma,[58] trichoepithelioma,[59] dermatosis papulosa nigra, xanthelasma,[60] adenoma sebaceum,[61] and sebaceous hyperplasia, have traditionally been treated with the conventional CO_2 laser.[62] However, use of a resurfacing CO_2 laser may lead to a reduction in the healing time and the risk of scarring by reducing the extent of unwanted thermal damage. Sometimes a combined approach can be employed. For example, rhinophyma can be debulked using the CO_2 laser in the superpulsed mode and then the remaining rhinophyma removed using the resurfacing mode of the laser. In the treatment of epidermal nevi, it is important that damage extend into the papillary dermis, with residual hypopigmentation expected (Fig. 13-8B). Failure to cause some degree of dermal fibrosis often results in nevus recurrence.[56,57]

Wound Care

During the first few days after laser resurfacing there is a significant amount of exudate, with some sloughing of thermally denatured collagen (see Fig. 13-1C). The variable amount of edema that develops in the first 48 hours can be controlled with ice packs, head elevation at night, and corticosteroids. Reepithelialization takes 3 to 10 days, taking more time the greater the number of laser passes and less time in patients whose skin has been "primed" with Retin-A. We encourage the use of occlusive dressings, such as Vigilon, during at least the

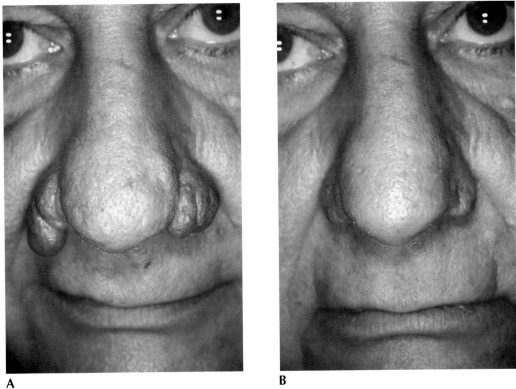

Fig. 13-7. Rhinophyma treated with the Sharplan SilkTouch CO_2 laser using 18 to 40 W, a 6.5-mm scan size, and multiple passes. (A) Before and (B) 5 months after the procedure.

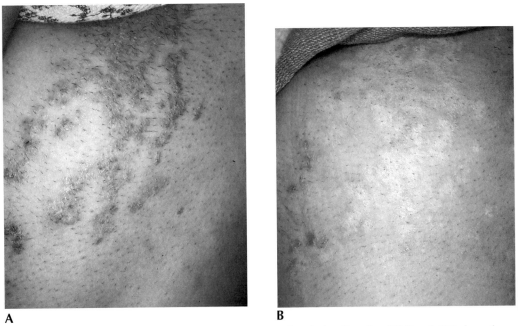

Fig. 13-8. Inflammatory linear epidermal nevus treated with the Sharplan SilkTouch CO_2 laser for severe pruritus using 20 W and a 6.5-mm scan size in the painting mode. (A) Before and (B) 7 months after the procedure, showing hypopigmentation. The injury has to extend into the dermis with resulting dermal fibrosis to prevent lesion recurrence. See Fig. 13-8 in color section.

first 24 to 48 hours, because this has been shown to speed reepithelialization after regular dermabrasion.[63] Continued moist wound healing is achieved with frequent soaks with 0.25% acetic acid, normal saline, or cool tap water, followed by the application of Aquaphor (xipamide) healing ointment. We have stopped using Polysporin (polymyxin B–bacitracin) ointment and petrolatum because Polysporin ointment seems to frequently cause allergic contact dermatitis in these patients and petrolatum may cause folliculitis, especially if it is not stopped immediately after reepithelialization is complete.[27]

The moderate burning discomfort experienced by some patients during the first 24 hours after laser resurfacing is controlled most effectively with ice packs, cold compresses, and acetaminophen, alone or with codeine. Pruritus often develops in patients during the first few weeks after resurfacing but is usually self-limited and controlled with antihistamines.

Almost universally, patients experience a feeling of tightening of the treated skin that may last for several weeks to several months, but this is generally thought to be a beneficial rather than an adverse effect of laser resurfacing.

After reepithelialization there is a variable period of erythema, lasting from 1 to 4 months (see Fig. 13-1D). The erythema can be successfully camouflaged with makeup containing a green foundation. Patients should be told to avoid exposure to the sun after laser resurfacing for the entire period of postlaser erythema to reduce the risk of postinflammatory erythema.

Occasionally milia develop in patients 1 to 3 months after resurfacing, but this is far less common after laser treatment than after dermabrasion. Pretreatment with Retin-A further reduces the likelihood of milia formation. The milia usually resolve spontaneously, but Retin-A treatment can speed their resolution, with milia extraction needed only on rare occasions.

Results of Rhytid Resurfacing

To evaluate the severity of wrinkling and photodamage present, and therefore somewhat predict a patient's response to resurfacing, a clinical classification and numeric scoring system has been devised.[3,8] Though other wrinkling and photodamage assessment scales exist, a system based purely on visible wrinkling and textural changes secondary to solar elastosis was thought to be more relevant to the topic of wrinkle eradication.

In this scoring system, wrinkling is broadly classified into mild, moderate, and severe categories and also rated with a more objective numerical severity score. In a study in which patients were assessed both before and after treatment for an average follow-up of about 90 days, it was found that the average patient's preoperative score decreased by approximately 50% after resurfacing.[3,8,30,31] This means that mild wrinkles generally resolve completely and moderate and severe wrinkles improve by one class. These are realistic expectations for the patient, though occasionally even severe wrinkles may completely resolve. The treated area continues to improve for several months after laser resurfacing while collagen remodeling takes place (see Figs. 13-1 to 13-3).

Laser resurfacing is more effective than chemical peels in the eradication of wrinkles, while at the same time preserving normal skin texture and pigment. Superficial chemical peels such as Jessner's solution and alpha-hydroxy acids remove only a partial thickness of the epidermis and have no appreciable effect on wrinkling.[64] Laser resurfacing is generally not done on such a superficial level. Medium-depth chemical peels done with solid CO_2 or Jessner's solution plus 35% TCA can lessen textural irregularities and very superficial wrinkling but rarely have a significant effect on clinically visible wrinkling.[48,49,65] This same level of resurfacing can be achieved with a single UltraPulse laser pass using a 250- to 350-mJ pulse and 3-mm spot size or with one SilkTouch laser pass using a 6.5-mm scan size at 15 to 18 W. Though this level of chemical peeling is generally predictable and safe, the acids may penetrate to variable depths, not only between patients but also within the same patient. This variation in the depth of penetration may be related to the quantity of acid applied, the pressure exerted while rubbing the acid into the skin, the degree of cleansing and defatting of the skin surface, the degree of photodamage present, the number and density of adnexal structures, and other unidentifiable factors. Deeper-than-wanted penetration of the acid may cause scarring, hypopigmentation, and textural changes. If the proper laser-resurfacing technique is used, the depth of resurfacing can be much better predicted, with little risk of inadvertent deeper penetration, with its associated risk.

Deep chemical peels using Baker's phenol solution can remove even deep lines and may result in dramatic clinical improvement but virtually always result in hypopigmentation and an atrophically smooth, altered surface. It is difficult to obtain an even result on the upper lip. In addition, lines at the vermilion border often persist, whereas the central area of the lip clears completely. Further, because of the extreme depth of resurfacing, there is an extended period of erythema, often lasting for 6 months or longer, and a significant risk of scarring. The postoperative course in patients who undergo phenol peeling is painful, and it takes at least 2 weeks for the skin surface to reconstitute itself.[66–69]

The deep injury produced by Baker's phenol chemical peel treatment has not been reported for laser resurfacing, nor is it desired. Because of the combination of the amount of tissue removed, collagen contraction–skin tightening, and new collagen formation-remodeling, laser resurfacing achieves results comparable to those of chemical peel, but without the hypopigmentation and altered surface texture seen for phenol treatment. The virtually complete loss of pigment (depigmentation) that at times occurs in patients who undergo phenol treatment has not been reported for laser resurfacing.

From a technical viewpoint, dermabrasion is significantly more difficult to perform than laser resurfacing and carries with it the additional risks of possibly exposing the physician and assistant to bloodborne infectious agents[34] and accidentally injuring the patient as the result of the rapidly rotating wire brush or diamond fraise catching onto loose skin or gauze and being thrown into an eyelid, lip, tooth, or other area.[33] To obliterate wrinkles using dermabrasion requires a degree of expertise not easily achieved, and it always remains a challenge to treat the upper lip and the eyelids using this method. Uneven results and hypopigmentation are common in the perioral area,[70] as is seen in patients who undergo deep chemical peels, and often wrinkling clears centrally across the upper lip but persists at the vermilion border. The depth of resurfacing achieved with dermabrasion is usually comparable to that achieved with approximately two to five passes of the UltraPulse laser using 350 to 500 mJ per pulse or with two to three passes of the SilkTouch laser using a 6.5-mm scan size at 15 to 18 W.

Precautions

By far the most common adverse effect of laser resurfacing is post-inflammatory hyperpigmentation. It is most often seen in patients with Fitzpatrick's skin types III to VI. The incidence of hyperpigmentation is greatest and it is most severe in treated patients during the summer and year-round in those living in southern areas such as Florida and Southern California. At the first sign of hyperpigmentation, bleaching cream and Retin-A treatment is restarted. Any sun exposure, even that through window glass, at this time can be expected to prolong and worsen the hyperpigmentation. If treatment is started early enough, the hyperpigmentation usually resolves within a few months.[27,71]

The risk of herpes labialis and impetiginization can be minimized with prophylactic acyclovir and oral antibiotic treatment. Occasionally herpes labialis develops in patients after the acyclovir course has been completed. Another 7-day course usually takes care of the problem. Rarely, a *Candida* yeast superinfection develops that slows reepithelialization. Results of a potassium hydroxide examination or fungal culture of areas showing delayed reepithelialization can help to establish the diagnosis. Treatment with ketaconazole (200 mg per day) is effective in eradicating the infection.

Infrequently, perioral dermatitis develops in patients 1 to 3 months after resurfacing of the perioral region. This is easily controlled with tetracycline and is usually self-limited.

Permanent hypopigmentation is rarely seen and appears to be far less frequent than it is after dermabrasion or deep chemical peels.[70] However, a color mismatch between the pale new skin of the resurfaced area and the surrounding sun-damaged areas, which may include ephelides and lentigines, may develop in patients with significant actinic damage. This mismatch is minimized by resurfacing entire cosmetic units and feathering the treatment into the surrounding areas. Rarely a medium-depth chemical peel of the untreated areas is needed to even out the skin color. Future sun exposure also helps to blend the resurfaced skin by promoting the development of new lentigines and ephelides.

Scarring appears to be a rare consequence of laser resurfacing, but proper patient selection, together with being conservative in the number of laser passes and carrying out good posttreatment wound care, should reduce the risk. It is better to do a touch-up procedure down the road than to go too deeply the first time in an attempt to totally eradicate the offending rhytides. Any areas in which scar tissue may be developing should be promptly treated with topically and intralesionally administered corticosteroids.

Future Directions

INCISIONAL LASER SURGERY

For over a decade, claims have been made that the CO_2 laser offers advantages over cold steel surgery in the performance of procedures requiring precision, such as rhytidectomy[72] and blepharoplasty.[73–76] However, no properly performed controlled trials have ever been done that have substantiated this claim. With the recent development of short-pulsed CO_2 lasers, the claims have become louder and more frequent, despite the absence of controlled data.

The advantage of high-powered, short pulses is completely lost when a device, such as the UltraPulse CO_2 laser, is used in its cutting mode. The cutting mode is a continuous-wave CO_2 laser beam that cuts through the skin, leaving a zone of thermal damage anywhere from 200 to 600 μm deep, and not the 50 to 75 μm of thermal damage left behind after ablation with the UltraPulse CO_2 laser used for resurfacing. Although this laser is no doubt hemostatic in its effects and has the potential to decrease the amount of operative and postoperative hemorrhage and bruising associated with cold steel procedures, there is no scientific reason for its being any better for precision surgery such as blepharoplasty than cold steel surgery.

LASER HAIR TRANSPLANTATION

A potential advantage of using the laser for hair transplantation is that it can create round and slit minigrafts by producing slits in which some width of tissue is removed by vaporization.[77–80] These lasers can also create small recipient holes for 1- to 2-hair micrografts. One can achieve maximum density, minimal transitional clumpiness, and more naturalness, with a more natural looking hair density, after a single session. The incision depth is precisely controlled, and slit width and length can be precisely controlled using computer-scanning technology. Once the technology is further refined, the speed with which the slits can be made promises to be greater than that with which slits can be made using the manual cold steel technique. Already, however, micrograft recipient holes can be created very rapidly with the existing lasers. The greatest advantage of laser hair transplantation is the great reduction in intraoperative bleeding, which can greatly speed graft placement. Disadvantages of laser hair transplantation include the fact that a plume is produced, hair growth is delayed for at least 2 to 6 weeks, there is greater postoperative crusting, existing hairs are ablated, and possible thermal damage at the recipient site leads to decreased graft take and destroys nearby hair follicles. The slits or holes made during laser transplantation have to be kept farther apart than those made during cold steel hair transplantation to accommodate the residual thermal damage that can reduce the blood supply to the recipient sites.[77–80] Until carefully controlled studies of hair growth after laser hair transplantation have been completed and show results comparable or superior to those achieved with cold steel surgery, however, the procedure should be considered experimental.

NEW RESURFACING LASERS

One of the main limitations of CO_2 laser resurfacing is oozing and crusting from the site, which lasts anywhere from 7 to 14 days after treatment, as well as the extensive erythema that persists for at least 4 to 6 weeks, but sometimes more than 3 months.[3,8] Using technology developed at the Los Alamos National Physics Laboratory, a high peak power, short-pulse, but low average power, CO_2 laser has recently been developed by Tissue Technologies and approved for skin ablation by the U.S. Food and Drug Administration. This 6-W laser, called the *TruPulse*, produces high peak power pulses that can achieve fluences of more than 5 J/cm^2, which is the ablation threshold of human skin, at variable pulse durations of from 30 μsec to 1 msec (see Table 13-1). By using pulse durations in the range of 60 to 100 μsec, which are shorter than those possible with the UltraPulse CO_2 laser, this device removes less tissue per pass (on the order of 30 μm in depth). The TruPulse laser requires more passes to effectively ablate significantly photodamaged skin but leaves less residual thermal damage (on the order of 15 to 30 μm in depth). Early, and so far unsubstantiated, claims have been made that the crusting, oozing, and erythema occurring after CO_2 laser resurfacing with the TruPulse laser are substantially less than those resulting from treatment with the other CO_2 lasers.

Several other laser wavelengths have the capacity to resurface skin. The erbium:yttrium, aluminum, garnet (Er:YAG) laser produces light (at 2.94 nm) in the near-infrared portion of the electromagnetic spectrum. This broad water-absorption band extends from just under 2 μm to beyond 10 μm, ensuring the superficial absorption of near-infrared light. When it is Q-switched, however, the Er:YAG laser ablates approximately 5 to 15 μm of skin and leaves such a thin layer of thermal damage that it is not at all hemostatic. Once bleeding begins, the Q-switched Er:YAG laser can no longer ablate or cut tissue, because all the laser energy is absorbed by blood. In its normal mode, the Er:YAG laser produces a train of pulses that ablate more tissue and leave a greater zone of thermal damage, which is hemostatic.[81,82] It is in this mode that the Er:YAG laser is being studied to determine whether it is an effective resurfacing device.

The titanium:sapphire laser produces ultra-short, femtosecond pulses at a wavelength of 800 nm. However, because its pulse duration is so short, the amount of tissue ablated per pass may be so thin, as low as 0.1 μm,[83] as to not be clinically useful for resurfacing. Like the short pulses produced by the Q-switched Er:YAG laser, the short pulses produced by this laser are not hemostatic.

Conclusion

Because of the cosmetic implications, a huge amount of interest in CO_2 laser resurfacing has been raised. Early treatment results have been impressive, but many questions remain unanswered. For example: How does CO_2 laser resurfacing work? Is thermal damage essential for beneficial results to be achieved or is ablation the key to successful treatment? What role does collagen shrinkage and remodeling play? Are short-pulsed CO_2 lasers effective for resurfacing moderately or severely photodamaged skin, and if so, is the wound healing time actually shorter and does erythema persist for a shorter time than those associated with treatment using the longer-pulsed CO_2 lasers? It is essential that the answers to these and many more questions be found to gain a better understanding of this rapidly evolving field.

References

1. David LM, Lask GP, Glassberg E et al. Laser abrasion for cosmetic and medical treatment of facial actinic damage. Cutis 1989;43:583–587.
2. Fitzpatrick RE, Goldman MP. Advances in carbon dioxide laser surgery. Clin Dermatol 1995;13:35–47.
3. Fitzpatrick RE, Goldman MP, Satur NM, Tope WD. Pulsed carbon dioxide laser resurfacing of photoaged facial skin. Arch Dermatol 1996;132: 395–402.
4. Fitzpatrick RE, Tope WD, Goldman MP, Satur NM. Pulsed carbon dioxide laser, trichloroacetic acid, Baker-Gordon phenol, and dermabrasion: a comparative clinical and histologic study of cutaneous resurfacing in a porcine model. Arch Dermatol 1996;132:469–471.
5. Yang CC, Chai CY. Animal study of skin resurfacing using the UltraPulse carbon dioxide laser. Ann Plast Surg 1995;35:154–158.
6. Chernoff G, Slatkine M, Zair E, Mead D. SilkTouch: a new technology for skin resurfacing in aesthetic surgery. J Clin Laser Med Surg 1995;13: 97–100.

7. Chernoff WG, Schoenrock LD, Cramer H, Wand J. Cutaneous laser resurfacing. Int J Aesth Restor Surg 1995;3:57–68.

8. Waldorf HA, Kauvar ANB, Geronemus RG. Skin resurfacing of fine to deep rhytides using a char-free carbon dioxide laser in 47 patients. Dermatol Surg 1995;21:940–946.

9. Anderson RR, Parrish RR. Selective photothermolysis: precise microsurgery by selective absorption of pulsed radiation. Science 1983;220:524–527.

10. Green HA, Domankevitz Y, Nishioka NS. Pulsed carbon dioxide laser ablation of burned skin: in vitro and in vivo analysis. Lasers Surg Med 1990;10:476–484.

11. Green HA, Burd E, Nishioka NS et al. Middermal wound healing. A comparison between dermatomal excision and pulsed carbon dioxide laser ablation. Arch Dermatol 1992;128:639–645.

12. Walsh JJ, Deutsch TF. Pulsed CO_2 laser tissue ablation: measurement of the ablation rate. Lasers Surg Med 1988;8:264–275.

13. Schenk P, Ehrenberger K. Effect of CO_2 laser on skin lymphatics. An ultrastructural study. Langenbecks Arch Chir 1980;350:145–150.

14. Slutzki S, Shafir R, Bornstein LA. Use of the carbon dioxide laser for large excisions with minimal blood loss. Plast Reconstr Surg 1977;60:250–255.

15. Walsh JJ, Flotte TJ, Anderson RR, Deutsch TF. Pulsed CO_2 laser tissue ablation: effect of tissue type and pulse duration on thermal damage. Lasers Surg Med 1988;8:108–118.

16. Hobbs ER, Bailin PL, Wheeland RG, Ratz JL. Superpulsed lasers: minimizing thermal damage with short duration, high irradiance pulses. J Dermatol Surg Oncol 1987;13:955–964.

17. Fitzpatrick RE, Ruiz EJ, Goldman MP. The depth of thermal necrosis using the CO_2 laser: a comparison of the superpulsed mode and conventional mode. J Dermatol Surg Oncol 1991;17:340–344.

18. Fitzpatrick RE, Goldman MP, Ruiz-Esparza J. Clinical advantage of the CO_2 laser superpulsed mode. Treatment of verruca vulgaris, seborrheic keratoses, lentigines, and actinic cheilitis. J Dermatol Surg Oncol 1994;20:449–456.

19. Brugmans MJP, Kemper J, Gijsbers GHM et al. Temperature response of biological materials to pulsed non-ablative CO_2 laser irradiation. Lasers Surg Med 1991;11:587–594.

20. Kauvar AN, Geronemus RG, Waldorf HA. Char-free tissue ablation: a comparative histopathological analysis of new carbon dioxide (CO_2) laser systems. Lasers Surg Med 1995;16(suppl 7):50.

21. Hruza GJ. Skin resurfacing with lasers. Fitzpatrick's J Clin Dermatol 1995;3(4):38–41.

22. Schoenrock LD, Chernoff WG, Rubach BW. Cutaneous UltraPulse laser resurfacing of the eyelids. Int J Aesthetic Restor Surg 1995;3:31–36.

23. Rubenstein R, Roenigk HH Jr, Stegman SJ, Hanke WC. Atypical keloids after dermabrasion of patients taking isotretinoin. J Am Acad Dermatol 1986;15:280–285.

24. Hayes DK, Stambaugh KI. Viability of skin flaps subjected to simultaneous chemical peel with occlusive taping. Laryngoscope 1989;99:1016–1019.

25. Hayes DK, Berkland ME, Stambaugh KI. Dermal healing after local skin flaps and chemical peel. Arch Otolaryngol Head Neck Surg 1990;116:794–797.

26. Alt TH. Technical aids for dermabrasion. J Dermatol Surg Oncol 1987; 13:638–648.

27. Lowe NJ, Lask G, Griffin ME. Laser skin resurfacing: pre- and posttreatment guidelines. Dermatol Surg 1995;21:1017–1019.

28. Mullarky MB, Norris CW, Goldberg ID. The efficacy of the CO_2 laser in the sterilization of skin seeded with bacteria: survival at the skin surface and in the plume emissions. Laryngoscope 1985;95:186–187.

29. David LM, Sarne AJ, Unger WP. Rapid laser scanning for facial resurfacing. Dermatol Surg 1995;21:1031–1033.

30. Lowe NJ, Lask G, Griffin ME et al. Skin resurfacing with the UltraPulse carbon dioxide laser: observations on 100 patients. Dermatol Surg 1995;21:1025–1029.

31. Lask G, Keller G, Lowe N, Gormley D. Laser resurfacing with the Silk-Touch flashscanner for facial rhytides. Dermatol Surg 1995;21:1021–1024.

32. Yarborough JM Jr, Beeson WH. Dermabrasion. In: Beeson WH, McCollough EG, eds. Aesthetic surgery of the aging face. St. Louis: Mosby, 1986:142–181.

33. Yarborough JM Jr. Dermabrasion by wire brush. J Dermatol Surg Oncol 1987;13:610–615.

34. Wentzell JM, Robinson JK, Wentzell JM Jr et al. Physical properties of aerosols produced by dermabrasion. Arch Dermatol 1989;125:1637–1643.

35. Abergel RP, Dahlman CM. The CO_2 laser approach to the treatment of acne scarring. Cosmet Dermatol 1995;8:33–36.

36. Wheeland RG. Revision of full-thickness skin grafts using the carbon dioxide laser. J Dermatol Surg Oncol 1988;14:130–134.

37. Alamillos-Granados FJ, Naval-Gias L, Dean-Ferrer A, Alonso del Hoyo JR. Carbon dioxide laser vermilionectomy for actinic cheilitis. J Oral Maxillofac Surg 1993;51:118–121.

38. Stanley RJ, Roenigk RK. Actinic cheilitis: treatment with the carbon dioxide laser. Mayo Clin Proc 1988;63:230–235.

39. Robinson JK. Actinic cheilitis. A prospective study comparing four treatment methods. Arch Otolaryngol Head Neck Surg 1989;115:848–852.

40. Zelickson BD, Roenigk RK. Actinic cheilitis. Treatment with the carbon dioxide laser. Cancer 1990;65:1307–1311.

41. Dufresne RJ, Garrett AB, Bailin PL, Ratz JL. Carbon dioxide laser treatment of chronic actinic cheilitis. J Am Acad Dermatol 1988;19:876–878.

42. Johnson TM, Sebastien TS, Lowe L, Nelson BR. Carbon dioxide laser treatment of actinic cheilitis. Clinicohistopathologic correlation to determine the optimal depth of destruction. J Am Acad Dermatol 1992;27:737–740.

43. Ries WR, Duncavage JA, Ossoff RH. Carbon dioxide laser treatment of actinic cheilitis. Mayo Clin Proc 1988;63:294–296.

44. Scheinberg RS. Carbon dioxide laser treatment of actinic cheilitis. West J Med 1992;156:192–193.

45. Whitaker DC. Microscopically proven cure of actinic cheilitis by CO_2 laser. Lasers Surg Med 1987;7:520–523.

46. Frankel DH. Carbon dioxide laser vermilionectomy for chronic actinic cheilitis. Facial Plast Surg 1989;6:158–161.

47. David LM. Laser vermilion ablation for actinic cheilitis. J Dermatol Surg Oncol 1985;11:605–608.

48. Monheit GD. The Jessner's +TCA peel: a medium-depth chemical peel. J Dermatol Surg Oncol 1989;15:945–950.

49. Brody HJ, Hailey CW. Medium-depth chemical peeling of the skin: a variation of superficial chemosurgery. J Dermatol Surg Oncol 1986;12: 1268–1275.

50. Brauner GJ, Schliftman AB. Treatment of pigmented lesions of the skin with alexandrite laser. Lasers Surg Med 1992;12(suppl 4):72.

51. Fitzpatrick R, Goldman M. Laser treatment of benign pigmented lesions using a 300 nanosecond pulse and 510 nm wavelength. J Dermatol Surg Oncol 1993;19:341–346.

52. Goldberg D. Benign pigmented lesions of the skin: treatment with the Q-switched ruby laser. J Dermatol Surg Oncol 1993;19:376–379.

53. Taylor CR, Anderson RR. Ineffective treatment of refractory melasma and postinflammatory hyperpigmentation by Q-switched ruby laser. J Dermatol Surg Oncol 1994;20:592–597.

54. Greenbaum SS, Krull EA, Watnich K. Comparison of CO_2 laser and electrosurgery in the treatment of rhinophyma. J Am Acad Dermatol 1988; 18:363–368.

55. Wheeland RG, Bailin PL, Ratz JL. Combined carbon dioxide laser excision and vaporization in the treatment of rhinophyma. J Dermatol Surg Oncol 1987;13:172–177.

56. Ratz JL, Bailin PL, Wheeland RG. Carbon dioxide laser treatment of epidermal nevi. J Dermatol Surg Oncol 1986;12:567–570.

57. Hohenleutner U, Landthaler M. Laser therapy of verrucous epidermal naevi. Clin Exp Dermatol 1993;18:124–127.

58. Apfelberg DB, Maser MR, Lash H et al. Superpulse CO_2 laser treatment of facial syringomata. Lasers Surg Med 1987;7:533–537.

59. Wheeland RG, Bailin PL, Kronberg E. Carbon dioxide (CO_2) laser vaporization for the treatment of multiple trichoepithelioma. J Dermatol Surg Oncol 1984;10:470–475.

60. Apfelberg DB, Maser MR, Lash H, White DN. Treatment of xanthelasma palpebrum with the carbon dioxide laser. J Dermatol Surg Oncol 1987; 13:149–151.

61. Wheeland RG, Bailin PL, Kantor GR et al. Treatment of adenoma sebaceum with carbon dioxide laser vaporization. J Dermatol Surg Oncol 1985;11:861–864.

62. Olbricht SM. Use of the carbon dioxide laser in dermatologic surgery: a clinically relevant update. J Dermatol Surg Oncol 1993;19:364–369.

63. Pinski JB. Dressings for dermabrasion: occlusive dressings and wound healing. Cutis 1986;37:471–476.

64. Stagnone JJ. Superficial peeling. J Dermatol Surg Oncol 1989;15:924–930.

65. Brody HJ. Variations and comparisons in medium-depth chemical peeling. J Dermatol Surg Oncol 1989;15:953–963.

66. Stegman SJ. A comparative histologic study of the effects of three peeling agents and dermabrasion on normal and sundamaged skin. Aesthetic Plast Surg 1982;6:123–135.

67. Alt TH. Occluded Baker-Gordon chemical peel: review and update. J Dermatol Surg Oncol 1989;15:980–993.

68. Asken S. Unoccluded Baker-Gordon phenol peels—review and update. J Dermatol Surg Oncol 1989;15:998–1008.

69. Baker TJ, Gordon HL. Chemical peeling as a practical method for removing rhytides of the upper lip. Ann Plast Surg 1979;2:209–212.

70. Falabella R. Postdermabrasion leukoderma. J Dermatol Surg Oncol 1987;13:44–48.

71. Ho C, Nguyen Q, Lowe NJ et al. Laser resurfacing in pigmented skin. Dermatol Surg 1995;21:1035–1037.

72. Lent WM, David LM. Laser-assisted rhytidectomy: a preliminary report. Dermatol Surg 1995;21:1039–1041.

73. Morrow DM, Morrow LB. CO_2 laser blepharoplasty: a comparison with cold-steel surgery. J Dermatol Surg Oncol 1992;18:307–313.

74. Tobin HA. CO_2 laser blepharoplasty. J Dermatol Surg Oncol 1993;19:499.

75. David LM, Goodman G. Blepharoplasty for the laser dermatologic surgeon. Clin Dermatol 1995;13:49–53.

76. Glassberg E, Babapour R, Lask G. Current trends in laser blepharoplasty: results of a survey. Dermatol Surg 1995;21:1060–1063.

77. Unger WP, David LM. Laser hair transplantation. J Dermatol Surg Oncol 1994;20:515–521.

78. Fitzpatrick RE. Laser hair transplantation: tissue effects of laser parameters. Dermatol Surg 1995;21:1042–1046.

79. Unger WP. Laser hair transplantation. III: computer-assisted laser transplanting. Dermatol Surg 1995;21:1047–1055.

80. Ho C, Nguyen Q, Lask G, Lowe N. Mini-slit graft hair transplantation using the UltraPulse carbon dioxide laser handpiece. Dermatol Surg 1995;21:1056–1059.

81. Walsh JT Jr, Cummings JP. Effect of the dynamic optical properties of water on midinfrared laser ablation. Lasers Surg Med 1994;15:295–305.

82. Walsh JJ, Flotte TJ, Deutsch TF. Er:YAG laser ablation of tissue: effect of pulse duration and tissue type on thermal damage. Lasers Surg Med 1989;9:314–326.

83. Frederickson KS, White WE, Wheeland RG, Slaughter DR. Precise ablation of skin with reduced collateral damage using the femtosecond-pulsed, terawatt titanium-sapphire laser. Arch Dermatol 1993;129:989–993.

14 ___ Excimer Lasers

Thomas J. Flotte
Steven L. Jacques

Excimer lasers are a family of lasers that are predominantly used for research and industrial applications but whose medical applications are currently being explored. The term *excimer* is a contraction of the words "excited" and "dimer." The term was originally used to refer only to molecules consisting of two atoms of the same element, such as He_2, but has now come to refer to any molecule composed of two (and sometimes three) atoms that exist only in the excited state. The theoretical concept of excimer lasers was proposed in 1962,[1] and the first demonstration of them was reported in 1972.[2]

The physics of these lasers is complex and has been described in detail by Krauss and Mies.[3] The ground states of closed-shell atoms are generally repulsive, except for weak van der Walls and electrostatic forces; however, an excited-state atom can bond strongly to a ground-state atom. The relaxation of the excited molecule to the ground state is accompanied by radiation and dissociation of the molecule. These systems are interesting from the standpoint of the population inversion needed for lasing, because the relevant molecule only exists in the excited state. There are many types of excimer lasers, and they have been categorized into four main categories: rare gas–dimer, rare gas–halide, rare gas–group IV, and group II–group II excimers. The wavelengths of the laser radiation range from ultraviolet to infrared. Those lasers that are available commercially are almost exclusively of the rare gas–halide type, with the remainder of the rare gas–dimer type.

The wavelengths of the generally available lasers are given in Table 14-1. Their pulse duration is typically 10 to 15 nsec, the pulse-to-pulse variation in power is between 5% and 15%, and the average power ranges up to 100 W. The beam quality is generally multi-modal, guassian, and poor.

There are two operational issues regarding excimer lasers. First, the commercial lasers are all ultraviolet lasers and therefore the post-

This work was supported in part by the SDIO-MFEL Program under contract #N0001486K0117 and by the Arthur O. and Gullan M. Wellman Foundation.

Table 14-1. Commercially available excimer lasers

Gas	Wavelength (nm)	Residual damage (μm)
F_2	157	—
ArF	193	1
KrCl	222	—
KrF	248	100
XeCl	308	50
XeF	351	—

laser optical elements chosen must be made of ultraviolet compatible optical materials. The second issue pertains to safety matters. Because the ultraviolet radiation can damage the cornea, lens, and retina, adequate eye protection is necessary. In addition, the electric discharge is typically in the 10- to 14-kilovolt domain. As a result, the laser must be adequately protected and, when the laser is open, the capacitors must be fully discharged. Further, the halogen gases are inflammable and toxic, and adequate ventilation systems are necessary.

Dermatologic Applications of Excimer Lasers

The excimer lasers used for dermatologic applications have predominantly been used for their ablative ability, but several articles have also been published on the treatment of pigmented lesions using these lasers. The ultraviolet wavelengths of these lasers are absorbed predominantly by proteins, unlike the wavelengths of the more prevalent CO_2 and Er:YAG lasers, which are predominantly absorbed by water molecules. This absorption of the wavelengths by proteins of energetic photons leads to two processes. First, it causes enough energy to be generated to break intramolecular bonds, which may produce ablation by means of a photochemical process termed *photodecomposition*.[4] Second, the excited molecules can release energy by increased vibrational relaxation, producing ablation by means of a photothermal mechanism.[5] Most likely both mechanisms are operative in the energy domains commonly utilized.

The depth of penetration of ultraviolet light is determined by the degree of absorption of the light. The ArF laser light is the most absorbed and thus penetrates the least, only 1 to 2 μm. The high absorption of the light limits the extent of residual damage and thus makes the ablation achieved with this laser the most precise of that achieved by any laser[6–12] (see Table 14-1), and it is this precision that distinguishes it from other lasers. This concept is illustrated in Figure 14-1, which shows keratinocytes in which half of the cell has been removed. Figure 14-2 shows scanning electron micrographs of sites ablated with an ArF excimer laser and a CO_2 laser. The rate of tissue removal is quite slow relative to that of other lasers, however, and this makes it only practical for ablating small areas. Although no specific

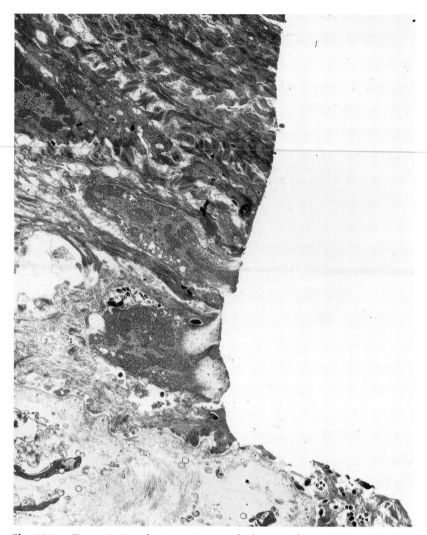

Fig. 14-1.   Transmission electron micrograph showing the precision of ArF excimer laser ablation. Note the ablation of portions of keratinocytes. (×7200)

skin condition has been identified for which this type of ablation is the method of choice, it may prove to be of particular use in the areas near the eyes and the mouth.

The ArF excimer laser may also be used to enhance percutaneous transport to allow the delivery and collection of compounds. The stratum corneum serves as a barrier to the percutaneous transport of many molecules. A segment of the medical device industry is now dedicated to the development of topical patch delivery systems. However, currently only lipid-soluble compounds and compounds that can be transported via hair follicles or sweat glands can be efficiently delivered by these devices. If the stratum corneum could be ablated by laser, this would make it possible to deliver a variety of pharmaceuticals by these topical devices.

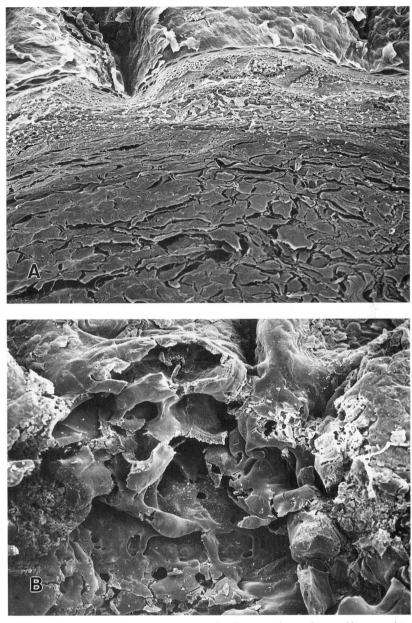

Fig. 14-2. Scanning electron micrographs showing the surfaces of human skin after ablation with an ArF excimer laser (A) and a CO_2 laser (B). Note the preserved architecture after excimer laser ablation and the altered dermis after CO_2 laser ablation. (Both specimens $\times 150$.)

Similarly, pharmacologic monitoring can be accomplished by the topical collection of compounds using patches placed on the skin. The patch collects material percutaneously, then is removed for laboratory analysis. Removal of the stratum corneum by laser ablation would make it possible to more efficiently collect compounds in this way.

These concepts have been tested in the laboratory. In one such investigation, the delivery of ^{3}H-labeled water and tetracycline across the stratum corneum to a receptor volume was demonstrated using in vitro epidermal samples.[11,13] The radiolabeled compound was introduced into a donor saline solution in contact with the surface of the stratum corneum of an isolated sample of epidermis, and diffusion of the compound across the sample into a receptor saline solution was monitored by the amount of radiolabel that accumulated in the receptor solution. The flux through a site of stratum corneum removed by laser ablation was then compared with the normal flux through an untreated site. The relative enhancements attributable to the effects of laser ablation are plotted in Figure 14-3A for water and tetracycline. They were found to be 124-fold and 47-fold, respectively.

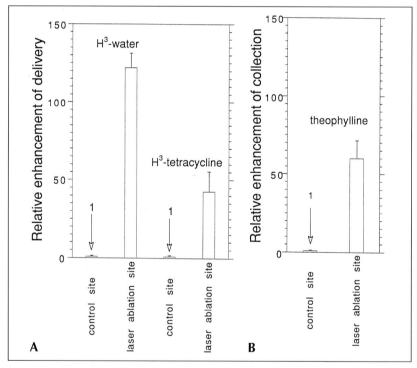

Fig. 14-3. Laser ablation enhancement of topical drug delivery and collection. The removal of the stratum corneum creates an entry site for the topical delivery and collection of compounds. (A) Laser-enhanced delivery is demonstrated with tritiated water and tetracycline, using in vitro epidermal samples.[11,13] (B) Laser-enhanced collection is demonstrated with theophylline, using an in vivo topical collection device (agar/charcoal patch) on hairless rats after the intravenous injection of theophylline.[14]

The collection of theophylline using topical patches has been demonstrated in vivo in hairless (*Fuzzy*) rats.[14] In this study, theophylline was injected intravenously and collected over a 6-hour period by a topical patch consisting of agarose and activated charcoal. The total amount of theophylline collected from a site of stratum corneum removed by laser ablation was compared with the amount collected from an untreated site. The relative enhancement of theophylline collection, which was found to be 60-fold, is plotted in Figure 14-3B.

The XeCl (351-nm) excimer laser has been shown to produce melanosome-specific injury in human skin.[15,16] The short pulsewidth emitted by this laser permits the temporal confinement of the energy to the melanosome. In fact, selective photothermolysis was first shown using this system.[17] Although this laser does work, more recent experience with the ruby,[18] Nd:YAG,[19] and tunable dye[20] lasers has indicated that longer wavelengths may be more appropriate for this purpose.

Complications of Excimer Laser Radiation

There are two undesirable consequences of excimer laser radiation—mutagenic and photoacoustic effects. Numerous studies have been performed to examine the extent and nature of the mutagenic effects, and it is now clear that the effects of the 248- and 308-nm lasers are mutagenic at the radiant exposures used for ablation.[21-25] The mutagenic potential of 193-nm light is a matter of controversy, however.[22-29] Several different assays have been performed to assess this potential but have generally shown no effect or only a small effect. These findings are surprising, because DNA absorbs this wavelength. The most likely explanation for this finding is that it is the cytoplasm that absorbs most of the light, thereby protecting the nucleus from damage, but if the radiation is sufficient to damage the nucleus, then the damage to the cytoplasm is fatal.[29]

A consequence of the use of short-pulse, high peak power lasers whose radiation is absorbed locally is the deposition of a large amount of energy in the tissue. The resultant rapid expansion of the tissue can then produce pressure waves that can propagate into the tissue much more deeply than the thermal or chemical processes. These effects have been seen after the ablation of skin using 193-nm light and must be considered during the design of a laser treatment for use in sensitive areas.[30-33]

Nondermatologic Applications of Excimer Lasers

The first clinical application proposed for the 193-nm ArF excimer laser was corneal refractive surgery, and this continues to be the leading medical application of this technology. Its precise ablative capability and the lack of residual damage after treatment make it of value for the ablation of the cornea for refractive correction.[34-37] Trials performed in human subjects have shown promising results in this regard.[38,39] An alternative approach to refractive corrective surgery is radial keratotomy.[40,41] Other ophthalmologic uses of the excimer lasers that have been proposed include its use for the treatment of corneal infections,[42] filtering procedures for glaucoma,[43] lens ablation,[44] trephination of donor and recipient corneas,[45] and ablation of corneal nodules.[46]

The other major application of excimer lasers has been in the treatment of atherosclerosis, particularly of coronary arteries. The laser used most frequently for this purpose is the XeCl excimer laser, emitting a 308-nm wavelength.[47] Clinical trials have been started to evaluate its merits in this setting, and results have been promising.[48–50] Endocardial ablation has also been proposed as a method for treating arrhythmias.[51]

A variety of other applications for excimer lasers have been proposed; these include ablation of the articular cartilage,[52] meniscus,[53] bone,[54] and teeth[55] and the disruption of biliary stones.[56] The XeCl excimer laser has also been proposed as a means to ablate the polymethylmethacrylate used in orthopedic procedures to hold a prosthesis in position.[54] Historically it has been difficult to revise this surgery because of the inability to remove this material. Finally, there has also been a preliminary effort to use excimer lasers to sterilize blood products.[57]

References

1. Houtermans FG. Über Maser-Wirkung im optischen Spektralgebiet und die Möglichkeit absolut negativer Absorption für einige Fälle von Molekülspektren (Licht-Lawine). Helv Phys Acta 1960;33:933–940.
2. Hoff PW, Rhodes CK. Introduction. In Rhodes CK, ed: Excimer lasers. Berlin: Springer-Verlag, 1984;1–4.
3. Krauss M, Mies FH. Electronic structure and radiative transitions of excimer systems. In: Rhodes CK, ed: Excimer lasers. Berlin: Springer-Verlag, 1984;5–46.
4. Srinivasan R. Ablation of polymers and biological tissue by ultraviolet lasers. Science 1986;234:559–565.
5. Clarke RH, Isner JM, Donaldson RF, Jones G II. Gas chromatographic-light microscopic correlative analysis of excimer laser photoablation of cardiovascular tissues: evidence for a thermal mechanism. Circ Res 1987;60:429–437.
6. Kaufmann R, Hibst R. Pulsed 2.94-microns erbium-YAG laser skin ablation—experimental results and first clinical application. Clin Exp Dermatol 1990;15:389–393.
7. Morelli JG, Kibbi AG, Boll J, Tan OT. 193 nm excimer laser selective ablation of in vivo guinea pig epidermis. J Invest Dermatol 1988;91:532–535.
8. Watanabe S, Flotte TJ, McAuliffe DJ, Jacques SL. Putative photoacoustic damage in skin induced by pulsed ArF excimer laser. J Invest Dermatol 1988;90:761–766.
9. Morelli J, Kibbi AG, Farinelli W, Boll J, Tan OT. Ultraviolet excimer laser ablation: the effect of wavelength and repetition rate on in vivo guinea pig skin. J Invest Dermatol 1987;88:769–773.
10. Lane RJ, Wynne JJ, Geronemus RG. Ultraviolet laser ablation of skin: healing studies and a thermal model. Lasers Surg Med 1987;6:504–513.

11. Jacques SL, McAuliffe DJ, Blank IH, Parrish JA. Controlled removal of human stratum corneum by pulsed laser. J Invest Dermatol 1987;88:88–93.

12. Lane RJ, Linsker R, Wynne JJ, Torres A, Geronemus RG. Ultraviolet-laser ablation of skin. Arch Dermatol 1985;121:609–617.

13. Jacques SL, McAuliffe DJ, Conner DP, Peck CC. Laser-enhanced percutaneous transport for topical drug delivery and collection. J Invest Dermatol 1988;91:216.

14. Conner DP, Jacques SL, Almirez RG et al. Laser-enhanced transcutaneous collection of theophylline. Clin Pharmacol Ther 1988;43:123.

15. Murphy GF, Shepard RS, Paul BS, Menkes A, Anderson RR, Parrish JA. Organelle-specific injury to melanin-containing cells in human skin by pulsed laser irradiation. Lab Invest 1983;49:680–685.

16. Parrish JA, Anderson RR, Harrist T, Paul B, Murphy GF. Selective thermal effects with pulsed irradiation from lasers: from organ to organelle. J Invest Dermatol 1983;80(suppl):75s–80s.

17. Anderson RR, Parrish JA. Selective photothermolysis: precise microsurgery by selective absorption of pulsed radiation. Science 1983;220:524–527.

18. Dover JS, Margolis RJ, Polla LL et al. Pigmented guinea pig skin irradiated with Q-switched ruby laser pulses. Morphologic and histologic findings. Arch Dermatol 1989;125:43–49.

19. Anderson RR, Margolis RJ, Watenabe S, Flotte T, Hruza GJ, Dover JS. Selective photothermolysis of cutaneous pigmentation by Q-switched Nd:YAG laser pulses at 1064, 532, and 355 nm. J Invest Dermatol 1989;93:28–32.

20. Tong AK, Tan OT, Boll J, Parrish JA, Murphy GF. Ultrastructure: effects of melanin pigment on target specificity using a pulsed dye laser (577 nm). J Invest Dermatol 1987;88:747–752.

21. Masnyk TW, Nguyen HT, Minton KW. Reduced formation of bipyrimidine photoproducts in DNA UV irradiated at high intensity. J Biol Chem 1989;264:2482–2488.

22. Green H, Boll J, Parrish JA, Kochevar IE, Oseroff AR. Cytotoxicity and mutagenicity of low intensity, 248 and 193 nm excimer laser radiation in mammalian cells. Cancer Res 1987;47:410–413.

23. Green HA, Margolis R, Boll J, Kochevar IE, Parrish JA, Oseroff AR. Unscheduled DNA synthesis in human skin after in vitro ultraviolet-excimer laser ablation. J Invest Dermatol 1987;89:201–204.

24. Kochevar IE. Cytotoxicity and mutagenicity of excimer laser radiation. Lasers Surg Med 1989;9:440–445.

25. Matchette LS, Waynant RW, Royston DD, Hitchins VM, Elespuru RK. Induction of lambda prophage near the site of focused UV laser radiation. Photochem Photobiol 1989;49:161–167.

26. Seiler T, Bende T, Winckler K, Wollensak J. Side effects in excimer corneal surgery. DNA damage as a result of 193 nm excimer laser radiation. Graefes Arch Clin Exp Ophthalmol 1988;226:273–276.

27. Trentacoste J, Thompson K, Parrish RK, Hajek A, Berman MR, Ganjei P. Mutagenic potential of a 193-nm excimer laser on fibroblasts in tissue culture. Ophthalmology 1987;94:125–129.

28. Kochevar IE, Buckley LA. Photochemistry of DNA using 193 nm excimer laser radiation. Photochem Photobiol 1990;51:527–532.

29. Kochevar IE, Walsh AA, Held KD, Gallo RL, Mirro J. Mechanism for 193-nm laser radiation-induced effects on mammalian cells. Radiat Res 1990;122:142–148.

30. Flotte TJ, Yashima Y, Watanabe S, McAuliffe DJ, Jacques SL. Morphological studies of laser-induced photoacoustic damage. SPIE 1990;1202:71–77.

31. Flotte TJ, Frisoli J, Goetschkes M, Doukas AG. Laser-induced shock wave effects on cells. SPIE 1991;1247:36–44.

32. Yashima Y, McAuliffe DJ, Flotte TJ. Cell selectivity to laser-induced photoacoustic injury of skin. Lasers Surg Med 1990;10:280–283.

33. Yashima Y, McAuliffe DJ, Jacques SL, Flotte TJ. Laser-induced photoacoustic injury of skin: effect of inertial confinement. Lasers Surg Med 1991;11:62–68.

34. Trokel SL, Srinivasan R, Braren B. Excimer laser surgery of the cornea. Am J Ophthalmol 1983;96:710–715.

35. Dehm EJ, Puliafito CA, Adler CM, Steinert RF. Corneal endothelial injury in rabbits following excimer laser ablation at 193 and 248 nm. Arch Ophthalmol 1986;104:1364–1368.

36. Marshall J, Trokel S, Rothery S, Krueger RR. A comparative study of corneal incisions induced by diamond and steel knives and two ultraviolet radiations from an excimer laser. Br J Ophthalmol 1986;70:482–501.

37. Puliafito CA, Wong K, Steinert RF. Quantitative and ultrastructural studies of excimer laser ablation of the cornea at 193 and 248 nanometers. Lasers Surg Med 1987;7:155–159.

38. Taylor DM, L'Esperance FJ, Del PR et al. Human excimer laser lamellar keratectomy. A clinical study. Ophthalmology 1989;96:654–664.

39. McDonald MB, Frantz JM, Klyce SD et al. Central photorefractive keratectomy for myopia. The blind eye study. Arch Ophthalmol 1990;108:799–808.

40. Cotliar AM, Schubert HD, Mandel ER, Trokel SL. Excimer laser radial keratotomy. Ophthalmology 1985;92:206–208.

41. Rosa DS, Boerner CF, Gross M, Timsit JC, Delacour M, Bath PE. Wound healing following excimer laser radial keratotomy. J Cataract Refract Surg 1988;14:173–179.

42. Serdarevic O, Darrell RW, Krueger RR, Trokel SL. Excimer laser therapy for experimental *Candida* keratitis. Am J Ophthalmol 1985;99:534–538.

43. Berlin MS, Rajacich G, Duffy M, Grundfest W, Goldenberg T. Excimer laser photoablation in glaucoma filtering surgery. Am J Ophthalmol 1987;103:713–714.

44. Nanevicz TM, Prince MR, Gawande AA, Puliafito CA. Excimer laser ablation of the lens. Arch Ophthalmol 1986;104:1825–1829.

45. Serdarevic ON, Hanna K, Gribomont AC, Savoldelli M, Renard G, Pouliquen Y. Excimer laser trephination in penetrating keratoplasty. Morphologic features and wound healing. Ophthalmology 1988;95:493–505.

46. Steinert RF, Puliafito CA. Excimer laser phototherapeutic keratectomy for a corneal nodule. Refract Corneal Surg 1990;6:352.

47. Grundfest WS, Litvack F, Forrester JS et al. Laser ablation of human atherosclerotic plaque without adjacent tissue injury. J Am Coll Cardiol 1985;5:929–933.

48. Litvack F, Grundfest WS, Goldenberg T, Laudenslager J, Forrester JS. Percutaneous excimer laser angioplasty of aortocoronary saphenous vein grafts. J Am Coll Cardiol 1989;14:803–808.

49. Karsch KR, Haase KK, Mauser M et al. Percutaneous coronary excimer laser angioplasty: initial clinical results. Lancet 1989;2:647–650.

50. Sanborn TA, Torre SR, Sharma SK et al. Percutaneous coronary excimer laser-assisted balloon angioplasty: initial clinical and quantitative angiographic results in 50 patients. J Am Coll Cardiol 1991;17:94–99.
51. Downar E, Butany J, Jares A, Stoicheff BP. Endocardial photoablation by excimer laser. J Am Coll Cardiol 1986;7:546–550.
52. Freedland Y. Use of the excimer laser in fibrocartilaginous excision from adjacent bony stroma: a preliminary investigation. J Foot Surg 1988;27:303–305.
53. Kroitzsch U, Laufer G, Egkher E, Wollenek G, Horvath R. Experimental photoablation of meniscus cartilage by excimer laser energy. A new aspect in meniscus surgery. Arch Orthop Trauma Surg 1989;108:44–48.
54. Yow L, Nelson JS, Berns MW. Ablation of bone and polymethylmethacrylate by an XeCl (308 nm) excimer laser. Lasers Surg Med 1989;9:141–147.
55. Pini R, Salimbeni R, Vannini M, Cavalieri S, Barone R, Clauser C. Laser dentistry: root canal diagnostic technique based on ultraviolet-induced fluorescence spectroscopy. Lasers Surg Med 1989;9:358–361.
56. Wrobel R, Bernage P, Niay P et al. XeCl laser in biliary calculus fragmentation: fluence threshold and ablation products. IEEE Trans Biomed Eng 1989;36:1202–1209.
57. Prodouz KN, Fratantoni JC, Boone EJ, Bonner RF. Use of laser-UV for inactivation of virus in blood products. Blood 1987;70:589–592.

III. Low-Energy Lasers and Other Light Energy Modalities

15 —— Biologic Effects of Low-Energy Lasers

Cynthia H. Halcin
Jouni Uitto

Low-energy lasers emit energy densities that are too low to cause temperature increases beyond 0.5°C in the target tissue.[1] Thus, the effects of low-energy laser irradiation are presumably not attributable to thermal events. The early literature on the effects of low-energy lasers, published mostly in eastern Europe some three decades ago, generally consisted of reports on largely anecdotal observations, and the scientific value of these lasers was not appreciated because the data could not hold up to the scrutiny of the research community. However, in the 1970s reports of more controlled clinical studies performed in both human and animal models and evaluating wound healing in response to treatment with low-energy lasers began to appear in the literature.[2–11] Subsequently, considerable interest grew in the biomodulation of tissue and cell metabolism produced by low-energy lasers, and during the past decade or so, findings from numerous studies assessing various aspects of the effects of low-energy lasers on biologic systems have been published.[12] Many of the recent studies deal with the effects of low-energy lasers on cellular metabolism, extracellular matrix production, tissue repair, and immune functions of the cells. Although these studies are in general carefully controlled and the laser parameters well defined, the results on the whole remain controversial and the efficacy of low-energy laser irradiation in the context of certain biologic functions remains in question.

A variety of different types of laser light sources have been used to deliver the laser energy at low levels (Table 15-1).[13] These lasers deliver energy at different wavelengths, which targets different structures, molecules, or both with different absorption spectra within the cells and tissues. The helium-neon (He-Ne), gallium-aluminum-arsenide (Ga-Al-As), and gallium-arsenide (Ga-As) lasers have been

The authors with to thank Valarie L. Benson for expert secretarial help. Dr. Edward J. Glassberg (UCLA School of Medicine) assisted in the preparation of this overview. Original studies performed by the authors were supported by U.S. Public Health Service, National Institutes of Health grant R01-AR41439 and by grants from the Dermatology Foundation.

Table 15-1.   Types of lasers used for delivery of low energy irradiation

Active medium	Wavelength (nm)
Argon	488, 514.5
Helium-neon	632.8
Krypton	647.1
Gallium-aluminum-arsenide	660, 820, 870, 880
Ruby crystal	694.3
Gallium-arsenide	904
Neodymium:yttrium-aluminum-garnet (Nd:YAG)	1064
CO_2	10,600

used in most of the recent studies, but the incident energy density used, the total dose delivered, and the treatment schedules followed have varied considerably from one study to another. This variability, combined with the fact that different cells and tissues have been used as targets for irradiation, may explain some of the variable and even controversial results yielded.

In this overview, we discuss the biologic effects of low-energy lasers, primarily concentrating on the characteristics of cell proliferation, the extracellular matrix production that occurs during wound healing, and immune modulation in vitro.

Effects of Low-Energy Laser Irradiation on Wound Healing

Clinical Observations

Results from the earlier, largely uncontrolled studies indicated that low-energy laser light may promote better wound healing in humans. For example, Mester and associates[9] found that wound healing appeared to be accelerated in six patients with skin ulcers treated with an He-Ne laser. Electron micrographs of tissue from the wound sites showed that the stimulation of healing was possibly primarily due to the activation of collagen production. Subsequently, other studies have pointed to normalization of the humoral immune responses, as measured by serum complement activity and immunoglobulin levels, as the mechanism responsible for the improved healing; this suggests that laser modulation of immune mechanisms may also play a role in enhancing healing.[10,11] It should be noted, however, that the cases studied represented a broad spectrum of leg ulcers of varying causes and in general studies consisting of such relatively small numbers of cases are difficult to control. It should also be noted that nonirradiated areas of the ulcers showed changes identical to, although less marked than, those seen in the irradiated area.[9,14] These observations indicate either that the ulcers healed spontaneously even in areas not subjected to direct laser irradiation or that the laser irradiation had systemic effects affecting sites not directly exposed to laser irradiation. The latter possibility was suggested by Bosatra and colleagues,[14] who noted that the healing of leg ulcers was enhanced after He-Ne laser irradiation but found no difference in the healing of the irradiated and nonirradiated halves of the wounds. This concurs with current data from studies[15–17] examining the interaction of various epidermal growth factors and cytokines found in healing wounds. However, conflicting findings were noted by Lundeberg and Malm, who reported on two series of patients, one consisting of 23 patients treated with an He-Ne laser[18] and the other consisting of 21 patients treated with a Ga-As laser.[19] The same number of patients in each series served as the control (placebo) group. They were treated with the same laser unit from which the specific laser energy had been removed. These two studies did not reveal any difference between either group of laser-treated patients and their placebo-treated counterparts. Thus, the clinical value of the He-Ne and Ga-As lasers in enhancing the healing of leg ulcers is uncertain.

ANIMAL MODELS OF WOUND HEALING

As noted earlier, clinical studies investigating the merits of low-energy lasers for the treatment of leg ulcers suffer from an inherent lack of matched controls. Furthermore, the healing of leg ulcers in general is unpredictable, and for this reason, differences in ulcers before and after laser treatment do not necessarily reflect the direct effect of the laser on the healing processes.

Because of these and other difficulties posed by clinical trials, several animal models have been developed for the purpose of examining the potential effects of laser irradiation on wound healing. A variety of models and animal species have been used in these studies. Several[20–24] have utilized the wounding of pig skin as the model system, with the reasoning that pig skin is more like human skin in terms of its thickness, epidermal turnover time, and subcutaneous attachments than, for example, rodent skin, which heals primarily with contraction of the wounds because of the laxity of the skin. Nevertheless, mice, rats, and rabbits have been used as the animal models in several studies.[2–8,20–33] In addition to differences in the animals studied, the types of wounds studied have varied considerably. For example, in some of the studies, burn wounds have been used as the model, whereas in others the healing of excisions or linear incisions of the skin have been studied. The variables monitored have included the time required for the wound closure, the tensile strength, the degree of epithelialization, and bacterial colonization.

However, even under these relatively controlled experimental conditions, the results yielded have been controversial. For example, findings from three studies[22,30,31] examining the healing of burns in rodent skin indicated that the rate of healing may be enhanced by

He-Ne lasers but pointed to different mechanisms. Specifically, one of these studies[30] showed that the lipid peroxide concentrations increased markedly in the serum of burned animals not treated with the laser, whereas the lipid peroxide concentrations in the laser-treated burned group remained relatively constant and were significantly lower than those in the control group. These observations indicated that the enhanced wound healing stemming from the effects of laser irradiation may relate to a reduction in the free oxygen radicals, which may perpetuate the tissue damage and impede the healing process. In contrast, another study[22] showed that wound healing was not enhanced if the irradiation was performed immediately after wounding. This suggested that the timing of the laser treatment in relation to the trauma was critical in determining the nature of wound healing after laser treatment. This may be of clinical significance, particularly in patients who undergo radiotherapy, in whom this modality could potentially be used to reduce or alleviate the late effects of ionizing irradiation in the dermis.

Other studies, however, have not shown laser treatment to have any significant effect on the healing of open wounds. For example, no beneficial effect from the low-energy laser treatment of skin flaps was seen in rat and porcine models of wound healing.[24] Furthermore, another study[28] did not show any difference in the bleeding time or the formation and loss of the crust of the healing wound between treated and untreated rats, and histologic examination revealed no obvious morphologic differences between the laser-treated and untreated wounds. It should be noted, however, that a contralateral wound in the same animal was used as the control in the latter study; therefore any systemic effect could have masked differences between the treated and untreated wounds.

Some studies have evaluated the tensile strength of incisional wounds in animals. In one such study, hairless mice were experimentally wounded, sutured, and subjected to He-Ne laser irradiation.[25] The wounds in the laser-treated animals were irradiated every other day for 2 months; the wounds in different (control) animals remained untreated. Tissue specimens from the wounds were obtained for histologic studies and for the purpose of assessing the tensile strength and total collagen content. The results of this study, shown in Figure 15-1, demonstrated that the tensile strength of the laser-irradiated wounds was considerably improved at 1 and 2 weeks of treatment, versus that in the control animals. The total collagen content was also significantly increased at 2 months in the wounds of the treated as opposed to the control animals. The findings from these studies agree with those from an earlier study performed by Mester's group,[5] in which a slight increase in tensile strength was demonstrable as early as the fifth day of treatment and the difference on the eighth day of treatment was highly significant. However, the increase in tensile strength on the twelfth day of treatment was closer to that in the untreated rats, suggesting that laser irradiation initially accelerates wound healing but eventually healing reaches the same level as that in

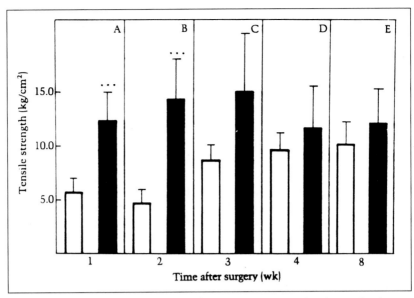

Fig. 15-1. Determination of tensile strength of the wounds subjected to laser irradiation (*solid bars*) in comparison with control wounds (*open bars*). The values are means ± SD of three parallel determinations. Three asterisks indicate that values are statistically different from the corresponding controls ($p < 0.001$). (Reproduced with permission from Lyons RF, et al. Biostimulation of wound healing *in vivo* by a helium-neon laser. Ann Plast Surg 1987;18:47–50.)

untreated wounds. Another study[29] in which an He-Ne laser was used also showed a significant increase in the tensile strength of laser-treated incisional wounds made in rabbit skin. However, the rate of wound healing and the amount of collagen formed, as determined by trichrome staining, were not significantly altered. Thus, several studies have shown that the tensile strength of incisional wounds is increased by treatment with the low-energy He-Ne laser. However, some of these have indicated that this may be due to an enhanced accumulation of collagen in the treated wounds, whereas one[29] in which the collagen content was found to be normal showed that perhaps other mechanisms, such as increased cross-linking of the existing collagen, contribute to the increased tensile properties of the healing wounds subjected to low-energy laser irradiation.

EFFECTS OF LOW-ENERGY LASERS ON COLLAGEN BIOSYNTHESIS IN VITRO

As already indicated, some of the animal studies in which collagen levels were directly measured as well as some of the clinical studies in which the collagen accumulation was estimated by semiquantitative electron microscopic means have shown that low-energy laser irradiation may increase the biosynthesis of collagen in treated wounds. To examine mechanistically the effects of low-energy laser irradiation on connective tissue metabolism, several studies were performed using established human skin fibroblasts in culture.[14,34–42] In one such study,[36] two low-energy lasers (He-Ne and Ga-As) were used to treat the cultured fibroblasts one or two times daily on several consecutive days using various fluences. These studies showed that collagen production, as quantified by the amount of radioactive hydroxyproline synthesized, was increased on average by approximately fourfold in different fibroblast cultures. However, the greatest enhancement, about 37-fold, was noted in cultures treated only once with the He-Ne laser and initially synthesizing collagen at a relatively low level; lesser effects were noted in cultures that were already actively synthesizing collagen (Table 15-2; Fig. 15-2). It was also noted that extended treatment with the Ga-As laser for up to 4 consecutive days resulted in a sustained increase in collagen production, with an energy density of ~2.0 J/cm² yielding maximal results (Fig. 15-3). In contrast, a treatment schedule consisting of two exposures on 1 day demonstrated a less than threefold increase using a maximal energy density of 0.2 J/cm². The lasers tested in this study (i.e., He-Ne and Ga-As lasers) had no effect on the activities of collagenase and gelatinase, two proteolytic enzymes that control the degradation of collagen. Therefore, the findings from these studies indicate that these two low-energy lasers may directly cause an increase in collagen biosynthesis as the result of a subtle biomodulation of collagen synthesis, either at the transcriptional or posttranscriptional levels of gene expression.

Molecular studies were performed that assessed the level of enhancement of collagen gene expression during accelerated wound healing resulting from laser treatment.[20,26] Collagen gene expression was determined by measuring the type I and III procollagen messenger RNA (mRNA) levels in full-thickness cutaneous wounds produced in the backs of pigs and treated with an He-Ne laser (Figs. 15-4 and 15-5). This study showed that the type I and III collagen mRNA levels, as determined by molecular hybridizations with the corresponding complementary DNA probes in slot-blot hybridiza-

Table 15-2. Stimulation of procollagen synthesis by He-Ne laser

| Fibroblast line | Collagen production in control cultures | | Stimulation by laser (-fold) |
	dpm × 10⁻¹ μg protein	Percentage of total protein	
A	0.15 ± 0.01	0.80	36.7 ($p < 0.001$)
B	1.55 ± 0.13	7.00	3.3 ($p < 0.001$)
C	20.68 ± 1.38	16.06	1.1 ($p = $ NS)

dpm = disintegrations per minute; NS = not significant.
Source: Modified with permission from Abergel RP, Meeker CA, Lam TS, Dwyer RM, Lesavoy MA, Uitto J. Control of connective tissue metabolism by lasers: recent developments and future prospects. J Am Acad Dermatol 1984;11:1142–1150.

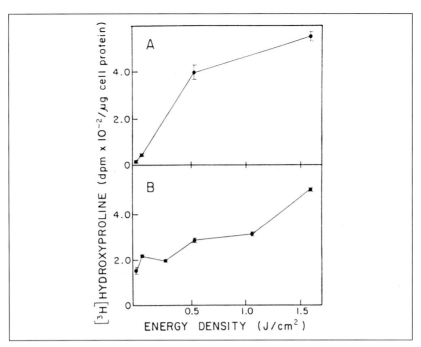

Fig. 15-2. Stimulation of procollagen production by a He-Ne laser in human skin fibroblast cultures. Cells were exposed to He-Ne laser irradiation, and [³H]hydroxyproline synthesis was assayed as an index of collagen production. The results are expressed as means ± SD of three parallel cultures. (A) This cell line was subjected to He-Ne laser irradiation once daily for 3 consecutive days. (B) This cell line was subjected to He-Ne laser irradiation once daily for 4 days. (Reproduced with permission from Lam TS, et al. Laser stimulation of collagen synthesis in human skin fibroblast cultures. Lasers Life Sci 1986;1:61–77.)

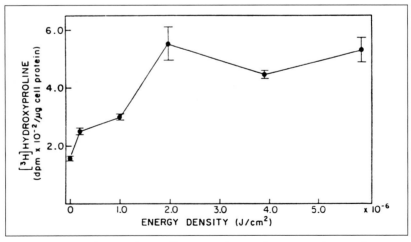

Fig. 15-3. Stimulation of procollagen production by a Ga-As laser in human skin fibroblast cultures. Cells were subjected to Ga-As laser irradiation once daily for 4 consecutive days and then assayed for collagen synthesis, as described in ref 36. The values are means ± SD of three parallel cultures. (Reproduced with permission from Lam TS, et al. Laser stimulation of collagen synthesis in human skin fibroblast cultures. Lasers Life Sci 1986;1:61–77.)

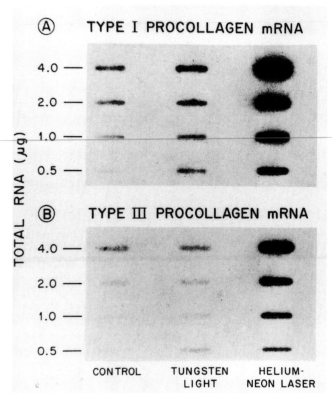

Fig. 15-4.   Assay of type I and type III procollagen messenger RNA (mRNA) levels in cutaneous wounds treated with the He-Ne laser or a tungsten light source, or left untreated as controls. Biopsy specimens were obtained from the wounds on day 17 of healing, and the total RNA was isolated by cesium chloride density gradient centrifugation. Varying amounts of RNA, in the range of 4.0 to 0.5 µg, as shown, were dotted onto nitrocellulose filters and hybridized with type I procollagen– (A) or type III procollagen– (B) specific complementary DNA (cDNA) probes, which were radioactively labeled by nick translation. The figure represents the autoradiograms of mRNA ^{32}P-cDNA hybrids. (Reproduced with permission from Saperia D, et al. Demonstration of elevated type I and type III procollagen mRNA levels in cutaneous wounds treated with helium-neon laser. Biochem Biophys Res Comm 1986;138:1123–1128.

tion assays, were increased at days 17 and 28 in the healing wounds treated with the laser, as compared with the levels in untreated control wounds or wounds treated with tungsten (nonlaser) light (see Fig. 15-5). These results indicate that some of the laser effects may take place at the pretranslational level.[26]

In another study,[35] cultured human skin fibroblasts were irradiated with a Ga-Al-As laser. Hydroxyproline formation, as determined by a chemical assay, was found to be significantly increased as a result of laser treatment. Beside the increase in the collagen synthesis noted, the uptake of ascorbic acid in laser-irradiated cells was also found to be markedly enhanced. Because ascorbic acid is a critical

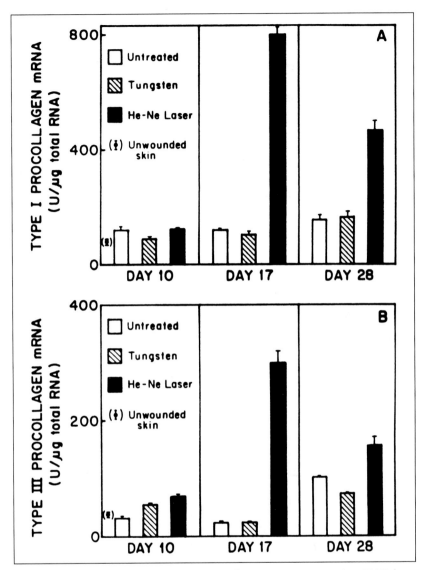

Fig. 15-5.   Type I (A) and type III (B) procollagen messenger RNA (mRNA) levels in cutaneous wounds. The wounds were treated with the He-Ne laser or tungsten light, or left untreated as control, as indicated in Figure 15-4. Biopsy specimens from the wounds, as well as from adjacent unwounded skin, were obtained at days 10, 17, and 28 of treatment. Type I and type III procollagen–specific mRNA levels were determined from the slot-blot hybridizations shown in Figure 15-4. The values are expressed as densitometric units per microgram of total RNA dotted (mean ± SD of three to four parallel determinations). (Reproduced with permission from Saperia D, et al. Demonstration of elevated type I and type III procollagen mRNA levels in cutaneous wounds treated with helium-neon laser. Biochem Biophys Res Comm 1986;138:1123–1128.)

cofactor for prolyl hydroxylase, the enzyme catalyzing the hydroxylation of prolyl residues, and therefore necessary for the synthesis of hydroxyproline,[43–46] the authors concluded that the increased uptake of ascorbic acid may be responsible for stimulating the collagen synthesis in laser-treated cells. This would point to an enhanced post-translational modification of prolyl residues as the event triggering the enhanced synthesis of hydroxyproline. Because hydroxyproline must be present for the formation and subsequent secretion of triple helical collagen molecules to occur,[43–46] this, together with the elevated levels of type I and III procollagen mRNA,[20] would mechanistically explain the enhanced collagen synthesis seen in vitro in laser-irradiated cells.

EFFECTS OF LOW-ENERGY LASERS ON EPIDERMAL WOUND HEALING

Most experimental studies that have examined the effects of low-energy lasers on wound healing have concentrated on the extracellular matrix, and primarily the collagen, the predominant component of normal skin and a critical constituent of healing wounds.[47,48] However, an essential component of cutaneous wound healing is the regeneration of the epidermis, particularly in pigs and humans, in whom wounds do not contract to the same extent as rodent wounds do. However, only a few studies have carefully examined the rate of epidermal healing in laser-treated wounds. An early study conducted by Braverman and colleagues[29] showed that the relative epidermal thickness was somewhat enhanced in the He-Ne laser–treated areas, as compared with the epidermal thickness of unexposed tissue, but the difference was not statistically significant. Nevertheless, this study did show that low-energy lasers may have effects on epidermal components. However, the comparison between the treated and untreated wounds was performed in the same animal, making it possible for systemic effects to also have been responsible for increasing the epidermal growth on the untreated contralateral wounds, and thus obscuring the true magnitude of the laser effect.

The effects of low-energy lasers on human epidermal keratinocytes have also been studied under carefully controlled in vitro conditions.[49,50] In these studies, He-Ne lasers were used to irradiate human epidermal keratinocytes, followed by a determination of the potential biostimulatory effects of the laser irradiation on cell motility and keratinocyte differentiation. In one set of experiments, the keratinocytes in confluent cultures were "wounded" by creating a 0.1-mm-long cellfree streak through the culture.[49] The motility of the cultured human keratinocytes was then documented by videocinemicroscopy, and cell movement toward the cellfree area was quantified sequentially for a 6-hour period 20 hours after the culture had been exposed to laser irradiation (0.8 J/cm^2 administered three times over a

20-hour period).[44] A significant difference was seen between the migration of the leading edge of the laser-irradiated cells, and that of the nonirradiated control cells (Fig. 15-6).

In the second set of experiments, subconfluent human keratinocyte cultures were irradiated with a single dose or multiple doses of laser energy at fluences varying from 0.4 to 7.2 J/cm^2.[50] Irradiated and nonirradiated keratinocyte cultures were also grown on a microporous membrane along with irradiated and nonirradiated fibroblasts to determine whether He-Ne laser irradiation might induce keratinocyte proliferation in a paracrine manner. None of these treatments was found to result in a significant increase in keratinocyte proliferation, indicating that the biostimulatory effect of He-Ne irradiation on keratinocyte motility is a result of a direct effect on these cells. Consequently, the authors suggested that the enhanced keratinocyte motility, as observed in vitro, may contribute to the effectiveness of He-Ne laser irradiation in promoting epidermal wound healing.[49]

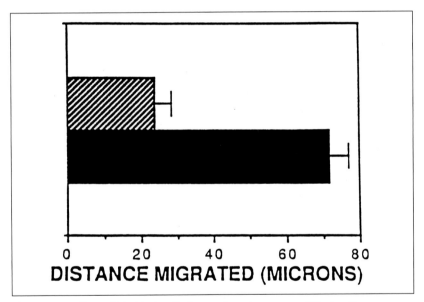

Fig. 15-6.   Effect of He-Ne irradiation on keratinocyte motility in vitro. "Wounded" monolayers of cultured keratinocytes received 3 × 0.8 J/cm^2 irradiation over a 20-hour period, after which the rate of migration of the wound margin was measured over a 6-hour period. The data are expressed as the means of 10 different measurements in two control and four irradiated separate experiments. Experimental values differed significantly from control values ($p <$ 0.0001), as shown by Student's t test. (*Hatched bar* = control, mock-irradiated culture [n = 20]; *solid bar* = irradiated cultures [n = 40].) (Reprinted by permission of Elsevier Science Publishing Co., Inc., from Low-energy helium-neon laser irradiation increases the motility of cultured human keratinocytes, by Haas S, et al. THE JOURNAL OF INVESTIGATIVE DERMATOLOGY, 194:822–826. Copyright 1990 by The Society of Investigative Dermatology, Inc.)

Because keratinocyte differentiation is an important feature of the formation of functional epidermis during human epidermal wound healing, these investigators also examined the effects of He-Ne laser irradiation on keratinocyte differentiation.[50] In this study, subconfluent keratinocyte cultures were irradiated three times within 24 hours using energy fluences varying from 0 to 7.2 J/cm². After the cultures had reached the postconfluence state, various aspects of cell growth and differentiation, including the number of cells, the status of cornified envelope formation, and the transglutaminase activity, were determined. No significant differences in these variables were noted between control and irradiated cultures. Furthermore, both cultures exhibited similar patterns of keratin gene expression, indicating that the He-Ne laser irradiation has no direct effect on keratinocyte differentiation. Thus, the chief effect of low-energy laser irradiation on epidermal wound healing appears to be the enhanced motility of the keratinocytes it stimulates. In addition, laser irradiation may not interfere with the normal processes leading to the terminal differentiation of keratinocytes in the epidermis. These findings are consistent with and may explain the increased epidermal thickness found in low-energy laser–irradiated wounds observed in the previously mentioned studies.

EFFECTS OF LOW-ENERGY LASERS ON CELL PROLIFERATION

Several studies have examined the effects of low-energy laser irradiation on the growth and replication of a variety of cell types.[4–8,36–42,51–54] These studies are important because the proliferation of fibroblasts or other cell types may play a major role in the reparative processes, such as wound healing, that could be accelerated by laser irradiation. Most of the studies reported on so far have shown that low-energy lasers may affect the rate of proliferation of cells in vitro. However, there are critical differences in terms of the response to different lasers and the magnitude of the effect produced. For example, Ga-As laser irradiation was noted in one study to suppress DNA replication in human skin fibroblast cultures (Fig. 15-7).[36,37] The DNA replication, measured by radioactive thymidine incorporation, was found to be already inhibited by approximately 80% after exposures in 1 day to ~0.3 J/cm².[36] However, the parallel incubation of cultures with an He-Ne laser using a similar experimental protocol did not reveal any significant changes in DNA replication. Nevertheless, both treatments, performed using the same parameters, caused collagen production to be increased in parallel cultures, indicating that the enhanced collagen synthesis cannot be explained by alterations in the rate of cell proliferation in the same cultures. These findings may be further elucidated, however, by the findings from a study performed by Noble and colleagues,[39] in which short bursts of He-Ne laser radiation were found to convert embryonic fibroblasts to a mature phenotype, inducing a "lethargic" locomotory phenotype of the

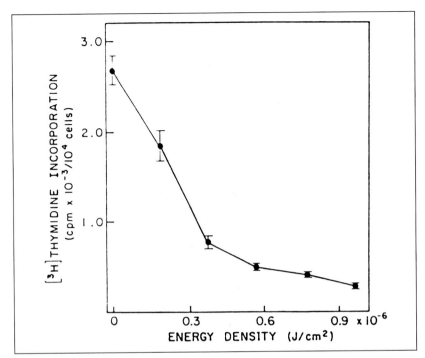

Fig. 15-7. Suppression by Ga-As laser of DNA replication in human skin fibroblast cultures. The cells were subjected to two exposures to laser treatment on the same day, using the energy densities indicated. [³H]Thymidine incorporation, an index of DNA replication, was then assayed, as described in ref 36. The values are means ± SD of three parallel cultures. (Reproduced with permission from Lam TS, et al. Laser stimulation of collagen synthesis in human skin fibroblast cultures. Lasers Life Sci 1976;1:61–77.)

treated fibroblasts. This decrease in locomotion indicates that the fibroblast may be unable to acquire enough resources to engage in locomotion while synthesizing collagen. These findings also correlate with those of Bard and Elsdale,[40] who showed an inverse relationship between the speed of fibroblast locomotion and collagen secretion. Low-energy laser irradiation has also been noted to enhance cell growth in human gingival fibroblast cultures.[41] This growth promotion was accompanied by the development of mitochondrial hyperplasia, cytoplasmic microfilaments, and a pericellular matrix, indicating that the accelerated cell growth was accompanied by an increase in the biosynthetic capacity of the same cells.

An interesting study examined the potential role of macrophages in enhanced wound repair from the standpoint of fibroblast proliferation.[52] Specifically, this study examined the effect of low-energy laser radiation at four different wavelengths (i.e., 660, 820, 870, and 880 nm) on the release of macrophage mediators that might cause the proliferation of fibroblasts in culture. The target cell was a macrophage-like cell line, U-937, which releases important cytokine mediators.[55–57] It was found that the lower wavelengths (660, 820, and 870 nm) triggered the release of factors from U-937 cells that stimulated fibroblast proliferation to levels greater than control levels.[52] In contrast, the 880-nm wavelength either inhibited the release of the stimulatory factors or triggered the release of some factors that inhibited fibroblast proliferation. This latter observation is consistent with the observation that the Ga-As laser, which emits radiation at 904 nm, causes fibroblast proliferation to be inhibited, while the 632.8-nm wavelength of the He-Ne laser has no effect on fibroblast proliferation in vitro.[36] It should be noted, however, that the latter study was performed using pure fibroblasts in culture, so it is unclear whether the laser energy might have caused the release of some autocrine factors that mimic the paracrine effects of radiation on macrophages in culture. Nevertheless, the release of factors from macrophages stimulating fibroblast proliferation in response to lower wavelengths, such as 660 nm (a wavelength that approaches the wavelength of He-Ne lasers, i.e., 632.8 nm), may play a role in enhancing the wound healing in intact animals and human skin. This may explain the findings from previous investigations in which spontaneous healing of the nonirradiated ulcers was noted to occur in low-energy laser–treated patients.

Finally, it should be noted that a controlled, randomized study in which cultured human skin fibroblasts were used as the target for low-energy He-Ne laser irradiation performed over a 5-day period failed to reveal significant changes in the replication of the cells.[42] This observation agrees with that from a previous study conducted by Lam and associates,[36] which also did not show that He-Ne laser radiation has any effect on DNA replication in fibroblast cultures. Collectively these studies show that the effects of low-energy lasers on cell proliferation and DNA replication may be wavelength specific and that the magnitude and nature of the effect may depend not only on the particular experimental conditions used but also on the laser used.

Immune Modulation of Cells by Low-Energy Lasers

As already discussed, some of the studies of wound healing have shown that various aspects of humoral immunity may be altered in laser-treated animals. This has been indicated by the systemic effects seen in studies in which contralateral wounds were used as controls. Some earlier studies also showed that complement and immunoglobulin levels may be normalized in the serum of patients with leg ulcers treated by low-energy laser irradiation.[10,11] This has been further borne out by the finding that the serum lipid peroxidase levels were normalized in mice with burn wounds treated by the He-Ne laser.[30]

Much work has also been done on the effects of low-energy laser irradiation on cellular immunity. The results obtained so far have indicated that cellular immunity is either stimulated or suppressed, depending on the particular experimental model used. For example, in one study,[54] cultured human lymphocytes were examined after irradiation with a Ga-As laser at fluences varying from 2.17 to 650 mJ/cm². The lymphocyte proliferation was assessed by radioactive thymidine incorporation. Spontaneous cell proliferation was found to be markedly inhibited by laser irradiation at a fluence as low as 10.85 mJ/cm² (Fig. 15-8). In addition, the proliferation of lymphocytes in response to the stimulation of mitogen by phytohemagglutinin (PHA) was found to be inhibited in cultures irradiated at the end of 4 days of incubation with PHA, whereas irradiation performed at the beginning of the 4-day period had no effect on the subsequent replication of cells in the presence of PHA (Fig. 15-9). Furthermore, the functional response of cells to antigenic stimulation in a one-way mixed lymphocyte reaction was also found to be

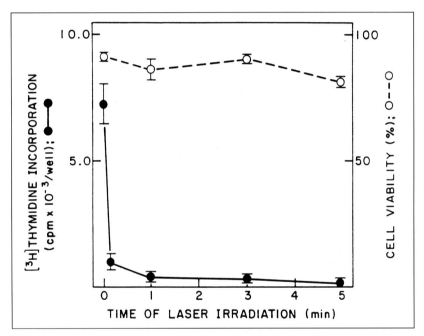

Fig. 15-8. Inhibition of spontaneous lymphocyte proliferation in vitro by a Ga-As laser. Lymphocytes (10⁵ cells/well) were subjected to laser irradiation in phosphate-buffered saline. Afterward the cells were recovered by centrifugation and placed in RPMI 1640 medium containing 10% fetal calf serum and [³H]thymidine. After a 7-hour incubation, the cells were harvested and the incorporation of radioactivity was determined as described in ref 54. Cell viability was assessed by the trypan blue exclusion test and expressed as the number of cells excluding the dye. The values are means ± SD of 4 to 12 parallel determinations. The laser inhibition of [³H]thymidine incorporation is statistically significant at all time points ($p < 0.001$), versus that in untreated controls, as shown by Student's t test. (Reproduced with permission from Ohta A, Abergel RP, Uitto J. Laser modulation of human immune system: inhibition of lymphocyte proliferation by a gallium-arsenide laser at low energy. Lasers Surg Med 1987;7:199–201.)

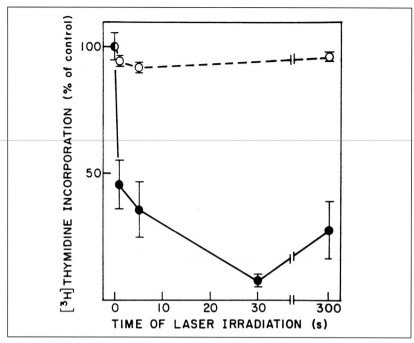

Fig. 15-9. The effect of Ga-As laser irradiation on the proliferation of human lymphocytes in culture in response to mitogenic stimulation by phytohemagglutinin. Lymphocytes (2×10^5 cell/well) were cultured in RPMI 1640 medium with 25 μg/ml of phytohemagglutinin for 4 days. The cell cultures were subjected to laser irradiation for the time periods indicated, either at the beginning (*open circles*) or at the end (*closed circles*) of the 4-day culture. The cell proliferation was determined by incubation with 2 μC of [³H]thymidine during the last 12 hours of culture. The incorporation of radioactivity was determined as described in ref 54, and the values (mean ± SEM of four to six parallel determinations) are expressed as the percentage of the corresponding control cultures without laser irradiation. The inhibition of [³H]thymidine incorporation by laser irradiation at the end of the 4-day culture was statistically significant at all time points ($p < 0.01$), as compared with that in untreated controls, as shown by Student's *t* test. (Reproduced with permission from Ohta A, Abergel RP, Uitto J. Laser modulation of human immune system: inhibition of lymphocyte proliferation by a gallium-arsenide laser at low energy. Lasers Surg Med 1987;7: 199–201.)

diminished as a result of laser irradiation (Table 15-3). Thus, it can be concluded that laser radiation does not interfere with the antigen recognition phase but does modulate the cell proliferation response to antigen stimulation. These results clearly indicate that low-energy laser radiation can interfere with the immune system in vitro and that similar modulation could occur in human subjects exposed to laser radiation in vivo.

In contrast to this, however, another study,[58] in which peripheral blood lymphocytes were irradiated in vivo, showed that the activity

Table 15-3.   Inhibition of one-way mixed lymphocyte reaction by
Ga-As laser irradiation

Cell donor[a]	Laser treatment[b]	Cell proliferation[c] (dpm $\times 10^{-3}$/well)	Laser inhibition[d] (%)	p value[e]
I	—	4.41 ± 1.06	—	—
I$^\diamond$	—	0.14 ± 0.03	—	—
II	—	0.59 ± 0.10	—	—
II$^\diamond$	—	0.12 ± 0.04	—	—
I + II$^\diamond$	—	32.26 ± 2.30	—	—
	+	22.02 ± 1.88	31.7	<0.01
I$^\diamond$ + II	—	6.22 ± 0.20	—	—
	+	4.22 ± 0.52	32.2	<0.05

[a]Lymphocytes from two subjects (I and II) were isolated and cultured either alone or in coculture (10^5 cells each per well) for 7 days. The cells indicated by a *diamond* ($\diamond$) were subjected to x-ray irradiation at 5000 rads at the beginning of the mixed lymphocyte reaction (MLR).
[b]The cultures indicated by a *plus* (+) were subjected to laser irradiation at 130.2 mJ/cm^2 at 6 days of coculture.
[c]Cell proliferation was determined by incorporation of [^{3}H]thymidine during the last 20 hours of the MLR. The values are the mean $\pm$ standard error of the mean of three to four parallel determinations.
[d]The laser inhibition was calculated as the percentage of the corresponding untreated cultures.
[e]Calculated by Student's *t* test.
Source: Modified from Ohta A, Abergel RP, Uitto J. Laser modulation of human immune system: inhibition of lymphocyte proliferation by a gallium-arsenide laser at low energy. Lasers Surg Med 1987;7:199–201.

of T and B lymphocytes was increased after exposure to the laser radiation, as determined by the activity of rosette-forming cells and immunofluorescence analysis. The maximum stimulation of rosette-forming cells was noted to occur after 10 minutes of irradiation. It should be noted, however, that the increases were relatively small. For example, the increase in the activity of rosette-forming cells after He-Ne irradiation was a maximum of only 1.56-fold at 5 hours after the irradiation.

Several other findings regarding alterations in immune functions in response to laser treatment have been yielded by different experimental models. For example, systemic immunostimulation was noted in 10 patients with retinitis pigmentosa who underwent a trial of scatter argon laser photocoagulation directed to the retina.[59] Specifically, the expression of certain lymphocyte activation epitopes associated with retinitis pigmentosa was noted to be significantly greater than pre–laser treatment values, and the soluble interleukin-2 receptor secretion was normalized after laser treatment. The doubling of the expression of cellular interleukin-2 receptors was particularly interesting, in that it suggested the stimulation of immune cells by a cytokine cascade, which might be associated with macrophage interleukin-1 secretion during the normal processing of foreign antigen. When a panel of viral antibodies was tested in these patients, the level of rubella antibodies was also found to be elevated in the early post–laser treatment period. These authors concluded that the immunostimulation occurring after laser-induced inflammation could be mediated by an antigenic stimulus originating from laser treatment–released retinal proteins, which might be of either an autoimmune or a latent infectious origin.[59]

Finally, an experimental model was developed to quantify bacteria-cell interactions using human peripheral blood lymphocytes and a mutant of *Salmonella,* and involved the irradiation of lymphocytes using an He-Ne laser.[60] This study was founded on the rationale that the laser therapy of wounds and decubitus ulcers could cause alterations in the lymphoid cell function, and this was borne out by the finding that the adherence of *Salmonella* to lymphocytes was enhanced after laser irradiation, indicating that the affinity or the number of lymphocyte receptor sites for *Salmonella* binding may have increased in response to laser radiation.

Effects of Low-Energy Lasers on Other Regenerative Processes

Neural Regeneration

Several other facets of tissue regeneration have been examined in the context of low-energy laser irradiation.[31,61] One of these is the recovery of injuries in the peripheral and central nervous system. One study[31] examined the effects of He-Ne laser radiation on injured sciatic nerves as well as on bilaterally inflicted crush injuries and revealed that healing appeared to be far more accelerated in the laser-treated group than in the control, nonirradiated group. A systemic effect was also found in the spinal cord segments corresponding to the crushed sciatic nerves. The findings from these studies indicated that bilateral retrograde degeneration of the motor neurons of the spinal cord, which is expected after bilateral crush injury of peripheral nerves, is greatly reduced in patients who undergo laser treatment.

Angiogenesis

Two studies involving the use of a rabbit ear chamber model, which allows the growth of blood vessels in response to laser irradiation to be directly observed, have shown that He-Ne laser irradiation may cause an increase in neovascularization during wound healing.[4,7] However, the precise mechanisms of neovascularization and the effects of laser energy on vascular endothelial and smooth muscle cells have not been studied in further detail.

Possible Mechanisms of Action of Low-Energy Lasers

Considering the complexity of the biologic systems that have been subjected to laser irradiation and the variability in the different experimental models studied, it has been somewhat difficult to formulate a unifying hypothesis concerning the mechanisms of low-energy lasers. However, several mechanisms of action of laser energy have been proposed.[35–37,52,54,62–64]

As mentioned earlier, the stimulation of collagen gene expression and an alteration in the protein synthesis at the transcriptional or posttranscriptional level are two mechanisms that have been postulated (Fig. 15-10).[65,66] These effects can be attributed to the direct modulation of regulatory elements within the cells, such as the promoter regions of type I and III collagen genes that have been shown to be overexpressed after laser irradiation.[36,37] Similarly, laser radiation may have a direct effect on cell proliferation by affecting the nuclear chromatin structure and other elements that regulate cell proliferation. The effects could also be more indirect, as suggested by the finding of an enhanced uptake of ascorbic acid after laser irradiation, this vitamin being a critical cofactor in the formation of collagen.[35] Furthermore, the effects can be indirectly elicited by paracrine factors, as indicated by the release of fibroblast stimulatory factors from macrophage-like U-937 cells after laser irradiation.[52]

Laser irradiation could affect immune function at several different levels, including alterations in the circulating factors that exert systemic effects at the tissue level (see, for example, ref. 52). On the other hand, alterations in the function of resident lymphocytes at the site of laser irradiation could also modulate the repair processes in such a way as to enhance wound healing.[54]

Karu[64] has proposed a unifying hypothesis embracing the various molecular events triggered by laser irradiation. The central theme of her proposal is that the components of the respiratory chain are the primary photoacceptors of laser energy (Fig. 15-11). The photosignal transduction and amplification that occur are then determined by the physiologic state of the cell at the time of laser irradiation. For example, if the redox potential in cells is low, the magnitude of the laser effect will be stronger than that in cells with a higher redox potential.[64] This suggestion is compatible with the observation that cells which constitutively show a low level of collagen production in culture are considerably more susceptible to up-regulation by laser energy than are cells that produce considerable collagen.[36]

The mechanistics of photosignal transduction have been proposed to involve the absorption of laser energy by enzymes that activate the mitochondrial respiratory chain (see Fig. 15-11). The resulting changes in the respiratory chain alter the redox potential by accelerating electron transfer, which in turn activates the electrical potential of mitochondria and increases the intracellular pool of ATP. These events

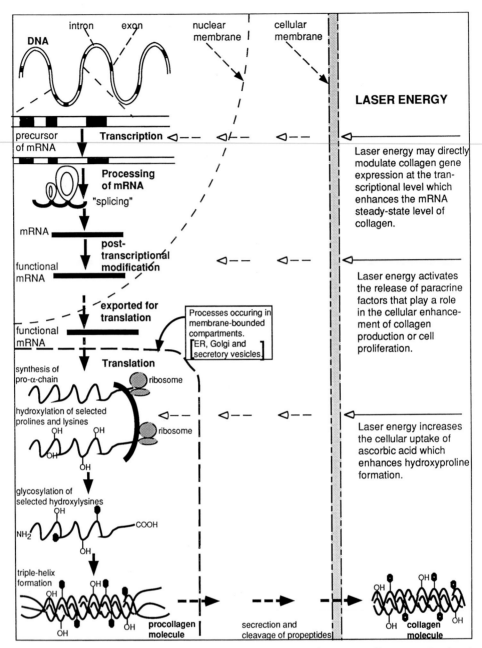

Fig. 15-10. Possible mechanisms of action of laser energy in enhancing collagen production in cells. The laser irradiation may increase the collagen production by fibroblasts by enhancing collagen gene expression on the transcriptional level through activation of the regulatory sequences of the corresponding genes, perhaps altering the chromatin structure by directed laser energy. Other effects of laser irradiation may occur directly at the translational or posttranslational level, or the effects could be more indirect; for example, they could activate the release of paracrine factors, which could elicit stimulatory mediators of collagen production, or increase the cellular uptake of ascorbic acid, which is an essential cofactor for the hydroxylation of proline and lysine at the ribosomal level and acts as a regulator of collagen synthesis. (For further details, see refs 65 and 66.)

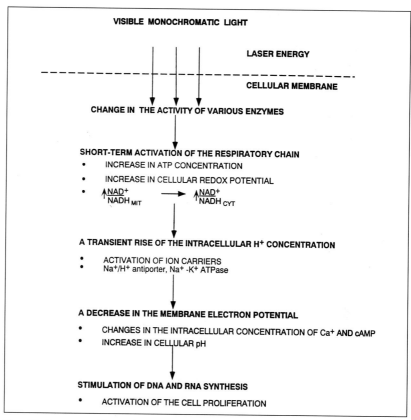

Fig. 15-11. Possible molecular mechanisms involved in photosignal transduction of low-energy laser for the activation of cellular proliferation. (For further explanation see ref 64.)

may lead to an increase in the intracellular hydrogen ion concentration, a necessary component for mitogenic signal transmission in the cells.[64] These events may also alter certain phenomena that activate the membrane ion transport systems, including the sodium-potassium pump and the activities of ATPase. The changes in the cellular redox potential can then alter proliferation, macromolecular synthesis, and the response of cells to immunologic modulator molecules.

Future Uses of Low-Energy Lasers

As is evident from this overview, there is an abundance of information on the biologic effects of low-energy lasers, but this information is often difficult to interpret, while the effects themselves have been described as "incredible and mysterious."[64] Although several carefully controlled studies have clearly shown that low-energy laser irradiation affects cellular metabolism, the test conditions and the laser parameters must be optimized and standardized before a careful analysis of the mechanistic details can be done. For example, the wavelength and energy density should be standardized to allow comparison between experimental models using either the same animal species or cells grown under comparable culture conditions. Furthermore, before low-energy lasers can be used in the clinical arena, studies must be done using rigorous controls, which allow parallel analysis of treated and untreated tissues. In this regard, it is particularly important to use as controls independent groups and not just tissue harvested from untreated areas of the skin from the same test subject, since, as noted throughout, systemic effects may be important in modulating the healing processes. Thus, rigorous guidelines for experimental protocols need to be established so that the efficacy of low-energy lasers can be documented under experimental conditions.

Low-energy lasers are extensively used in Europe for the treatment of various clinical conditions.[12,67–72] In the United States, however, these lasers have not been approved for use in humans, although clinical trials of their effectiveness in the treatment of rheumatoid arthritis are in progress under the Investigative Device Exemption, which is under the auspices of the U.S. Food and Drug Administration.[73] However, it may prove difficult to evaluate the efficacy of low-energy lasers in this diverse group of patients who have varying degrees of involvement and in whom the assessment of the clinical symptoms, such as joint swelling, morning stiffness, pain, and inflammation, is largely subjective. Nevertheless, controlled clinical trials are critical to eventually proving the merits of low-energy lasers in reducing the symptoms of diseases such as rheumatoid arthritis. These lasers may also eventually prove to be of value in repairing peripheral nerve injuries and in promoting the healing of chronic wounds.

References

1. Basford J. Low-energy laser therapy: controversies and new research findings. Lasers Surg Med 1989;9:1–5.
2. Mester E, Spiry T, Szende B, Tota JG. Effect of laser rays on wound healing. Am J Surg 1971;122:532–535.
3. Mester E, Szende B, Spiry T, Scher A. Stimulation of wound healing by laser rays. Acta Chir Acad Sci Hung 1972;13:315–324.
4. Kovacs IB, Mester E, Görög P. Laser-induced stimulation of the vascularization of the healing wound. An ear chamber experiment. Experientia 1974;4:341–343.
5. Kovacs IB, Mester E, Görög P. Stimulation of wound healing with laser beam in the rat. Experientia 1974;11:1275–1276.
6. Mester E, Bacsy E, Spiry T, Tisza S. Laser stimulation of wound healing. Enzyme-histochemical studies. Acta Chir Acad Sci Hung 1974;15:203–208.
7. Kovacs I, Mester E, Görög P. Stimulation of wound healing by laser rays as estimated by means of the rabbit ear chamber method. Acta Chir Acad Sci Hung 1974;15:427–432.
8. Namenyi J, Mester E, Földes I, Tisza S. Effect of laser irradiation and im-

munosuppressive treatment on survival of mouse skin allotransplants. Acta Chir Acad Sci Hung 1975;16:327–335.

9. Mester E, Korenyi-Both A, Spiry T, Scher A, Tisza S. Stimulation of wound healing by means of laser rays. Acta Chir Acad Sci Hung 1973;14:347–356.

10. Mester E, Nagylucskay S, Döklen A, Tisza S. Laser stimulation of wound healing. II. Immunological tests. Acta Chir Acad Sci Hung 1976;17: 49–55.

11. Mester E, Nagylucskay S, Tisza S, Mester A. Stimulation of wound healing by means of laser rays. Part III—investigation of the effect on immune competent cells. Acta Chir Acad Sci Hung 1978;19:163–170.

12. Ohshiro T, Calderhead RG, eds. Selected papers from the October 1990 ILTA Congress (Progress in Laser Therapy). New York: Wiley, 1991.

13. Dorros G, Seeley D. Understanding lasers. A basic manual for medical practitioners including an extensive bibliography of medical applications. Mount Kisco, NY: Futura, 1991.

14. Bosatra M, Jucci A, Olliaro P, Quacci D, Sacchi S. *In vitro* fibroblast and dermis fibroblast activation by laser irradiation at low-energy. Dermatologica 1984;168:157–162.

15. Mauviel A, Uitto J. The extracellular matrix in wound healing: role of the cytokine network. Wounds 1993;5:137.

16. Gailit J, Clark RAF. Wound repair in the context of extracellular matrix. Current Opin Cell Biol 1994;6:717–725.

17. Mauviel A, Lapiere J-C, Halcin C, Evans CH, Uitto J. Differential cytokine regulation of type I and type VII collagen gene expression in cultured human dermal fibroblasts. J Biol Chem 1994;269:25–28.

18. Lundeberg T, Malm M. Low-power He-Ne laser treatment of venous leg ulcers. Ann Plast Surg 1991;27:537–539.

19. Malm M, Lundebreg T. Effect of low power gallium arsenide laser on healing of venous ulcers. Scand J Plast Reconstr Hand Surg 1991;25: 249–251.

20. Saperia D, Glassberg E, Lyons RF et al. Demonstration of elevated type I and type III procollagen mRNA levels in cutaneous wounds treated with helium-neon laser. Biochem Biophys Res Commun 1986;138:1123–1128.

21. Basford JR, Hallman HO, Sheffield CG, Mackey GL. Comparison of cold-quartz ultraviolet, low-energy laser, and occlusion in wound healing in a swine model. Arch Phys Med Rehabil 1986;67:151–154.

22. Resvani M, Nissan M, Hopewell JW, van den Aardweg GJMJ, Robbins MEC, Whitehouse EM. Prevention of X-ray-induced late dermal necrosis in the pig by treatment with multi-wavelength light. Lasers Surg Med 1992;12:288–293.

23. Hunter J, Leonard L, Wilson R, Snider G, Dixon J. Effects of low-energy on wound healing in a porcine model. Lasers Surg Med 1984;3:285–290.

24. Smith RJ, Birndorf M, Gluck G, Hammond D, Moore WD. The effect of low-energy laser on skin-flap survival in the rat and porcine animal models. Plast Reconstr Surg 1992;89:306–310.

25. Lyons RF, Abergel RP, White RA, Dwyer RM, Castel JC, Uitto J. Biostimulation of wound healing *in vivo* by a helium-neon laser. Ann Plast Surg 1987;18:47–50.

26. Abergel RP, Lyons RF, Castel JC, Dwyer RM, Uitto J. Biostimulation of wound healing by lasers: experimental approaches in animal models and in fibroblast cultures. J Dermatol Surg Oncol 1987;13:127–133.

27. Kana JS, Hutschenreiter G, Haina D, Waidelich W. Effect of low-power density laser radiation on healing of open skin wounds in rats. Arch Surg 1981;116:293–296.

28. Anneroth G, Hall G, Ryden H, Zetterqvist L. The effect of low-energy infra-red laser radiation on wound healing in rats. Br J Oral Maxillofac Surg 1988;26:12–17.

29. Braverman B, McCarthy RJ, Ivankovich AD, Forde DE, Overfield M, Bapna MS. Effect of helium-neon and infrared laser irradiation on wound healing in rabbits. Lasers Surg Med 1989;9:50–58.

30. Zhang D, Chen T, Wang C, Wu S, Fu C. Effect of helium-neon laser irradiation on serum lipid peroxide concentrations in burnt mice. Lasers Surg Med 1992;12:180–183.

31. Rochkind S, Rousso M, Nissan M, Villarreal M, Barr-Nea L, Rees DG. Systemic effects of low-power laser irradiation on the peripheral and central nervous system, cutaneous wounds, and burns. Lasers Surg Med 1989;9:174–182.

32. Zarkovic N, Manev H, Pericic D et al. Effect of semiconductor GaAs laser irradiation on pain perception in mice. Lasers Surg Med 1989;9:63–66.

33. Berki T, Nemeth P. Photo-immunotargeting with haematoporphyrin conjugates activated by a low-power He-Ne laser. Cancer Immunol Immunother 1992;35:69–74.

34. Pourreau-Schneider N, Ahmed A, Soudry M et al. Helium-neon laser treatment transforms fibroblasts into myofibroblasts. Am J Pathol 1990;137:171–178.

35. Labbe RF, Skogerboe KJ, Davis HA, Rettmer RL. Laser photobioactivation mechanisms: *in vitro* studies using ascorbic acid uptake and hydroxyproline formation as biochemical markers of irradiation response. Lasers Surg Med 1990;10:201–207.

36. Lam TS, Abergel RP, Meeker CA, Castel JC, Dwyer RM, Uitto J. Laser stimulation of collagen synthesis in human skin fibroblast cultures. Lasers Life Sci 1986;1:61–77.

37. Abergel RP, Meeker CA, Lam TS, Dwyer RM, Lesavoy MA, Uitto J. Control of connective tissue metabolism by lasers: recent developments and future prospects. J Am Acad Dermatol 1984;11:1142–1150.

38. van Breugel HHFI, Bär PRD. Power density and exposure time of He-Ne laser irradiation are more important than total energy dose in photobiomodulation of human fibroblasts *in vitro*. Lasers Surg Med 1992;12:528–537.

39. Noble PB, Shields ED, Blecher PDM, Bentley KC. Locomotory characteristics of fibroblasts within a three-dimensional collagen lattice: modulation by a helium-neon soft laser. Lasers Surg Med 1992;12:669–674.

40. Bard J, Elsdale T. Growth regulation in multilayered cultures of human diploid fibroblasts: the roles of contact, movement and matrix production. Cell Tissue Kinet 1986;19:141–154.

41. Pourreau-Schneider N, Soudry M, Remusat M, Franquin JC, Martin PM. Modification of growth dynamics and ultrastructure after helium-neon laser treatment of human gingival fibroblasts. Quintessense Int 1989;20:887–893.

42. Hallman HO, Basford JR, O'Brien JF, Cummins LA. Does low-energy helium-neon laser irradiation alter *"in vitro"* replication of human fibroblasts? Lasers Surg Med 1988;8:125–129.

43. Schneir M, Golub L, Ramamurthy N. Dietary ascorbic acid increases nascent collagen production in skins of diabetic rats by reversing procol-

lagen underhydroxylation and concomitant intracellular degradation. In: Fleischmajer R, Olsen BR, Kühn K, eds. Biology, chemistry, and pathology of collagen. New York: The New York Academy of Sciences, 1985;500–502.

44. Geesin JC, Darr D, Kaufman R, Murad S, Pinnell SR. Ascorbic acid specifically increases type I and type III procollagen messenger RNA levels in human skin fibroblasts. J Invest Dermatol 1988;90:420–424.

45. Pinnell SR. Regulation of collagen biosynthesis by ascorbic acid: a review. Yale J Biol Med 1985;58:553–559.

46. Murad S, Grove D, Lindberg KA, Reynolds G, Sivarajah A, Pinnell SR. Regulation of collagen synthesis by ascorbic acid. Proc Natl Acad Sci USA 1981;78:2879–2882.

47. Structural and Contractile Proteins. Part A: Extracellular Matrix. In: Cunningham LW, Frederiksen DW, eds. Methods in enzymology. New York: Academic, 1982;82.

48. Clark RAF. Cutaneous wound repair. In: Goldsmith LA, ed. Physiology, biochemistry, and molecular biology of the skin. New York: Oxford University Press, 1991;576–601.

49. Haas AF, Isseroff RR, Wheeland RG, Rood PA, Graves PJ. Low-energy helium-neon laser irradiation increases the motility of cultured human keratinocytes. J Invest Dermatol 1990;94:822–826.

50. Rood PA, Haas AF, Graves PJ, Wheeland RG, Isseroff RR. Low-energy helium-neon laser irradiation does not alter human keratinocyte differentiation. J Invest Dermatol 1992;99:445–448.

51. Mester E, Jaszsagi-Nagy E. Biological effects of laser radiation. Radiobiologia Radiotherapia 1971;12:377–385.

52. Young S, Bolton P, Dyson M, Harvey W, Diamantopoulos C. Macrophage responsiveness to light therapy. Lasers Surg Med 1989;9:497–505.

53. Marchesini R, Dasdia T, Melloni E, Rocca E. Effect of low-energy laser irradiation on colony formation capability in different human tumor cells *in vitro*. Lasers Surg Med 1989;9:59–62.

54. Ohta A, Abergel RP, Uitto J. Laser modulation of human immune system: inhibition of lymphocyte proliferation by a gallium-arsenide laser at low energy. Lasers Surg Med 1987;7:199–201.

55. Sundström C, Nilsson K. Establishment and characterization of a human histiocytic lymphoma cell line (U-937). Int J Cancer 1976;17:565–577.

56. Higashiyama S, Abraham JA, Miller J, Fiddes JC, Klagsbrun M. A heparin-binding growth factor secreted by macrophage-like cells that is related to EGF. Science 1991;251:936–939.

57. Kong ZL, Miwa M, Murakami H, Shinohara K. Establishment of a macrophage-like cell line derived from U-937, human histiocytic lymphoma, grown serum-free. In Vitro Cell Dev Biol 1990;26:949–954.

58. Kupin VI, Bykov VS, Ivanov AV, Larichev VY. Potentiating effects of laser radiation on some immunological traits. Neoplasma 1982;29:403–406.

59. Williams LL, Shannon BT, Chambers RB, Leguire LE, Davidorf FH. Systemic immunostimulation after retinal laser treatment in retinitis pigmentosa. Clin Immunol Immunopathol 1992;64:78–83.

60. Passarella S, Casamassima E, Quagliariello E, Caretto G, Jirillo E. Quantitative analysis of lymphocyte-salmonella interaction and effect of lymphocyte irradiation by helium-neon laser. Biochem Biophys Res Commun 1985;130:546–552.

61. Belkin M, Schwartz M. New biological phenomena associated with laser radiation. Health Phys 1989;56:687–690.

62. Enwemeka CS. Laser biostimulation of healing wounds: specific effects and mechanisms of action. J Orthop Sports Phys Ther 1988;9:333–338.

63. Tiphlova O, Karu T. Role of primary photoacceptors in low-power laser effects: action of he-ne laser radiation on bacteriophage *T4-Escherichia coli* interaction. Lasers Surg Med 1989;9:67–69.

64. Karu T. Photobiology of low-power laser effects. Health Phys 1989;56: 691–704.

65. Uitto J, Ryhämen L, Tam EML. Collagen: its structure, function, and pathology. In: Fleischmajer R, ed. Progress in the diseases of the skin, vol. 1. New York: Grune & Stratton, 1981;103–141.

66. Alberts B, Bray D, Lewis J, Raff M, Roberts K, Watson JD. Cell adhesion, cell junctions, and the extracellular matrix. In: Molecular biology of the cell, ed 2. New York: Garland, 1989;814.

67. Minekov AA, Konchugova TV, Kul'chitskaia DB. Clinicoexperimental prerequisites for the physiotherapeutic use of laser radiation. Vopr Kurortol Fizioter Lech Fiz Kult 1992;2:11–14.

68. Grubnik W, So BH, Shipulin PP, Beliakov AV. Use of laser irradiation for the prevention and treatment of complications following surgery of the lungs and pleura. Klin Khir 1992;4:16–19.

69. Komarova LA, Radenko GV. Laser therapy efficacy in patients with osteoarthrosis deformans of the knee and hip joints. Vopr Kurortol Fizioter Lech Fiz Kult 1990;6:45–46.

70. Haker E, Lundeberg T. Is low-energy laser treatment effective in lateral epicondylalgia? J Pain Symptom Manage 1991;6:241–246.

71. Hansen HJ, Thoroe U. Low power laser biostimulation of chronic orofacial pain. A double-blind placebo controlled cross-over study in 40 patients. Pain 1990;43:169–179.

72. Amano A, Miyagi K, Azuma T et al. Histological studies on the rheumatoid synovial membrane irradiated with a low energy laser. Lasers Surg Med 1994;15:290–294.

73. Fact sheet: laser biostimulation. Clin Manage 1985;5:52.

16 —— The Infrared Coagulator

Graham B. Colver

Physicians often use controlled heat to treat skin lesions. Cautery and diathermy are established methods, but more recently practitioners have turned to using lasers. All of these methods have their own special advantages and disadvantages. On the down side, many are hard to control precisely; others are extremely expensive; none is perfect. All aspects of laser-induced tissue alterations are explored in this book, and it is clear from this discussion that the precise energy output and therefore precise and repeatable tissue injury are important properties of laser therapy.

These are also properties of the infrared coagulator, however. Although the coagulator does not damage specific targets in the skin, it can yield good clinical results in the treatment of a variety of cutaneous disorders. This points up the fact that it is as important for laser operators to appreciate the merits of nonlaser technology as it is for nonlaser operators to appreciate the therapeutic options offered by lasers. The structure and physics of the coagulator are described in this chapter, and its properties are compared with some properties of lasers. A series of laboratory experiments are also described that have shown the depth of coagulation achieved by different exposures, and the repeatability of the pulses, as assessed by a light-sensitive diode and measuring their effect on tissues, is discussed as well. Work on human skin is also discussed, including observations on the value of the coagulator in the treatment of patients with tattoos, port-wine stains (PWSs), venous lakes, angiomas, and Kaposi's sarcoma.

The Infrared Coagulator

The infrared coagulator most often used is the one made by Lumatec of Munich, Germany (Figs. 16-1 and 16-2). It is approved by the U.S. Food and Drug Administration and available in the United States from the Redfield Corporation, Montvale, New Jersey. It has two chief components. One is a pistol-shaped device that contains the bulb, light guide, and trigger. This handheld piece is attached by an electric cable to the second chief component, or power unit, which

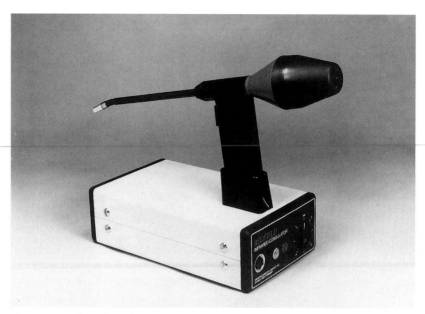

Fig. 16-1. The infrared coagulator.

houses the transformer and timer. The energy source is a tungsten-halogen bulb, and when activated, its emission passes, both directly and by reflection, down the light guide. The bulb lies within a parabolic, gold-coated reflector, and the reflected radiation focuses onto the end of the light guide. The preferential reflection of the near-infrared light is ensured by the gold foil coating of the parabola. When the light guide contact tip is placed on skin, the intense radiation emerging from the guide penetrates and coagulates the tissue. A hissing noise, made by the steam that forms from tissue water, is usually heard after an exposure of 1.0 second or longer. The voltage is

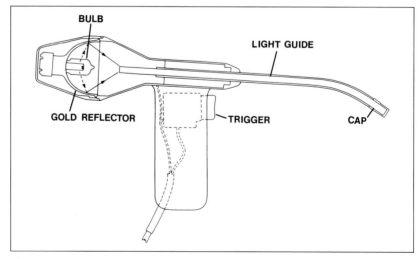

Fig. 16-2. Cross-section of the infrared coagulator.

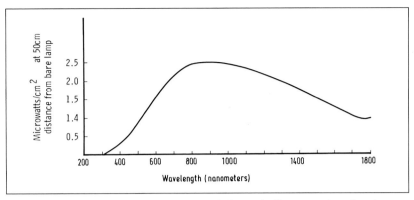

Fig. 16-3. Spectral output of a tungsten-halogen bulb. (Reproduced with permission from Colver GB. The infrared coagulator in dermatology. Dermatol Clin 1989;7:157.)

reduced to 12 V by a transformer. Exposure times are set on an electronic timer, with the standard ranging from 0.5 to 3.0 seconds, but alternative timers can be fitted to the unit for more accurate adjustment. A switch, or trigger, is incorporated into the handpiece.

The tungsten-halogen bulb has a maximum output at 900 to 960 nm in the near-infrared range (Figs. 16-3 and 16-4). The peak, however, changes as the temperature of the filament rises, starting near 1300 nm and approaching 800 nm with increasing temperatures.

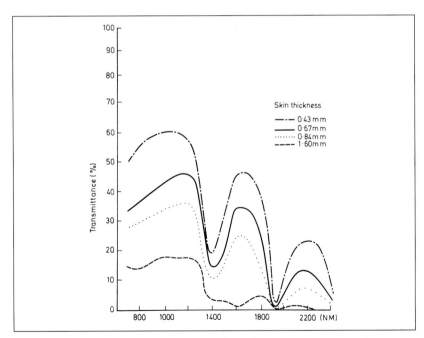

Fig. 16-4. Spectral transmittance of excised white human skin. (Modified from Hardy JD, Hammel HT, Murgatroyd D. Spectral transmittance and reflectance of excised human skin. J Appl Physiol 1956;9:257–264.)

The wavelength of the maximum spectral power at any temperature can be calculated from the equation $M = 2898/T$, where M is the wavelength (in nanometers) and T is the temperature (in kelvin). The intensity of the radiation is clearly sufficient to coagulate skin, but it can also easily damage the eye. This does not happen, however, because of the intense visible light that is also emitted, which evokes the blink reflex, papillary constriction, and avoidance by moving the head.

Quartz glass transmits visible and infrared light and can withstand rapid changes in temperature. It is used to make the solid light guides that screw into the bulb housing. The radiation passes down the guide by total internal reflection and can negotiate bends. Three diameters of light guides are manufactured: 2, 6, and 10 mm. These light guides come in various lengths and are formed in various angles for use in different specialties. The technique of using the light guide is shown in Figure 16-5.

The contact tip is one of the most important components, because it endows the coagulator with special properties. Screwed onto the distal end of the light guide is a small cylinder (2, 6, or 10 mm in diameter according to the diameter of the light guide) into which is set a flat circular sapphire disk that is transparent in the near-infrared range. When the contact tip is in contact with the skin, the transmitted energy is absorbed by the tissue and causes coagulation. The intense heat on the surface is in part removed by the contact tip, which has a high thermal conductivity. This heat sparing delays the onset of carbonization and keeps the tip from sticking to the coagulated surfaces.

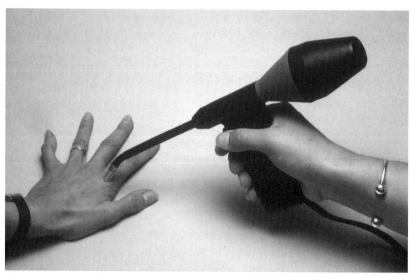

Fig. 16-5.   Normal use of coagulator with light guide applied to skin. (Reproduced with permission from Colver GB, Cherry GW, Dawber RPR, Ryan TJ. Tattoo removal using infrared coagulation. Br J Dermatol 1985;112:482.)

The sapphire tip has some special properties. Manufactured sapphire monocrystals (chemical formula Al_2O_3) can take a high polish, so the contact surface is therefore perfectly even. A melting point of 2050°C enables it to withstand the heat generated in all clinical applications, plus the heat of autoclaving. It is virtually inert chemically and extremely hard, surpassed only by the diamond in both regards. It is therefore quite safe to clean the sapphire with a scalpel blade and so dislodge any adherent material.

Laboratory Assessments

It is clear that infrared coagulation is an effective way to coagulate blood vessels and destroy a small zone of tissue. The work of Gruneberger and associates,[1] who used the coagulator to treat benign alterations of the cervix, also revealed that longer exposures lead to deeper coagulation. This finding was not necessarily predictable, in that, if carbonization had occurred at an early stage, as it does after exposure to CO_2 laser light, there would have been significant attenuation of the thermal effect, because carbon is a poor conductor of heat and a poor transmitter of near-infrared radiation.

These studies were therefore helpful but not a substitute for in vivo assessments on skin. In one such experiment on pig skin, two squares each received a single pulse of 0.5, 0.625, 0.75, 0.875, 1.0, or 1.125 seconds, using a light guide with a sapphire tip. Biopsy samples were taken from each area between 20 and 30 minutes later and the dermal and epidermal injury measured. This experiment confirmed that longer pulses are associated with greater tissue injury, both in terms of the depth and the diameter of the epidermal and dermal injury. The shrinkage of tissue caused by the heat may cause the depth to be underestimated, however, partly accounting for the leveling off in the depth-dose response. A slight variation in the tissue effects of consecutive pulses was seen, perhaps resulting from changes in the pressure with which the coagulator was applied to the skin from one exposure to the next (Figs. 16-6 to 16-8).

Although the diameter of the sapphire tip was 6 mm, the diameter of the injured dermis was never more than 4.8 mm. Therefore overlapping adjacent circles must be used in any clinical treatment to avoid leaving untreated skin. Although the clinical benefits of using a contact tip with a larger surface area seem obvious, this has been ruled out by experiments that have shown that a larger-diameter light guide and tip produce a deep saucer-shaped injury.

The repeatability of this method is due to the ability of the coagulator to emit the same energy repeatedly for a given exposure. This was shown by a study[2] in which the emission from the coagulator was first passed through a 50-μm spatial filter and then a neutral-density filter, before impinging onto a photodiode with built-in amplifier. The diode was connected to an oscilloscope so that the light incident

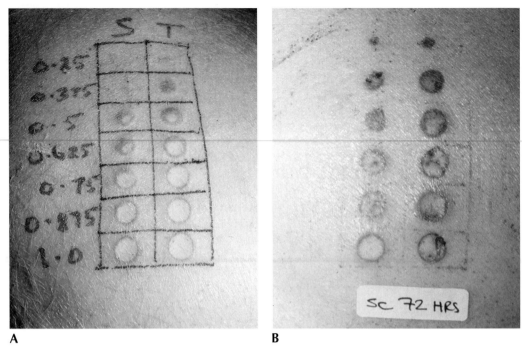

A **B**

Fig. 16-6. Pig skin coagulated using a 1-mm light guide. (A) 20 minutes after coagulation. (B) 72 hours after coagulation. (*S* = sapphire; *T* = Teflon tip.)

on the diode would register as a negative deflection. Using this system it was clear that, for a given exposure, repeated pulses produce similar curves, both in reaching the maximum power and with decay. The area under the curve (i.e., energy) was noted to diminish with decreasing pulses, but the maximum deflection (i.e., power) did not diminish until pulses around 0.5 second were used. It was also found that the maximum deflection did not vary with the interval between pulses.

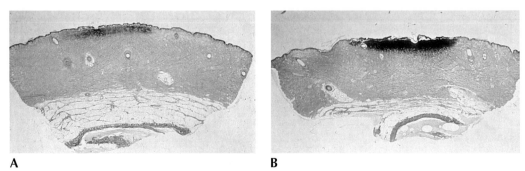

A **B**

Fig. 16-7. Photomicrographs of pig skin. Biopsies taken 20 minutes after 0.75-second coagulation pulse with (A) sapphire tip and (B) Teflon tip. (Verhoeff–van Gieson; ×5.)

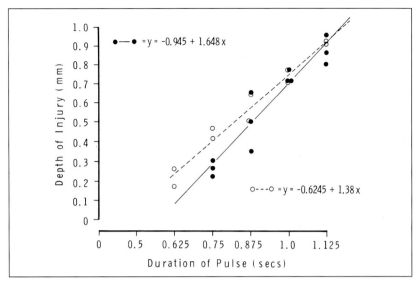

Fig. 16-8.   Relationship between depth of injury and pulse duration in pig skin. (*Solid circles* = flank; *open circles* = chest.) (Reproduced with permission from Colver GB, Cherry GW, Dawber RPR, Ryan TJ. Precise dermal damage with an infrared coagulator. Br J Dermatol 1986;114:606.)

Value of the Coagulator in Cutaneous Surgery

The infrared coagulator is able to produce repeatable and predictably uniform tissue injury, and several common benign cutaneous lesions are suitable to treatment producing superficial thermal effects, such as those of infrared coagulators. The uniformity of the resulting scar is also of considerable importance in the treatment of such lesions, and the coagulator seems well suited to the task.

TATTOOS

In an initial trial, 36 tattoos on 21 patients were treated using the infrared coagulator.[3] Only two were larger than 2 × 5 cm, and all but two were amateur. The skin was anesthetized using 1% lidocaine hydrochloride. The length of the coagulating pulse was constant for each tattoo but varied from 1.125 to 1.375 seconds between tattoos. Starting at the periphery (Fig. 16-9), the sapphire tip was placed on the skin and a single pulse emitted. After a 5-second interval this was repeated on a contiguous area, and the process was repeated until the desired area had been covered. An ice cube was applied to the site for 5 seconds before the first pulse and after each subsequent second or third pulse. Patients with residual pigment at 6 weeks received further treatment using the same pulse as that used before.

The treated skin became white immediately after treatment, irrespective of the pulse length. A hissing noise or even a pop was heard

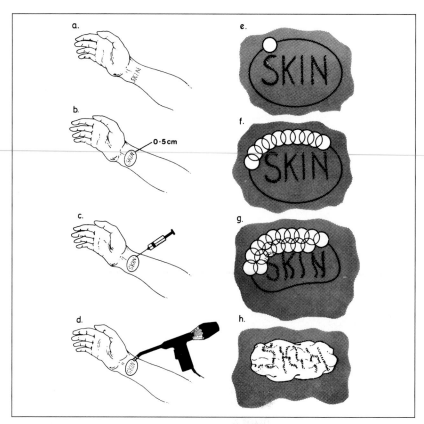

Fig. 16-9. Technique of infrared coagulation for tattoos. (A) Tattoo on volar aspect of forearm reading "SKIN." (B) Line drawn around tattoo with 0.5-cm clearance. (C) Local anesthetic injected. (D) Coagulator applied to skin. (E) Single pulse given on periphery. (F) Further overlapping pulses. (G) Further pulses. (H) Remaining tattoo shrinking. (Reproduced with permission from Colver GB. The infrared coagulator in dermatology. Dermatol Clin 1989;7:161.)

when longer exposures were used. Tissue desiccation also led to shrinkage, apparent early as a distortion of the pattern of the untreated area. Blisters developed in 5 patients, but all resolved within 48 hours. When pulses of 1.125 seconds were used, a crust formed within 4 days and was shed by 2 weeks. These times were 10 days and 1 month, respectively, when pulses exceeding 1.25 seconds were used. The initial crust contained most of the ink, but sometimes a second thinner crust formed and a little ink was found in it. The resulting scar was red at first but became pale over 1 to 1.5 years. Often during the first 6 months it was surrounded by a thin line of hyperpigmentation.

Two of three tattoos treated early in the trial with 1.5-second pulses became infected; they took 6 weeks to heal, and the patients were left with poor scars. Although ink removal was complete, this exposure was not used again and no further infections developed. These early patients were not included in the final results. Four patients with five tattoos were not available for follow-up. In the remaining group of patients with a total of 31 tattoos, ink removal was satisfactory in 21 tattoos after a single treatment. Two other tattoos had residual pigment at the periphery because the treatment area had been too conservative; both responded fully to retreatment. The remaining eight had residual ink within the treated area, and only five of these responded well to retreatment. Six of these eight had been treated with pulses of less than 1.125 second. Three scars became hypertrophic (Figs. 16-10 to 16-13).

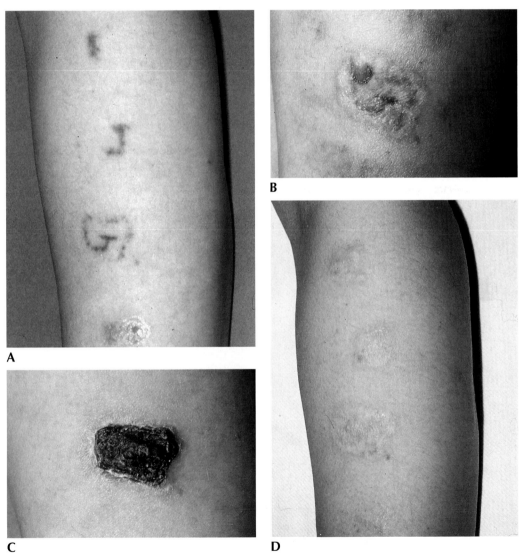

Fig. 16-10.   Tattoo on forearm. (A) Before coagulation. (B) After 1 week. (C) After 1 month. (D) After 6 months.

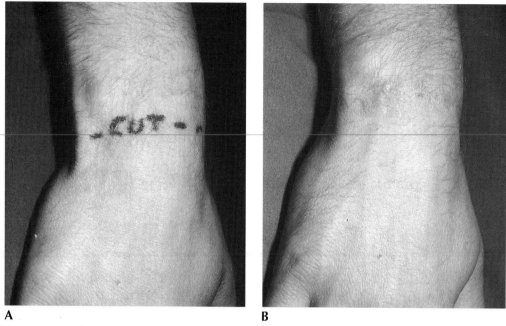

A   B

Fig. 16-11. Tattoo on wrist. (A) Before coagulation. (B) Good result 15 months later.

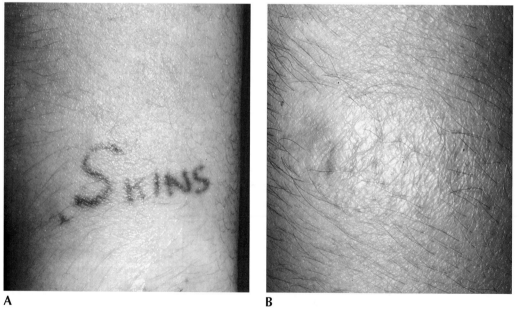

A   B

Fig. 16-12. Tattoo on forearm. (A) Before coagulation. (B) Atrophic, hypopigmented scar 1 year later.

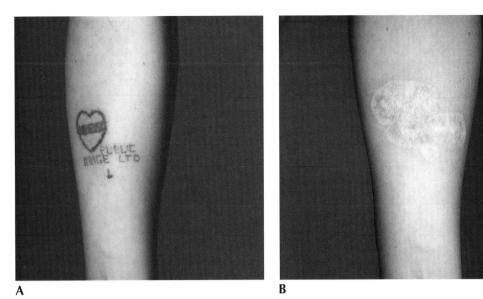

A   **B**

Fig. 16-13.   Tattoo on volar aspect of forearm. (A) Before coagulation. (B) Depressed, depigmented scar 1 year later.

It was not clear from this trial whether the failure to remove ink in some tattoos treated with pulses of less than 1.25 seconds was due to the nature of the tattoos or to the lesser injury inflicted using shorter pulses. To elucidate the reasons for this, another group of 19 patients with 42 tattoos was studied who were treated using pulses of 1.125 seconds.[3] The tattoos were all on the hand or forearm. The appearance 3 months after treatment was scored as good, fair, or poor.

Results in 82% were classified as good and the other five as fair. All of the patients except one were pleased with the results. Three scars were slightly lumpy, and two were depressed. Flecks of peripheral ink remained in 13 tattoos, but all responded well to localized retreatment. Central ink remained in seven and was considerable in three. Retreatment was less effective in this group.

Healing was quite rapid in those treated tattoos not biopsied: a dry crust formed in 19 of the 20, which was sloughed after a mean of 25 days. Lumpy scars formed in four of the treated tattoos (including two of the professional tattoos). Flecks of residual ink were left at the periphery of five tattoos, which responded fully to retreatment. Swelling of the hand occurred in one of the eight patients in whom no biopsy specimen was taken; another patient in this group required antibiotics for a wound infection. The patients with the seven tattoos which were biopsied fared less well, wound pain occurred in two tattoos and wound infections developed in four. However, overall results confirm the value of infrared coagulation in the treatment of amateur tattoos. The persistence of ink in the periphery of many treated tattoos highlighted the importance of treating 0.5 cm of normal skin outside the ink design.

It is difficult to remove tattoos on the digits because the skin is not loose enough to allow excision and closure; also, any such wound is liable to trauma and infection. Therefore, in a further study, the infrared coagulator was used in 14 patients with amateur tattoos on the dorsum of the fingers to assess its effectiveness in this setting. In most, only four fingers of one hand were involved, but in one patient four fingers of both hands were tattooed. Only one finger was affected in two patients. The method of treatment was identical to that described earlier for other tattoos; the exposure time used in all patients was 1.125 seconds. Treatment led to the removal of all or most of the ink in every patient. Healing was quite rapid, and the crust had finally been sloughed by 3 weeks in all patients (Figs. 16-14 and 16-15). Only the two patients in whom wound infections developed took time off work. All others found little problem with the healing wounds, which were fairly dry throughout.[3]

In a further study, 10 patients with small tattoos (nine amateur, one professional) were selected to test the effectiveness of EMLA cream as an anesthetic agent during laser treatment. Up to 5 gm of EMLA cream was applied to cover a maximum area of 3 × 3 cm, which was then covered with an occlusive dressing (Tegaderm) and left for 90 to 120 minutes before removal. The tattoos were then treated with the infrared coagulator using 1.125-second exposures. If the discomfort was great, an ice cube was applied to the site for 5 seconds before the next pulse. Application of the cream proved unsatisfactory for the removal of two tattoos on fingers, and neither patient could tolerate treatment. A further two patients managed to tolerate only one or two pulses but were able to tolerate additional treatment after ice was applied. Six patients were able to tolerate the full treatment of their tattoos (maximum of 16 pulses), but even they found that the application of ice diminished the discomfort of a subsequent pulse.

On the basis of our findings from these studies, we have reached the following conclusions regarding the treatment of tattoos with the infrared coagulator:

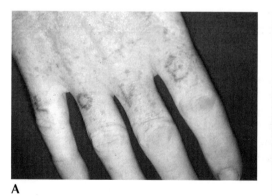
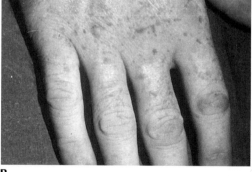

A   B

Fig. 16-14.   Digital tattoos. (A) Before coagulation. (B) Depigmentation 1 year later. See Fig. 16-14 in color section.

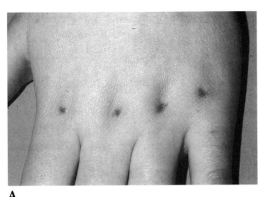
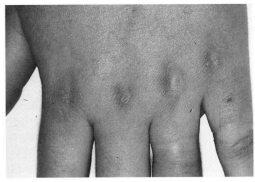

A   **B**

Fig. 16-15.   Tattoos on knuckles. (A) Before coagulation. (B) 6 months later. See Fig. 16-15 in color section.

1. The infrared coagulator offers a simple, inexpensive means of removing amateur tattoos: the dry wound that results saves patient and nursing time.
2. 1.125-second pulses accomplish the most complete removal with the least number of complications.
3. The density of the pigment, rather than its depth, is probably the main limitation to the complete removal of ink in professional tattoos.
4. Infrared coagulation seems to be an effective method for treating tattoos on fingers.
5. Most tattoos can be treated using EMLA as a topical anesthetic agent, with or without the additional application of ice between pulses.
6. It is important to keep the treated site clean, to apply an antibiotic ointment twice daily, and to keep the wound covered until healing is complete.

PORT-WINE STAINS

Infrared coagulation has some features in common with continuous-wave laser treatment, making it of possible use in the treatment of PWSs. Therefore we undertook a study to assess its effectiveness in this setting. All patients were selected carefully to optimize the chance of a successful outcome. Specifically, children with light pink PWSs that blanched easily and refilled quickly were selected and those with extensive PWSs were not. In an initial study, only those with facial lesions were treated.[4] Further criteria selection included high motivation on the part of the patient, a clear understanding of the treatment as explained, and residence near the hospital. Patients with slightly elevated, dark purple lesions were also favored.

Routine diagrammatic records were kept and color photographs taken of all patients studied. The initial test area was 1 cm in diameter, and the area treated at any visit did not exceed 3 × 3 cm. A

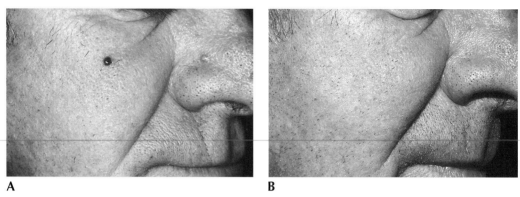

A   **B**

Fig. 16-19. Venous lake on cheek. (A) Before coagulation. (B) 4 months after coagulation.

months. The healing time compares well with the 4 weeks reported for cryotherapy.[9]

OTHER COMPRESSIBLE VASCULAR TUMORS

Excision is often the treatment of choice for acquired vascular tumors, but both glomus tumors and lesions of the blue rubber bleb nevus syndrome (BRBNS) may recur around an excision scar. Because of its effectiveness in the treatment of other vascular lesions and the problems associated with the surgical excision of these tumors, attempts have been made to excise these tumors using the infrared coagulator. Specifically, deep coagulating doses of infrared light were used in three patients with BRBNS and one with multiple glomus tumors. After several seconds of compression, 1.25-second pulses were applied, which inevitably led to a wound that healed slowly. However, the results in the three patients were satisfactory, with no recurrence

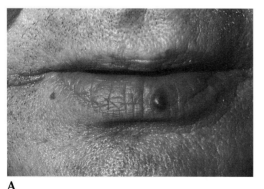
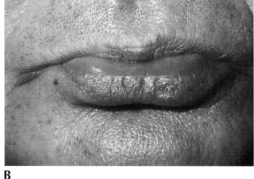

A   **B**

Fig. 16-20. Venous lake on lower lip. (A) Before coagulation. (B) 4 months after coagulation, showing a small depressed scar.

and a marked reduction in pain at 6 months' follow-up. The palmar lesions of one patient with BRBNS did not respond to treatment.

General Discussion and Conclusions

It has been possible to show in the laboratory that the depth of coagulation induced by the infrared coagulator can be measured accurately and that the injury is very repeatable for each pulse duration. Clinical studies have shown how different depths of coagulation can be used to remove tattoos, ameliorate PWSs, and treat other lesions. On the basis of these findings and others yielded by comparisons with other modalities, the coagulator appears to have a useful role in the treatment of various skin conditions.

To overcome this problem, it is essential to adopt a standard method for selecting the optimal pulse for treatment. There may be a small decrease in the output over many months as the bulb ages. Very small variations in the bulb filament, in the position of the bulb within the reflector plate, and in the distance of the bulb from the proximal end of the light guide can create differences in the power output of up to 20%.

Infrared treatment is suitable for the removal of amateur tattoos on the distal forearms, wrist, and hands. It is quick, and apart from those very small tattoos which can be readily excised, it produces cosmetic results comparable to those yielded by the best of other single-session treatments, but not as effective as treatment with the newer short-pulsed lasers. Professional tattoos, however, do not respond well. Mature PWSs on the face generally respond well to this therapy, and marked lightening can be expected without textural changes. The reports of Krumrey[7] and Dorn and associates[8] on the treatment of PWSs show that neither group was daunted by large birthmarks: several of their patients had a lesion covering half the face. Krumrey describes some honeycomb patterning of the residual lesions, which was retreated at a later date; however, both groups express overall satisfaction with the results. Venous lakes are very suited to coagulation treatment and respond consistently well to a single pulse of radiation, whereas the response of blue rubber bleb nevi and some other thicker lesions has proved to be less consistent.

The technique with the infrared coagulator is simple, but inattention to a few minor details may affect the outcome. The method for tattoo treatment can be quickly mastered, but confidence in the use of this device for the treatment of PWSs is less easily achieved. Safety is important, but there appears to be no risk of igniting flammable liquids or gases, nor is there an optical hazard because the intense visible light causes the user and others to avert their eyes. There is also no risk to patients with pacemakers. Further, there is no plume of smoke or spray of blood and tissue, so the risk of transmitting human immunodeficiency virus or hepatitis B virus is reduced.

Sparing of the epidermis could be improved in two ways. First, thicker sapphires might be used to conduct heat more efficiently: in this way it should be possible to create a thermal burn in the reticular dermis without damaging the epidermis or papillary dermis. Second, the area of the surface heating, much of which is induced by rays in the visible spectrum, could be reduced. Suitable filters could be developed that would lessen the surface injury, but care would have to be taken not to block the visible component completely, because the protective mechanism of eye aversion is a response to the visible, not infrared, radiation.

The infrared coagulator is a controlled heat source that produces thermal damage of the skin in a relatively reproducible fashion. Although not selective in its ability to damage cutaneous targets—contrary to pulsed laser light sources—the infrared coagulator is able to clear tattoos and improve some vascular lesions by thermal destruction. Because of its nonselective effect, however, risk/benefit ratio of treating these lesions with the device is higher than that of pulsed lasers. Because there is a risk of scarring from all treatments with the infrared coagulator, it cannot be considered a first-line treatment for any dermatological conditions.

References

1. Gruneberger W, Kubista E, Ulm R. Clinical experience with infrared coagulation in treating benign alterations of the cervix. Gynakol Praxis 1983;7:115–121.
2. Colver GB, Cherry GW, Dawber RPR, Ryan TJ. Precise dermal damage with an infrared coagulator. Br J Dermatol 1986;114:603–608.
3. Colver GB, Cherry GW, Dawber RPR, Ryan TJ. Tattoo removal using infrared coagulation. Br J Dermatol 1985;112:481–485.
4. Colver GB, Cherry GW, Dawber RPR, Ryan TJ. The treatment of cutaneous vascular lesions with infrared coagulation. Br J Plast Surg 1986;39:131–135.
5. Muhlbauer W, Nath, Kreitmair A. Lichtbehandlung capillarer Hemangiome und Naevi flammei. Langenbecks Arch Klin Chir 1976;(suppl 1):91–94.
6. Schmoll M. Treatment of capillary hemangioma by infrared contact coagulator. Hautarzt 1981;32:588–591.
7. Krumrey KW. Die Behandlung des Naevus flambeaus lateralis durch Infrarot-kontaktkoagulation. Z Kautkr 1983;59:1070–1072.
8. Dorn B, Christophers E, Kietzmann H. Treatment of port wine stains and hemangiomas by infrared contact coagulation [abstract]. Paper presented at the 17th World Congress of Dermatology, Berlin, 1987;ii:307.
9. Bean WB, Walsh JR. Venous lakes. Arch Dermatol 1956;74:459–463.
10. Castro-Ron G. Cryosurgery of angiomas and birth defects. In: Zacarian SA, ed. Cryosurgery for skin cancer and cutaneous disorders. St. Louis: Mosby, 1985:77–97.
11. Landthaler M, Haina D, Waidelich W, Braun Falco O. Laser therapy of venous lakes (Bean Walsh) and telangiectasis. Plast Reconstr Surg 1984;73:78–83.
12. Colver GB, Hunter JAA. Venous lakes: treatment by infrared coagulation. Br J Plast Surg 1987;40:451–453.

17 ___ Principles and Applications of Photodynamic Therapy in Dermatology

J. Stuart Nelson
Jerry L. McCullough
Michael W. Berns

The basic concept of photodynamic therapy (PDT) is that certain molecules can function as photosensitizers. The presence of these photosensitizers in biologic tissues makes the tissue vulnerable to light at wavelengths absorbed by the chromophore. Although such photosensitizers can be naturally occurring constituents of cells or tissues, in the case of PDT, they are introduced into the organism as a first step in treatment. In the second step, the tissue-localized photosensitizer is exposed to light of a wavelength predominantly absorbed by the photosensitizer and is elevated to an excited state. The excited photosensitizer then reacts with a substrate, such as oxygen, to produce highly reactive singlet molecular oxygen, which causes irreversible oxidative damage to biologically important molecules and structures. The phototoxic reaction is a local phenomenon that takes place within the cell in microseconds. Irradiation at the appropriate wavelength absorbed by the photosensitizer provides the energy to drive photodynamic reactions without the generation of heat. Although this therapeutic strategy is generally referred to as *PDT,* other terms, such as *photoradiation therapy, phototherapy,* and *photochemotherapy,* have also been used in the literature.

This chapter provides a review of historical and current research related to various aspects of PDT. Specifically, we will concentrate on the photochemistry and photobiology of photosensitizers, in vitro and in vivo preclinical tests of PDT, and the clinical use of PDT. Although this review concentrates primarily on the use of photosensitizers and visible light for the treatment of malignant tumors, the reader should be aware that PDT is also being used for the clinical management of selected nonmalignant dermatoses.

History

The origins of PDT go back to 1900, when Raab[1] made the now much-cited observation that exposure to an acridine dye and light can be lethal to paramecia. Neither light nor dye alone had any apparent effect on the paramecia, but together they were effectively cytotoxic. Since that time, numerous examples of the "photodynamic effect" have been noted for a wide range of photosensitizers, both in vitro and in vivo. The first use of photosensitization to treat human cancer was described in 1903 by von Tappenier and Jesionek.[2] In their technique, a 5% aqueous solution of eosin dye was applied to skin tumors, and in some cases supplemented with an injection of the dye into the center of the tumor. Subsequent illumination of the tumor with sunlight or an arc lamp was found to produce tumor necrosis. The authors also included clinical data from their experimental use of eosin-sensitized phototherapy for the management of several skin conditions, including pityriasis versicolor, herpes, molluscum contagiosum, psoriasis, and lupus. The same investigators[3] later reported on their use of eosin at various concentrations, as well as other potential photosensitizing dyes, including fluorescein, sodium dichloroanthracene disulfonate, and Grubler's magdaline red, activated by light to treat human tumors.

Porphyrins have received the most attention as photosensitizers since the demonstration by Policard[4] of a reddish fluorescence in certain malignant tumors in animals and human subjects illuminated with a Wood's lamp, which he attributed to the accumulation of endogenous porphyrins resulting from secondary infection by hemolytic bacteria. Auler and Banzer[5] noted this characteristic fluorescence in implanted carcinomas and sarcomas as well as in the lymph nodes of rats after the systemic injection of hematoporphyrin (Hp). The authors also found that necrosis occurred in tumors implanted in a small series of animals injected with Hp and then exposed to radiation from a quartz lamp. The latter effect was confirmed by Figge and co-workers,[6] who studied a wide range of induced and transplanted tumors in mice.

In an attempt to purify Hp by the addition of a mixture of sulfuric and acetic acids, Lipson and co-workers[7] developed a new product called *hematoporphyrin derivative* (HpD) for the fluorescence and localization of tumors. HpD, a complex mixture of porphyrins prepared by the alkaline hydrolysis of acetylated Hp, showed increased localization in human tumors, with a good correlation between the finding of fluorescence and a biopsy-proven malignant tumor, as compared with that seen for Hp. In 1966, HpD-sensitized PDT was used to treat a patient with a large ulcerating, recurrent breast tumor using filtered red light from a xenon arc lamp, with positive results.[8]

During the early 1970s, two groups of investigators independently began to examine HpD-PDT as a potential cancer therapy. Diamond and co-workers[9] found that glioma tumors implanted subcutaneously in rats were destroyed upon illumination after the administration of commercial HpD. Dougherty and co-workers,[10] at Roswell Park, showed that the systemic administration of HpD, activated by light from a xenon arc lamp, could cause complete eradication of a transplanted mouse mammary tumor without appreciable damage to the overlying skin. Their technique involved the intraperitoneal injection of HpD, followed 1 to 2 days later by illumination with highly penetrating red light (630 nm). After the appropriate toxicologic and preclinical studies were completed, this group began a full-scale clinical trial of this technique.[11]

Both the scope and the intensity of basic research into the nature and uses of PDT, as well as the number of clinical applications of PDT, have grown considerably during the past few years, and this has been thoroughly reviewed in several recently published symposia proceedings.[12,13] The development of instrumentation for exploiting the localization of photosensitizers in neoplastic lesions has provided a further incentive for continued clinical studies. Although the porphyrins have been the principal photosensitizers studied to date in clinical trials, other promising agents are now being studied in vitro and in vivo, and in some cases in early clinical trials.

Mechanism of Photodynamic Therapy

The concept of PDT is relatively simple, in that only three components need to be present for cytotoxicity to occur: a photosensitizer, light, and oxygen. As mentioned earlier, this technique consists of the following steps. First, a photosensitizer that is selectively retained in tumors to a greater extent than the surrounding normal tissue is administered to the patient. Sufficient time is then allowed to pass to optimize the ratio of the drug in the tumor to that in normal tissue. The photosensitizer, now preferentially localized in the tumor, is exposed to light of a wavelength predominantly absorbed by the photosensitizer, which is then elevated to an excited state. The excited photosensitizer subsequently reacts with oxygen, to produce highly reactive singlet molecular oxygen, which causes irreversible oxidative damage to the tumor (Fig. 17-1).

PHOTOSENSITIZER

HpD is a complex mixture of several porphyrins, including Hp, hydroxyvinyldeuteroporphyrin (HVD), protoporphyrin (Pp), and a chromatographically poorly resolved hydrophobic component. Attempts to ascertain which of the porphyrins are active have been frustrated, however, by the difficulty in determining the relative purity of the various components. Even apparently pure preparations have been found to contain impurities that often complicated the interpretation of data. Dougherty and colleagues,[14] who used fast atom bombardment, mass spectrometry, and nuclear magnetic resonance spectra to study these substances, concluded that the active component was most likely a structural isomer of dihematoporphyrin ether. However, it is now known that dihematoporphyrin ether is not the only important photosensitizer within the HpD mixture, which consists primarily of oligomers of two to eight Hp molecules.[15]

The concentration of the "active" ingredient led to the commercial introduction of Photofrin (formerly called *Photofrin II*), or porfimer

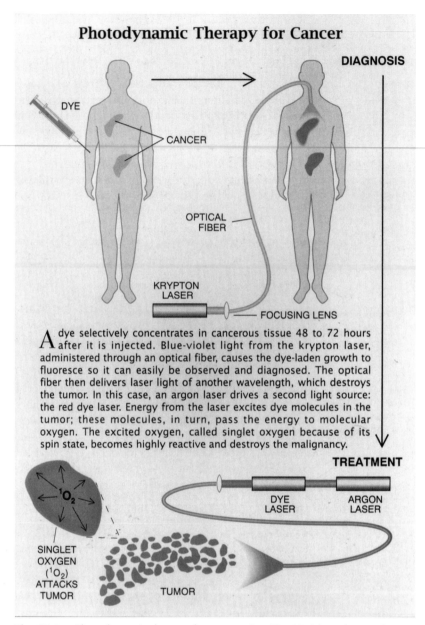

Photodynamic Therapy for Cancer

A dye selectively concentrates in cancerous tissue 48 to 72 hours after it is injected. Blue-violet light from the krypton laser, administered through an optical fiber, causes the dye-laden growth to fluoresce so it can easily be observed and diagnosed. The optical fiber then delivers laser light of another wavelength, which destroys the tumor. In this case, an argon laser drives a second light source: the red dye laser. Energy from the laser excites dye molecules in the tumor; these molecules, in turn, pass the energy to molecular oxygen. The excited oxygen, called singlet oxygen because of its spin state, becomes highly reactive and destroys the malignancy.

Fig. 17-1. Photodynamic therapy for cancer. See Fig. 17-1 in color section. (Reproduced from Scientific American 1991;June.)

sodium (approved generic name), and its evaluation in clinical trials in the mid-1980s. Photofrin consists of an 80% to 90% mixture of the ether linkages and is commercially available from QLT Phototherapeutics Inc., in Vancouver, BC, Canada. However, other porphyrins make up the remaining 10% to 20%; these include Hp, HVD, Pp, and a variety of monoacetates and diacetates that may interact in various ways with cells and tumors, depending on a wide range of environmental and physiologic factors. Photofrin exhibits the strongest absorption in the violet-blue region of the spectrum (400–420 nm), with weaker absorption bands seen at 514, 540, 580, and 630 nm. Paradoxically, the weakest band, at 630 nm, is the one most often used clinically because of the deeper tissue penetration of red light at this longer wavelength than of the violet-blue or green light.

Although Photofrin is currently the only drug approved by the U.S. Food and Drug Administration for phase 3 clinical trials, it is far from ideal. Specifically, Photofrin is known to be a mixture of monomeric and aggregated porphyrins; it is very weakly absorbed at wavelengths above 600 nm; and it is retained in numerous normal tissues, particularly skin, for extended periods. The second generation of photosensitizers developed to replace Photofrin should ideally be chemically pure and show minimal dark toxicity, a major excitation peak (large extinction coefficient) at a wavelength above 650 nm, a high quantum yield for the generation of singlet oxygen, preferential accumulation in target tissue, and rapid uptake in the targeted tissue and speedy clearance from normal tissue.[16] Because of the limited treatment depth possible in the removal of bulky lesions infused with Photofrin, efforts are under way to develop other classes of photosensitizers that absorb strongly at longer wavelengths. It has to be kept in mind, however, that the uptake of exogenous photosensitizers by tissue and the absorption of light therein can limit tissue light penetration. This phenomenon has been termed *self-shielding* and is particularly pronounced for photosensitizers that absorb very strongly at the appropriate treatment wavelength.[17,18]

Benzoporphyrin derivative–monoacid ring A (BPD-MA) is a chemically pure second-generation semisynthetic porphyrin made from protoporphyrin that is currently being evaluated in phase I clinical trials. BPD-MA is composed of two regioisomers differing in the location of the methyl ester group at either position three or four of the porphyrin ring. It has a maximum light absorption at 690 nm, a wavelength well suited to tissue penetration.[19,20] Treatment with BPD-MA can also be carried out on the same day as the drug is infused, in contrast to treatment with HpD or Photofrin. Most importantly, because the drug is cleared from normal tissues relatively faster than other porphyrins, skin photosensitivity rapidly disappears after PDT in which BPD-MA has been used. This has been shown in animals, and preliminary clinical results indicate that the skin photosensitivity occurring after treatment with BPD-MA (at the clinically relevant drug doses) lasts for less than 1 week.

Chlorins (650–700 nm), phthalocyanines (600–700 nm), purpurins and verdins (690–700 nm), bacteriochlorophyll-a (780 nm), and naphthalocyanine (776 nm) are also being evaluated as potential photosensitizers for use in PDT.[21] Preclinical experience has indicated that chlorins, phthalocyanines, purpurins, and verdins have favorable differential sensitizer uptake or retention, or both, in target tissue and little intrinsic, light-independent toxicity. Many of the other compounds being evaluated may do the same, but the information available is as yet sparse. The continuing development of small, simple diode lasers that emit light within the 750- to 800-nm range has made these wavelengths particularly attractive.

LIGHT

PDT requires sufficient light to produce effective photosensitization, and any source having the appropriate spectral characteristics can be used. The amount of light delivered, or energy (expressed in joules), represents the product of the light power in watts (joules per second) and the duration of irradiation (in seconds). Light dosages are also expressed in terms of energy density, or fluence, which is defined as the energy delivered to an area of target tissue in joules per square centimeter.

Most commonly, light is obtained from an argon-ion pumped dye laser, which emits light in a continuous wave. More recently the gold vapor laser has been used as the light source. The gold vapor laser produces short pulses of 30 nsec at high peak powers of 50 to 200 kW and is an inherently simpler system. However, reports of tumor response to the gold vapor laser have been conflicting. One group of investigators reported that much deeper necrosis in an experimental animal tumor was achieved using the gold vapor laser than the dye laser at the same average energy density,[22] whereas other investigators have found no difference between these two lasers, either in the photoinactivation of HpD-labeled cells in vitro or in the induction of tumor necrosis in vivo.[23,24]

Laser light is coupled into quartz or fused silica fibers. The output end of the fiber has a microlens at its terminus that focuses the laser radiation into a circular field of uniform light intensity (Fig. 17-2). Multiple fibers can be used for the treatment of large tumors. Uniform superficial illumination may be difficult to achieve, however, when irradiating skin folds or curved surfaces using such fibers. Interstitial fibers that emit light in a cylindrical distribution can be used for deeper infiltrating lesions (Fig. 17-3).

The use of the laser for PDT differs somewhat from its use for other forms of medical therapy, in that its primary purpose in PDT is to provide many photons at the desired wavelength in order to efficiently excite the photosensitizer present in the target tissue. A further advantage to its use in this setting is that the high laser output at the appropriate drug-activating wavelength minimizes the exposure times needed. The thermal effects of laser light used for other treatments, although potentially present in varying degrees depending on the technique of light delivery, are not of particular use. More conventional light sources (such as an incandescent or xenon arc lamp with appropriate filter) have also been shown effective. In early studies, slide projectors and solar simulators were used as light sources.

Clearly, a key element in the ability of PDT to completely eradicate the target tissue is the adequate delivery of light to all parts of the tu-

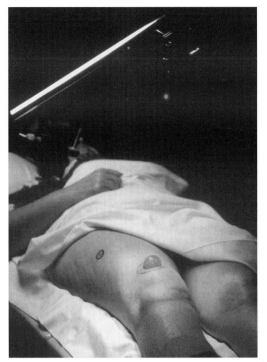

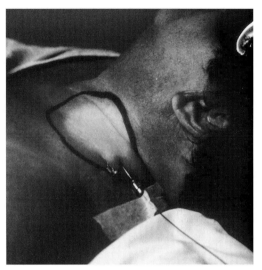

Fig. 17-2.   During PDT, laser light is coupled into quartz or fused silica fibers. The output end of the fiber is terminated with a microlens that focuses the laser radiation into a circular field of uniform light intensity.

Fig. 17-3.   Interstitial fibers that emit light in a cylindrical distribution can be used for PDT of deeper infiltrating lesions.

mor. Svaasand[25] measured light penetration in skin at several wavelengths and fitted the data to theoretically derived equations based on diffusion theory. Light fluence in tissue decreases exponentially with distance; the effective penetration depth, α, is inversely proportional to the effective attenuation coefficient, $\varepsilon (\alpha = 1/\varepsilon)$. The latter is influenced by the optical absorption (owing to endogenous tissue chromophores, especially oxyhemoglobin) and by optical scattering in the tissue. On the average, α in skin is 1 to 3 mm at 630 nm, the wavelength used for Photofrin therapy, while penetration is approximately twice as deep at 750 to 800 nm. The increased penetration depth of longer wavelengths is the major incentive for the development of photosensitizers excited by such wavelengths.

OXYGEN

Underlying the biologic response to PDT is the ability of photosensitizing agents to undergo various photochemical reactions when they absorb light.[26] These photochemical reactions are initiated when the photosensitizer molecule is converted into a series of highly reactive, excited electronic states—the short-lived singlet state—which can either return to the ground state by emitting the photons as fluorescence or progress through intersystem crossover to the longer-lived triplet state (Fig. 17-4). A molecule in the triplet state can interact directly with the biologic substrate, producing substrate and sensitizer radicals, which can further interact with oxygen to produce various reactive oxygen species, such as hydroxyl radicals, superoxides, and peroxides (type I reaction). By undergoing a spin-state transition, it can also transfer its excitation energy directly to oxygen, thereby producing highly reactive singlet oxygen (type II reaction). Type I and II reactions may occur simultaneously, and the ratio between the two is influenced by the sensitizer, substrate, and oxygen concentrations as well as the binding of sensitizer to substrate. However, singlet oxygen appears to be the major cytotoxic agent produced by most photosensitizers, as shown by the fact that the removal of singlet oxygen by traps or chemical quenchers confers almost complete cellular protection from damage in vitro.[27] Although there is also evidence indicating the formation of other highly reactive oxygen species (hydroxyl radicals, superoxides, and peroxides), these appear to play only a minor role in the PDT-induced inactivation of cells. Nevertheless, the

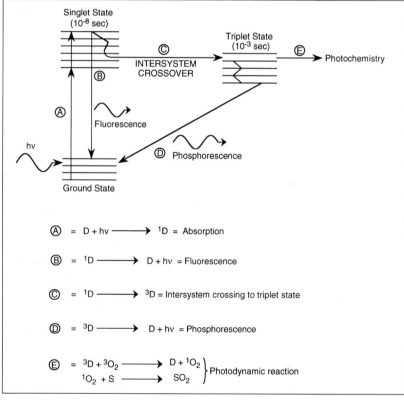

Fig. 17-4.   Transitions between energy levels of a photosensitizer during PDT.

effects of PDT are oxygen dependent, as shown by the fact that no photosensitization is observed in the absence of measurable oxygen. That is, when there is no or only a 2% or less concentration of oxygen in the system, cells are resistant to PDT-induced cytotoxicity.[28] This has also been shown by the finding that the induction of tissue hypoxia in vivo by clamping the arterial oxygenated blood supply abolishes any PDT effects in animals.[29]

De-excitation of activated sensitizer to ground state can also occur through photon emission, a process termed *fluorescence* or *phosphorescence,* depending on the spin state of the excited sensitizer. Although fluorescence yields are low, it has been shown that the fluorescent properties of porphyrins can be used to detect and localize tumors not detected by more conventional techniques.[30,31] In the case of Photofrin, fluorescence yields light in the visible red range with an emission wavelength of between 600 and 700 nm. Excitation with ultraviolet or blue light produces pinkish red fluorescence in tissue that contains localized photosensitizer (Fig. 17-5). Unfortunately, autofluorescence in normal tissues often causes contrast to be poor, especially in small, thin tumors. However, instrumentation has recently been developed that can subtract the background fluorescence and greatly enhance the contrast. A clinical trial is now in progress at our institution in which the effectiveness of this equipment in the fluorescent detection and localization of skin tumors is being evaluated.

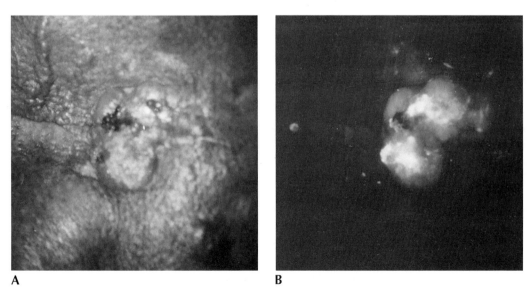

A　　　　　　　　　　　　　**B**

Fig. 17-5. Patient with dermal recurrence of breast cancer on anterior chest wall injected previously with Photofrin. Excitation with blue light (A) from a krypton-ion laser ($\lambda = 405$ nm) is used, and red fluorescence can be observed in the malignant cells (B) with appropriate filters. See Fig. 17-5 in color section.

In Vitro Cellular Effects of PDT

The lifetime and diffusion distance of singlet oxygen molecules in the cellular environment are limited by their avid reactivity and their quenching by cell constituents, such as histidine, tryptophan, and cholesterol. Moan[32] has estimated the diffusion distance of singlet oxygen in cells to be about 0.1 μm. Therefore the cell damage mediated by singlet oxygen occurs close to its site of generation. Experiments conducted by Oseroff and colleagues,[33] using a photosensitizer linked to monoclonal antibodies, in which the quantity of sensitizer at the cell surface was known, have shown that on the order of 10^{10} singlet oxygen molecules are necessary to lethally damage a single cell.

The search to identify the specific, primary cellular target site of PDT damage is still ongoing; but this may well be futile, considering the varied distribution of photosensitizers in cells. The distribution strongly depends on the chemical nature of the sensitizing compound and the specific experimental conditions, as borne out by the numerous studies that have shown some degree of PDT-induced destruction in nearly every subcellular component. The predominant role of membrane disturbance in PDT-induced cell destruction has been particularly well documented by microscopical observations and the correlation between the onset of membrane lysis and cell death.[34,35] Most obvious of the microscopical findings are changes in the cell membrane, which cause permeability and transport functions to be impaired. Other intracellular membranes may also be at risk, including the nucleus, mitochondria, lysosomes, Golgi apparatus, and endoplasmic reticulum. The mitochondrial damage produced by PDT has been shown by the specific inhibition of oxidative phosphorylation and electron transport systems and a reduction in the cellular adenosine triphosphate levels.[36,37]

Irrespective of the locus, the consequence of PDT-induced damage is a rapid loss of cell integrity, together with the release of inflammatory and immune mediators, such as eicosanoids and histamine. All of these substances are potent, fast acting, and vasoactive (either constrictive or dilatory), and there is evidence implicating them in the development of PDT-induced vascular damage, which is discussed in the next section.

In Vivo Tissue Effects of PDT

One of the beneficial effects of PDT stems from the ability of tumor tissue to retain substantial amounts of photosensitizer for a longer period than normal tissue. However, the mechanism responsible for causing this preferential localization of porphyrins in tumors remains incompletely understood, and the extent to which porphyrin directly damages tumor cells in vivo is also unclear. There is little doubt that there is a difference in the fluorescence and cytotoxicity that occur in tumor and certain normal tissues in both animals and patients; this has been reported by many independent investigators. Nevertheless, differences in the localization of porphyrins in tumors and normal tissue appear to occur at the tissue rather than at the cellular level and probably depend on several factors.

The macroscopic tumor response to PDT consists in a rapidly developing coagulation necrosis, which becomes apparent within hours after treatment (Fig. 17-6). When treated effectively, the tumor forms a nonpalpable scab that is sloughed within a few days. Previous basic science studies performed by our group at the University of California, Irvine, were conducted in an attempt to elucidate the mechanism of tumor destruction after PDT. Histopathologic studies of PDT-treated tumors have shown that internal hemorrhage and red cell extravasation are common findings after PDT, not only in experimental animal tumors but also in the tumors of patients.[38,39] This indicates that the effects of PDT that cause the necrosis of tumor tissue are not the result of the direct killing of tumor cells but are secondary to destruction of the tumor microvasculature. This has been further shown by the finding that tumor blood flow stops shortly after the initiation of PDT.[40,41] In the latter study, it was observed that complete cessation of tumor circulation was required to effect complete eradication of the tumor. Conversely, noncurative treatments frequently resulted in the resumption of intratumoral blood flow. Another study showed a definite correlation between the degree of in vivo tumor fluorescence localization and the amount of tumor microvasculature.[42] Further, oxygen radicals are known to cause vascular damage,[43] and singlet oxygen may be similarly toxic to the tumor vasculature. In addition, the localization of isotopically labeled HpD using autoradiography showed that the distribution of tritiated HpD in the surrounding perivascular stroma and tumor cells occurred at a

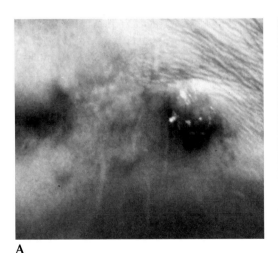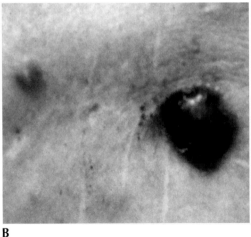

A   **B**

Fig. 17-6.   Patient with dermal recurrence of breast cancer on anterior chest wall (A) before PDT and (B) 24 hours after PDT. Note the black, necrotic tumor nodules.

ratio of 5 : 1.[44] Using tumor cell clonogenicity following PDT to assess in vitro colony formation, it was found that clonogenicity was unaffected by PDT if the tumor tissue was excised and explanted immediately.[45] If, however, tumor cells were left in situ for varying lengths of time after PDT (1–24 hours), tumor cell death was found to occur rapidly and progressively, implying that one of the major factors contributing to tumor destruction may be damage to the tumor circulation and the consequences of treatment-induced changes in tumor physiology. Taken together, the findings from these studies suggest that the vascular compartment represents an important target for PDT in the treatment of malignant tumors. Direct toxic effects to malignant cells undoubtedly also occur, but they are probably of secondary importance in terms of the overall clinical effect.

Why might the tumor microvasculature be a unique target for the localization and photochemical reaction of porphyrins? This may be at least partly explained by the fact that there are several characteristic differences between normal vessels and tumor vessels. For example, the neovasculature of the proliferating tumor is much "leakier" than the vasculature of most normal tissues.[46] This has been shown by the finding that azo dyes, such as Evans blue, pontamine sky blue, vital new red, and Congo red, move rapidly out through tumor capillaries and stain the tumor stroma, whereas they do not penetrate normal vasculature.[47] Similarly, many plasma components, including proteins and other colloids, penetrate easily through tumor capillaries into the interstitial compartment of tumors. In addition, blood vessels in normal tissues contain endothelial cells that are damaged or missing in tumors.[48] That tumor collagen is produced by the host and its synthesis is governed by the tumor cells is particularly noteworthy.[49] Tumor collagen fibers also resemble the types of fibers seen in embryonic tissue and in wounds during healing. That these fibers, recently made in the neovascularization of tumors, would not be as highly cross-linked as those in more mature tissues is to be expected. One study has shown that newly formed collagen, and perhaps elastin and fibrin as well, have a substantially greater binding capacity for porphyrins than does mature collagen; as a result they may constitute potentially important binding sites for porphyrin localization and retention.[50] In addition, poorly developed tumor lymphatics, lower tumor pH, the binding of porphyrins to lipoproteins, and subsequent receptor-mediated endocytosis may all contribute to the selective retention of porphyrins in tumors.

Clinical PDT of Malignant Skin Tumors

Clinically, PDT is carried out in a two-step procedure. First, the photosensitizer is administered intravenously as a bolus. After a delay of 48 to 72 hours (to allow for accumulation of the photosensitizer in the target tissue and its clearing from most normal tissues), the target is irradiated with visible red light at wavelengths corresponding to the longest absorption peak of the photosensitizer. Such a schedule for the treatment of skin lesions was developed empirically on the basis of the observation that this interval between photosensitizer administration and laser irradiation was associated with the greatest tumor destruction but minimal destruction to the surrounding normal skin. Unfortunately, there is often appreciable uptake of the drug in normal skin, such that necrosis of irradiated peritumoral skin occurs at the light doses necessary for tumor eradication. The recent discovery of photobleaching during illumination was an important development in the treatment of skin lesions. This has led to reductions in the dose of the photosensitizer injected, so that the drug concentration in the normal skin surrounding tumors may be low enough when irradiated that only residual drug is photobleached and destroyed during light delivery. This permits increased light doses to be delivered to tumors (which still contain active photosensitizer), but with much less risk of injury to normal skin.

Most of the clinical experience with PDT acquired to date has involved the use of either HpD or Photofrin. However, HpD is no longer commercially available in the United States, and Photofrin is currently available only as an investigational drug. PDT using these agents has been used effectively to treat surface lesions, both primary skin cancers (basal and squamous cell carcinomas, malignant melanomas, mycosis fungoides, and Kaposi's sarcoma) and metastatic tumors from a primary source (breast). The disease in most patients had not been controlled by prior surgery, chemotherapy, ionizing radiation, or some combination thereof. Although investigators have used different criteria to judge response, it is clear that responses have been obtained, even in patients who have undergone extensive prior treatment that failed to produce a response. All reporting investigators have noted the difference in the response of tumor and adjacent normal tissue within the light field. Unfortunately, the results of PDT in the management of skin tumors that have been reported in the literature have varied widely, owing in part to differences in the treatment parameters used (i.e., the drug used, the light source, the drug and light dose, and the interval between drug administration and irradiation).

CLINICAL TRIALS

Several clinical trials evaluating the effectiveness of PDT in the control of malignant skin tumors have been performed. Bandieramonte and colleagues[51] treated seven patients with 61 lesions, 43 of which were basal cell carcinomas and 18 of which were metastatic breast cancer lesions. Patients received an injection of HpD (3 mg/kg body weight) and light doses of 60 to 120 J/cm^2. Clinically, complete responses were observed in 26 of 61 lesions (no visible tumor), whereas 16 of the lesions showed only a partial response. The follow-up in this study ranged from 4 to 16 months. Side effects noted were photosensitivity and pain during and after treatment secondary to tumor necrosis; the treatment of larger and more deeply infiltrating lesions caused more pain than did the treatment of smaller lesions.

Waldow and colleagues[52] reported on the treatment of nine patients with various forms of skin cancer: six had basal cell carcinomas and three had Bowen's disease or squamous cell carcinomas. Patients were treated 24 to 72 hours after injection (HpD, 3 mg/kg; or Photofrin, 2 mg/kg) with light doses of 40 to 60 J/cm². All primary skin cancer lesions showed a visually complete response by 3 months during a total follow-up of 8 to 24 months.

Pennington and colleagues[53] reported on the treatment of six patients with a total of 53 primary basal cell or squamous cell skin tumors. Patients were treated 3 to 5 days after the injection of HpD (5 mg/kg body weight) at a fluence of 30 J/cm². Complete responses were achieved in 52% of the basal cell lesions and 81% of the squamous cell lesions. However, half of the squamous cell lesions and most of the basal cell lesions had recurred by the 6-month follow-up visit. No attempts were made to determine whether alterations in the drug or light dose would have affected the treatment outcome.

The most careful studies of the dermatologic use of PDT with systemically administered Photofrin have been carried out at the Roswell Park Cancer Institute. Wilson and colleagues[54] reported on the treatment of 37 patients with a total of 151 basal cell lesions. Total light dosages of 180 to 233 J/cm² were delivered 48 to 72 hours after the patients received 1 mg/kg of Photofrin. Patients with extensive disease were treated at different sessions over a period of 2 or 3 days after injection or approximately 4 to 6 weeks later after a second injection. A complete response was observed in 133 of the tumors and a partial response in 18. At a minimum of 12 months of follow-up, 13 of the 133 tumors initially showing a complete response had recurred. Most patients who had recurrences had morpheoform basal cell epitheliomas or extensive disease or the disease was located on the nose, which the researchers suggested is more effectively treated with greater light doses or intralesional fiberoptic implantation. If the nose lesions are excluded, the complete response rate was 92%. Eleven of the 18 lesions showing a partial response were retreated, and all showed a complete response to PDT and remained free of disease 12 months later. Excellent cosmetic effects were obtained in most patients and disfiguring surgery was avoided in some. No adverse effects of therapy were reported.

The multiple lesions of Bowen's disease (intraepidermal carcinoma) have shown an excellent response to PDT, but more than one course of treatment is required for the tumors to be completely eradicated. Robinson and colleagues[55] described the treatment of two patients with Bowen's disease who together had more than 500 lesions. Irradiation (25 J/cm²) was performed 72 hours after the injection of Photofrin (2 mg/kg). Treatment was performed in up to a total of five sessions, and complete clearing of the lesions was seen by 6 months after treatment.

Excellent results have been reported for the treatment of multiple basal cell carcinomas in patients with nevoid basal cell carcinoma syndrome. Tse and colleagues[56] reported on the treatment of three patients with a total of 40 such lesions. Light doses ranging from 38 to 180 J/cm² were given 72 and 96 hours after the injection of HpD (3 mg/kg). A complete response was seen in 82.5% of the lesions treated. A higher complete response rate was seen in lesions receiving light doses greater than 70 J/cm². Patients showing a complete response were followed for 12 to 14 months, and four recurrences (10.7%) were observed during that time.

Pigmented melanomas are almost completely unresponsive to PDT. Work by our group at the University of California, Irvine, in an animal tumor model showed that phototoxicity was inefficient during PDT as the result of interference by the melanin in melanotic melanoma.[57] This may happen because melanin competes with the photosensitizer for the absorption of photons or because the excitation energy of the photosensitizer in the excited triplet state is transferred to melanin instead of cellular oxygen. Furthermore, at least one study showed that melanin may in fact be a very effective quencher of singlet oxygen in aerobic photosensitization.[58] As already noted, nonpigmented lesions, however, can be effectively controlled by PDT.

Because PDT damages the tumor microvasculature, it is logical to expect it to be effective in the treatment of Kaposi's sarcoma. In this vein, Schweitzer and colleagues[59] reported on the treatment of five patients with oral HIV-associated Kaposi's sarcoma. In one patient, a lesion as large as 3 cm in diameter was effectively controlled using PDT. One advantage of PDT over other ablative forms of therapy is that it does not cause the aerosolization or volatilization of tissue or viral products.

Cutaneous lesions on the chest wall resulting from metastatic breast cancer have also been treated using PDT. Schuh and colleagues[60] reported on 14 such patients, all of whom had been previously treated using other means. Patients received 2.0 mg/kg of Photofrin, followed 24 to 96 hours later by irradiation at fluences of 36 to 288 J/cm². Two patients were considered to show complete responses; nine, partial responses, and two, no responses. Recurrent disease developed within 4 months in one of the patients considered initially to show a complete response, but the other patient remained free of disease at 6 months after treatment. A significant reduction in the amount of chest wall disease was obtained in patients showing a partial response. The average response lasted from 8 to 12 weeks but ranged from 8 weeks to 8 months. Thus, the treatment of recurrent breast cancer on the chest wall with PDT appears to produce brief partial responses. The authors concluded that PDT is best for the control of superficial lesions confined to relatively small areas and that its use for extensive and bulky disease, although responsive, is not of particular benefit. Most patients experience moderate to severe pain for several days after treatment, requiring narcotics for control in some cases. Clearly, PDT is most beneficial to these patients before the disease is out of control and its use will probably be limited to selected patients with focal areas of small nodular recurrences.

Gilson and co-authors[61] reported on the effects of various doses of Photofrin and radiation in the treatment of six patients with a total of 34 cutaneous and subcutaneous cancers, such as squamous cell cancer, small-cell lung cancer, large-cell anaplastic lung cancer, malignant melanoma, anaplastic parotid carcinoma, and metastatic or recurrent skin lesions resulting from breast adenocarcinoma. Patients received 1, 1.5, or 2 mg/kg of Photofrin, and lesions were treated with total light doses of 25, 50, 75, or 100 J/cm^2 48 to 72 hours after injection. All tumors were less than 1.5 cm thick. None of the light doses used resulted in a complete response in the patients receiving 1 mg/kg of Photofrin. At a Photofrin dose of 1.5 mg/kg, a complete response was observed in one of six lesions treated with 25 J/cm^2, six of ten lesions treated with 50 J/cm^2, and the four lesions treated with 75 J/cm^2 (no sites were treated with 100 J/cm^2 at this sensitizer dose). At a Photofrin dose of 2.0 mg/kg, a complete response was observed in the one lesion treated with 25 J/cm^2, two of the three lesions treated with 50 J/cm^2, and the two lesions treated with 75 J/cm^2. Therefore, it appears that a dose of Photofrin as low as 1.5 mg/kg may produce good results in patients with these tumors, provided that a sufficient light dose is applied. Lower drug doses offer the advantage of producing greater sparing of normal tissue and superior depth of treatment, because of the photobleaching of the photosensitizer that occurs. However, such reductions in the dose of the photosensitizer necessitate increases in the light dose for treatment to be effective, which may pose a practical problem in the treatment of large lesions.

Lui and colleagues[62] recently reported on the use of PDT for the treatment of malignant skin tumors using as the photosensitizer BPD-MA, a second-generation semisynthetic porphyrin described earlier. These investigators treated 64 lesions in 15 patients, nine with basal cell carcinomas, three with metastatic breast cancer, two with metastatic gastrointestinal carcinoma, and one with metastatic amelanotic melanoma. Patients received an injection of BPD-MA (0.25–0.50 mg/kg) 3 to 4 hours before receiving a total dose of from 50 to 150 J/cm^2 of 690-nm laser light. A complete response was noted in 63% of the tumors treated, a partial response in 1%, and no response in 36%. In addition, daily serial photosensitivity testing was carried out before and after BPD-MA injection to determine the duration of photosensitivity produced by the drug, and it was found to range from an average of 2.4 days for the 0.25-mg/kg dose to 5.4 days for the 0.5-mg/kg dose.

Summary

Studies of various doses of photosensitizers (HpD, Photofrin, BPD-MA) and light are being performed to determine the optimum treatment parameters for the management of a variety of skin tumors. Although PDT can be used to eradicate relatively large skin tumors, it appears to be especially advantageous for patients with early disease or early recurrence. On the basis of the clinical experience accumulated thus far, PDT has been found to be most effective for the management of those malignant tumors that are localized and extend to a depth of less than 1 cm. PDT may prove to be curative in appropriately selected cases of primary nonmelanotic skin cancers. The high therapeutic ratio and relative safety of the method could make this a very attractive therapy. Treatment parameters have been refined such that now therapy can be undertaken with a reasonable expectation of good results. In some patients, such therapy may be a viable alternative to debilitating surgery; in others, it may be the treatment of choice. In addition, the use of PDT is not precluded in patients who have already undergone surgery, radiation therapy, or chemotherapy, and in fact many of the patients making up the study populations in the clinical studies reported on to date have previously failed some or all other available therapies.

One of the most exciting applications of PDT is its use in combination with other therapies. Published results of studies have already shown a synergistic response is produced by the combination of PDT and chemotherapeutic agents, and this has been seen under both in vitro and in vivo conditions.[63,64] Additionally, several investigators have examined the contribution of hyperthermia to the overall tumoricidal effect of PDT. They have found that there can be a hyperthermic contribution to cytotoxicity when high light irradiances are employed during PDT.[65] Among the major determinants of this contribution are the rate of blood flow and the optical absorption properties of the tissue.[66] Recent studies using an animal tumor model have also shown a possible synergism between hyperthermia and PDT.[67,68] Specifically, it has been demonstrated that temperatures in the 40° to 45°C range, induced by the thermal effects of laser radiation, have a synergistic effect on tumor kill if the heat treatment immediately follows PDT. If, however, the interval between light and heat treatments is increased, this interaction is lost. Additional data on animal and tissue toxicity of the single and combined treatments are being obtained in preparation for clinical trials.

Adverse Effects of PDT

Persistent generalized skin photosensitivity is the most relevant side effect in patients after the administration of HpD or Photofrin and usually lasts for 6 to 8 weeks, although on occasion it lasts as long as

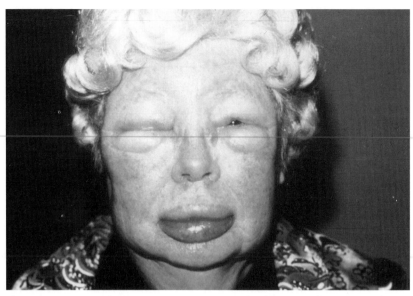

Fig. 17-7. Severe phototoxic reaction as a result of unwanted exposure of a patient to bright artificial light 2 weeks after hematoporphyrin derivative injection.

several months (Fig. 17-7). A prospective study in which detailed written and verbal instructions regarding photoprotection were given to patients undergoing PDT revealed that three out of every four patients reported cutaneous photosensitivity.[69] Of these patients, 17% experienced blister formation. It appears that lower doses of HpD or Photofrin do lead to a reduction in the severity and the incidence of photosensitivity reactions. Aside from wearing protective clothing and strictly avoiding exposure to bright direct light (even through window glass), there are no effective strategies for alleviating this complication. Conventional sunscreens are of no benefit, because the action spectrum of these agents lies only within the visible light region and their use may also give patients a false sense of protection.

Burning, stinging, or pain is common during extensive treatments (either a single large lesion or multiple sites) and likely results from direct nerve stimulation or damage by singlet oxygen and released mediators. Such discomfort is generally moderate, however, and can be controlled with mild analgesics. Local edema may occur for several days after therapy, particularly after the treatment of multiple sites on the face. Other porphyrin-related complications include skin hyperpigmentation, ocular discomfort, itching, nausea, pain at the injection site, and a metallic taste.[70]

New Approaches

A significant disadvantage of PDT is persistent generalized skin photosensitivity stemming from the systemic administration of porphyrin photosensitizers. Methods of topically applying photosensitizers are under active investigation in an effort to minimize this complication. An additional advantage of the topical application of photosensitizers is that it eliminates the need for intravenous injection. Although the topical application of HpD and Photofrin has not worked well,[71] the topical application of two different photosensitizers has proved successful in large clinical trials.

In one of these trials, Santoro and colleagues[72] evaluated the effectiveness of topically administered mesotetraphenylporphinesulfonate (TPPS) in the treatment of 292 patients with basal cell carcinomas seen over a 5-year period. Patients received three applications of a 2% topical solution of TPPS (isopropyl alcohol/water/azone) 24, 6, and 3 hours before laser treatment using total light doses of 120 to 150 J/cm². A 93.5% complete response rate with a 20% recurrence rate was seen in these patients during 2 years of follow-up. Approximately half of the recurrences arose in the margins of the treatment field. Almost all of these patients underwent a second treatment, and 73% showed a complete response.

Kennedy and colleagues[73] proposed a novel approach to the topical application of a photosensitizer: the application of a metabolic precursor to an endogenous photosensitizer rather than the sensitizer itself. This was based on the knowledge that the administration of δ-aminolevulinic acid (ALA) leads to the accumulation of the endogenous photosensitizer protoporphyrin IX (PpIX) in certain tissues. PpIX is a porphyrin in the biosynthetic pathway of heme (Fig. 17-8). Normally the endogenous synthesis of ALA by the rate-limiting enzyme ALA synthetase is the control point in this pathway. However, this control point can be bypassed if excess ALA is administered, with the result that the cells make excess PpIX that is then converted to heme. If ALA is converted to PpIX faster than PpIX is converted to heme, then this very potent photosensitizer temporarily accumulates.

Two factors make PDT with endogenous PpIX, formed from topical ALA, selective. First, PpIX induces photosensitization in epidermally derived cells, including malignancies, but not in the dermis. Second, because ALA in aqueous solution passes more readily through abnormal keratin than intact stratum corneum, the topical application of such ALA to actinic keratoses or superficial basal cell or squamous cell carcinomas induces a photosensitization that is restricted primarily to the abnormal epithelium.

Not only is PpIX an efficient photosensitizer, it is also very easily photobleached. Therefore, prolonged photosensitivity should not be a problem because the endogenously produced PpIX decays by means of both light-independent conversion to heme and light-dependent conversion to "bleached PpIX." PpIX is cleared from the skin within 24 hours of topical administration.

Kennedy and colleagues[73] treated 80 patients with basal cell carcinoma, squamous cell carcinoma, Bowen's disease, or actinic keratoses using topically applied 20% ALA. After a 3-hour interval, presumably to allow for ALA uptake and its conversion to PpIX, the tumor was

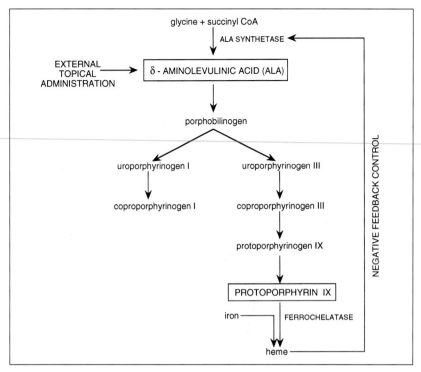

Fig. 17-8. Administration of δ-aminolevulinic acid leads to the accumulation of the endogenous photosensitizer protoporphyrin IX through the biosynthetic pathway of heme.

irradiated with total light doses of 54 to 540 J/cm² using a Kodak slide projector and red filter. Ninety percent of the basal cell carcinomas responded completely and 7.5% responded partially. Every thin lesion that was covered by an abnormal keratin layer showed a complete response. Conversely, the treatment failures occurred in deeper, thicker, or nodular lesions that had a relatively normal stratum corneum.

Wolf and Kerl[74] treated 13 patients with 70 lesions, of which 37 were superficial basal carcinomas, 10 were nodular, ulcerative basal cell carcinomas, 9 were solar keratoses, 6 were superficial squamous cell carcinomas, and 8 were cutaneous metastatic tumors of malignant melanomas. A 20% solution of ALA was topically applied to patients 4 to 8 hours before phototherapy using light doses of 30 to 60 J/cm². All 9 solar keratoses, 5 of the 6 superficial squamous cell carcinomas, and 36 of the 37 superficial basal cell carcinomas showed a complete response after a single treatment. Only 1 of the 10 nodular, ulcerative basal cell carcinomas resolved completely. All cutaneous metastatic tumors of malignant melanoma were considered treatment failures. The authors concluded on the basis of these results that PDT after topical application of ALA is effective for the eradication of superficial epithelial skin tumors.

Our group at the University of California, Irvine, has conducted a pilot dose-ranging study to evaluate the safety and clinical efficacy of PDT using topically administered ALA in the treatment of actinic keratoses. Forty patients were selected, each with six clinically typical actinic keratoses. ALA emollient cream in concentrations of 0%, 10%, 20%, or 30% was applied to the lesions, which were then covered with an occlusive dressing. Three hours after ALA application, immediately before PDT, the treatment sites were examined by ultraviolet (UV) light to determine whether they showed ALA-induced porphyrin fluorescence. The sites were then irradiated with 630-nm red light from an argon-ion pumped dye laser at total light doses ranging from 10 to 150 J/cm^2. The safety of the procedure and the clinical response were assessed immediately after PDT, at 24 and 72 hours, and at weeks 1, 4, 8, and 16.

Actinic keratoses showed moderate red fluorescence 3 hours after ALA application, with a less intense fluorescence observed in the surrounding normal skin. Cutaneous photosensitization of actinic keratoses, characterized by localized erythema and edema, peaked at 72 hours after PDT and was more intense and prolonged after the use of higher concentrations of ALA. There was less photosensitization of the adjacent normal skin. Some patients experienced mild discomfort during treatment, which was also a function of the concentration of ALA. The clinical responses were also found to correlate with the ALA concentration, with better responses seen in patients in whom 20% to 30% ALA was used. At 8 weeks after a single treatment using 30% ALA, there was total clearing of 61% of actinic keratoses (n = 100). These results indicate that the topical application of ALA for use in PDT is an effective treatment for actinic keratoses and that the ALA concentration is important in determining the response to PDT. Complete clearing of typical actinic keratoses can be achieved using 20% to 30% ALA, with minimal patient discomfort (Fig. 17-9).

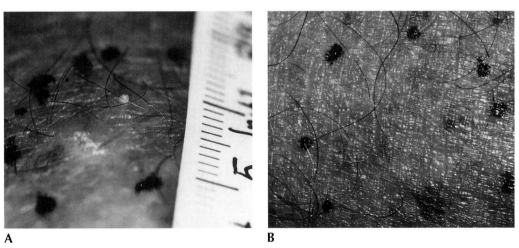

A   **B**

Fig. 17-9. Patient with actinic keratosis on forearm (A) before PDT and (B) 8 weeks after PDT, done using topically administered δ-aminolevulinic acid.

PDT for Nonmalignant Lesions

Preliminary studies have shown that benign hyperproliferative and vascular conditions such as psoriasis, papillomavirus infections, and port-wine stains can be effectively treated using PDT.

An intriguing use of PDT has been in the treatment of psoriasis. However, it should be noted that the therapeutic objectives in the clinical management of psoriasis and cancer are quite different (Table 17-1), that, in psoriasis, selective photosensitization may be related to the increased vascularity of psoriatic plaques. Silver,[75] in 1937, was the first to report on the use of PDT to treat psoriasis and this involved the use of both orally and intramuscularly administered hematoporphyrin and UV light. In 1980 Diezel and colleagues[76] reported on the effectiveness of systemic hematoporphyrin and UV light in the treatment of psoriasis. They treated 20 patients with a single intravenous dose of 1 mg/kg of HpD and daily whole-body UVA light irradiations using light doses of 0.8 to 2.8 J/cm^2. The psoriatic lesions disappeared in 15 of 20 patients after 15 treatments.

Our group at the University of California, Irvine, used systemic HpD (3 mg/kg) and 20 to 40 J/cm^2 of red light to treat a patient with vulvar neoplasia who had concurrent psoriasis.[77] The irradiated psoriatic skin eroded and became necrotic after exposure and showed some clearing 17 days after PDT. Subsequently, we have used systemic Photofrin (3 mg/kg) plus light to treat plaques in patients with malignancies who had psoriasis as a secondary disease. The photosensitivity of both the psoriatic lesions and clinically normal skin was concurrently assessed in these patients. Light doses of 20 to 40 J/cm^2 were found to produce tissue necrosis in the psoriatic lesions by 24 hours after treatment, similar to the eschar response of tumors. In marked contrast, there was only a slight erythema in the clinically normal skin after exposure to the highest dose of 40 J/cm^2, demonstrating the selectivity of Photofrin-induced photosensitivity in psoriasis. After 4 to 6 weeks the treated psoriatic lesions resolved, producing normal-appearing skin (Fig. 17-10). In view of the extreme selectivity of Photofrin in psoriasis, it would appear that a much lower dose could be given and the photosensitivity of the psoriatic

Table 17-1. Therapeutic objectives in the clinical management of cancer and psoriasis

Disease	Goal of therapy
Cancer: a discrete population of cells with a parasitic relationship to the host	Total destruction of neoplastic cells
Psoriasis: epidermal hyperplasia; inherent abnormalities in epidermal regeneration	Suppression or interruption of the proliferative process ↓ Normal epidermal proliferation

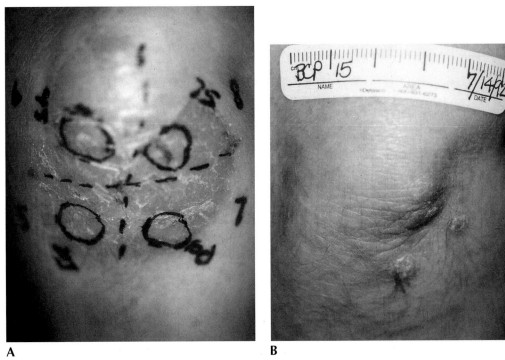

A   **B**

Fig. 17-10.   Patient with psoriasis on elbow injected previously with Photofrin (A) before PDT and (B) 3 months after PDT. See Fig. 17-10 in color section.

skin still be maintained, while minimizing or even eliminating the sensitivity of normal skin.

In a recent dose-ranging pilot study,[78] we investigated the effectiveness of PDT using low-dose systemically administered Photofrin (0.5–1.0 mg/kg) in the treatment of psoriasis and evaluated whether the residual photosensitivity of normal skin was minimized. Patients received a single intravenous dose (0.5 mg/kg) of Photofrin and then, 4 to 48 hours later, had several sites of lesional and normal skin treated with various doses of visible light in various schedules, as follows: a single treatment with the argon-ion pumped dye laser (wavelength, 630 nm) or the krypton-ion laser (wavelength, 405 nm); or multiple irradiations with UVA light (9–20 treatments over 3–4 weeks). Treatment sites were evaluated weekly for 7 weeks to assess lesion severity and the photosensitivity of normal skin. Eight patients have completed the study, and the clinical responses have been found to be dose related. The lowest doses used for the krypton-ion laser (0.5 J/cm^2), argon-ion pumped dye laser (5 J/cm^2), and cumulative UVA light exposure (75 J/cm^2) were clinically ineffective. For this reason, light doses were sequentially escalated in succeeding patients to maximize the clinical response. Two patients showed 85% to 100% clearing 3 weeks after a single treatment with 15 J/cm^2 using the argon-ion pumped dye laser. The maximum response obtained with the krypton-ion laser (1–30 J/cm^2) was 25% clearing of the psoriatic plaque, and 20% clearing was seen in the sites exposed to UVA light (cumulative dose, 97–394 J/cm²). Maximum therapeutic effects were obtained when laser treatment was performed 48 hours after Photofrin administration, with no response obtained when laser treatment was performed 4 or 24 hours after Photofrin administration. Selective fluorescence could be detected in psoriatic sites as opposed to normal skin 24 to 48 hours after Photofrin administration. There was only transient mild to moderate erythema in both psoriatic and normal skin 24 hours after treatment. With the low dose of 0.5 mg/kg of Photofrin, there were no episodes of prolonged cutaneous photosensitivity in patients who used reasonable protection.

These preliminary results indicate that PDT using Photofrin and visible light may constitute a safe and useful alternative treatment for psoriasis. However, there are several factors that currently limit the successful clinical development of this therapy. First, the surface areas that can be irradiated with the laser are extremely small (approximately 2 cm in diameter in the current study). Irradiation would have to be so prolonged in the treatment of larger fields as to be impractical. Second, the use of expensive, bulky lasers to treat patients with the kind of extensive skin involvement commonly seen in psoriasis is also impractical. Therefore we have recently initiated studies designed to develop alternative visible light sources (laser diodes and nonlaser sources) to treat large skin areas, which could be used for the PDT of both psoriasis and other cutaneous lesions.

We have also conducted a dose-ranging study to investigate the safety, patient tolerance, and clinical efficacy of the topical application of ALA in combination with UVA irradiation for the PDT of psoriasis. ALA (2%, 10%, 20%, or nondrug control) emollient cream was applied topically to six psoriatic sites in each of 14 patients, and then covered with an occlusive dressing for 3 hours. The sites were then treated with UVA (1–30 J/cm²). PDT using this protocol was performed either in a single treatment or once weekly for 4 consecutive weeks.

Immediately before PDT, treatment sites were examined by UV light to assess for ALA-induced PpIX fluorescence. All concentrations of ALA were found to produce intense red fluorescence in the psoriatic lesions, with minimal fluorescence in the surrounding normal skin (Fig. 17-11). Localized erythema and edema developed after treatment with UVA and peaked 24 to 72 hours later. In comparison, there was only mild photosensitization of the adjacent normal skin.

Although even a single treatment with 10% or 20% ALA plus PDT resulted in clinical improvement in some subjects with psoriatic lesions, multiple PDT treatments were found to be more effective. More than 50% clearing of the lesion was obtained with both 10% ALA and a total cumulative UVA light exposure of 80 to 120 J/cm² and 20% ALA and UVA light exposure of 1 to 39 J/cm². In contrast, less than 10% improvement was seen in patients receiving 2% ALA and control patients who underwent nondrug PDT. Patients experienced some discomfort during treatment, the degree of which corre-

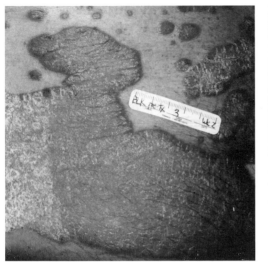 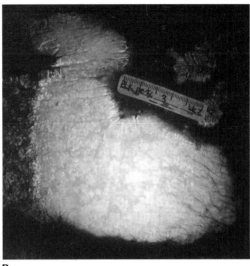

A **B**

Fig. 17-11. Patient with psoriasis, 3 hours after topical administration of ALA (A). Excitation with UV light is used, and red fluorescence can be observed in the psoriatic plaques with appropriate filters (B). See Fig. 17-11 in color section.

lated with the ALA concentration and the total UVA dose. Patients treated with 10% or 20% ALA were unable to tolerate the higher scheduled doses of UVA. In contrast, patients treated with 2% ALA were able to tolerate all doses of UVA. This study showed that topical ALA and UVA PDT is effective in alleviating psoriasis, and the data indicate that multiple PDT sessions may be necessary to optimize therapy.

Extensive human papillomavirus infections of the upper respiratory tract have been observed to regress after PDT using Photofrin. Abramson and colleagues[79] noted a 50% decrease in the average rate of laryngeal papilloma growth in 33 patients treated with PDT. PDT did not eradicate latent HPV infection, as evidenced by persistence of the vital DNA in clinically normal tissue, but because therapeutic alternatives are scarce, this appears to be an appropriate indication for such therapy.

A pilot study was carried out by members of our group to evaluate the potential efficacy of PDT using BPD-MA as the photosensitizer in the treatment of the Shope rabbit papillomavirus disease.[80] To establish proof-of-principle for BPD-MA treatment, however, a comparative study was first performed using systemically administered BPD-MA or Photofrin (the latter shown to be efficacious in previous studies). In this study, BPD-MA (2 mg/kg) or Photofrin (10 mg/kg) was administered intravenously, and then up to six warts were exposed to light 3 hours after BPD administration (wavelength, 690 nm) or 24 hours after Photofrin administration (wavelength, 630 nm). Control warts were not exposed to laser light. It was found that both the BPD-MA and Photofrin were effective in the treatment of papillomavirus disease.

78. Weinstein GD, McCullough JL, Nelson JS, Berns MW, McCormick A. Low dose Photofrin II photodynamic therapy of psoriasis. Clin Res 1991;39:409A.
79. Abramson AL, Shikowitz MJ, Mullooly VM, Steinberg BM, Amella CA, Rothstein HR. Clinical effects of photodynamic therapy on recurrent laryngeal papillomas. Arch Otolaryngol Head Neck Surg 1992;118:25–29.
80. Logan PM, Mayer LD, Comiskey S et al. Photodynamic therapy of papillomavirus disease using topical benzoporphyrin derivative. Photochem Photobiol 1992;55:30A–31S.
81. Orenstein A, Nelson JS, Liaw L-H, Kaplan R, Kimel S, Berns MW. Photochemotherapy of hypervascular dermal lesions: a possible alternative to photothermal therapy? Lasers Surg Med 1990;10:334–343.
82. Nelson JS. Photodynamic therapy of port wine stain: preliminary clinical studies. SPIE 1993;1876:142–146.
83. Mew D, Lum V, Wat C-K et al. The ability of specific monoclonal antibodies and conventional antisera conjugated to hematoporphyrin to label and kill selected cell lines subsequent to light activation. Cancer Res 1985;45:4380–4386.
84. Jori G, Reddi G, Cozzani I, Tomio L. Controlled targeting of different subcellular sites by porphyrins in tumor bearing mice. Br J Cancer 1986;53:615–621.

IV. Lasers in Clinical Practice

that only 20% of his malpractice suits were due to physician negligence, while 100% stemmed from physician-patient misunderstandings that led to unrealistic patient expectations.[11] He suggested that by making the additional effort to ensure patient comprehension and a shared understanding, physicians could significantly reduce the risk of litigation. In view of the increased patient satisfaction and better health outcome observed when careful informed consent has been achieved,[10,11] the cost-effectiveness of taking the time to ensure it seems irrefutable.

Issues of Body Image and Disfigurement

Many patients who undergo laser treatments expect an aesthetic change in the appearance of their skin, and some seek the amelioration of a long-standing disfigurement. Patients with PWSs are prominent members of the latter subgroup. To best serve patients who undergo treatment for a disfigurement, it is helpful to be somewhat familiar with the social and developmental stresses of a flawed appearance, as well as with the psychosocial effects of laser treatment. After summarizing what is currently known about disfigurement and social development, we will discuss patients' psychosocial responses to the laser treatment of PWSs as well as their long-term adaptation to the results.

GROWING UP DISFIGURED

A large body of research literature on the psychosocial effects of physical attractiveness has documented a panoply of benefits of looking attractive and detriments of looking unattractive.[18–20] Children as young as 3 years of age have been found to judge other children's attractiveness and be influenced by this judgment in their choice of companions in a manner comparable to that of adults.[21]

Numerous researchers interested in the effects of appearance have assessed the responses to people with a disfigurement. In one such study, an actress who appeared to have either a PWS or bruise on one cheek or who had no lesion at all was stationed at a busy downtown street corner.[22] Among the 450 pedestrians who waited for a light and unwittingly served as subjects in the study, it was observed that those who saw the actress with a PWS stood significantly farther away from the woman than those who saw the actress with the bruise and nearly twice as far from the actress with the PWS than those who saw the actress who had neither lesion. Pedestrians tended to stand on the unblemished side of the actress with the PWS to avoid looking at the disfigurement. In another study, actors who wore makeup resembling a PWS and pretended to collapse on a subway train were found to be significantly less likely to receive assistance from other riders than the same actors without a PWS.[23] These findings offer a glimpse of the kind of social exclusion that people with a defect such as a PWS may encounter.

Parallel findings have been observed in children. For example, a research team arranged a 3-week session at a summer camp for 121 children aged 7 through 14, 28 of whom had a variety of obvious physical defects.[24] At the end of the session, the children with physical defects were found to be significantly less preferred as friends than the physically normal children. Other research performed using children between 5 and 12 years of age has revealed that children become more accepting of children with functional impairments (e.g., leg braces) as they grow older but become more rejecting toward children with facial disfigurements.[25] From an intrapsychic perspective, researchers at Boston's Children's Hospital Medical Center have observed that "the continuing stimulus of deformity can interfere with normal psychological maturation and result in the persistence of a primitive and maladaptive defensive structure."[26]

The degree of psychological damage caused by a disfigurement varies considerably from person to person, and parents' behavior toward a disfigured child may account for much of the variation. The parental coping style identified as most conductive to a healthy adaptation is a realistic acknowledgment of the impairment, a willingness to discuss it with the child, and an effort to treat the child in other respects exactly like any other member of the family.[27] Less beneficial coping styles include parental denial of the impairment or an attempt to compensate for it by pampering or sheltering the child.

Parents have increasingly sought to ameliorate their children's impairments through corrective surgery. Studies of patients with a range of maxillofacial and craniofacial impairments have shown that corrective surgery tends to bring about considerable improvements in appearance,[28,29] self-esteem,[28,30] and social functioning.[31] In one study, 91% of patients under 12 years of age and 55% of patients between 12 and 18 years of age were found to feel more confident and self-assured during social interactions after their surgery.[31] Surgery may therefore be most effective when performed at the earliest feasible age, simply because it forestalls the trauma incurred during years of living with a disfigurement.

Pertschuk and Whitaker[32] have reported their findings in patients aged 6 to 50 years who had craniofacial abnormalities. They found that the psychosocial damage resulting from a disfigurement increases and accumulates through at least the young adult years. Their series of patients included two distinct groups of children aged 6 to 13. One group had had major reconstructive surgery before the age of 4 (the "earlier" group) and the other group was scheduled to undergo major reconstructive surgery (the "later" group). Testing revealed that the "earlier" group, who at that time had had their procedures several years before, closely resembled normal, nondisfigured children on a variety of psychosocial measures. In contrast, the later group showed a series of small but measurable deficiencies, including poorer self-concept, greater anxiety, more introversion, and more behavior problems at home and in the classroom. It was found during follow-up that, although surgery led to psychological improvements, it did not obliterate the deficiencies in these children. These findings indicate that disfigurements may cause progressive and increasingly difficult-to-reverse psychosocial damage across the childhood maturational years.

Patients requesting laser treatment for disfigurements will have encountered many of the psychosocial hazards that faced Pertschuk and Whittaker's patients, so that they will frequently be hoping to alleviate not only the physical flaws but also the psychological distress. It is therefore important for laser practitioners to have some idea of the extent of psychosocial improvement that might be expected in disfigured patients. In the sections that follow, we discuss the findings from psychosocial research performed in patients who have undergone laser procedures for the treatment of facial disfigurements.

RESPONSES OF PATIENTS WITH PWSs TO LASER TREATMENT

Although some conditions treated by the laser (e.g., some PWSs) can be quite disfiguring, patients with PWSs who undergo laser treatment are likely to be less disfigured than the patients with craniofacial impairments just discussed. In addition, patients perceive the laser as being quite distinct from conventional surgery, and their expectations of treatment tend to differ accordingly.

Patients' expectations and responses have been examined by Kalick and associates,[33,34] who studied a group of patients with PWSs and their experiences with laser treatment. This study was begun in 1978, when practitioners at Boston's Beth Israel Hospital started using an argon laser to treat PWSs. The psychosocial research sample consisted of 82 consenting patients out of the first hundred who underwent treatment. Patients were asked to complete psychological test instruments after their initial interview with a plastic surgeon and also to return survey materials regarding their experience with having a PWS and their expectations of treatment. Patients were then surveyed several additional times, up until about 18 months after their final treatment (or after dropping out), and retook the psychological tests shortly after the final treatment. A total of 39 patients supplied information at the 18-month follow-up. The initial sample of patients ranged from 7 to 66 years of age, with a median age of 24. Only two of the patients were preadolescents. The sample included 31 male and 51 female patients.

During the pretreatment interview with the surgeon, patients were informed that the risks of treatment included scarring, uneven lightening of the PWS, and failure of the treatment. They were also told that the treatments would cause scabbing and other manifestations of a local wound. (Some of these hazards have been much reduced as the result of subsequent improvements in laser technology and the methods used.) In the survey form patients filled out after they returned home from the initial interview with the plastic surgeon, patients were asked what the surgeon had told them regarding potential hazards of treatment. A quarter of the patients could recall no hazards, and only a few could recall more than one of those just listed. Subsequent surveys revealed that many patients had viewed the laser as producing a magic ray that would do only good and no harm. Patients' difficulty thinking of the laser as an instrument that functions, in effect, by causing controlled tissue damage points to the need for physicians to take pains to educate patients sufficiently regarding the workings of the laser to ensure meaningful informed consent.

The psychological tests given to patients included standardized instruments measuring extroversion, neuroticism, depression, hostility, self-esteem, and several forms of anxiety. The patient sample was not found to be significantly more troubled than normal comparison groups on any of these measures. This finding indicates that PWSs probably constitute somewhat less of a life stress than craniofacial disfigurements or other flaws in appearance that have been studied.[35,36] Furthermore, the severity of the PWSs, defined as a composite of the lesion size and color, was not found to correlate significantly with any of the personality measures. It should be noted, however, that the normal test scores for the group as a whole do not imply that the group was free of individual patients with psychological impairments.[37]

Most patients in the research sample required laser treatments spaced several months apart and performed over 1 year or more, with the final degree of lightening apparent only some months after treatment. A follow-up assessment was therefore conducted 18 months after completion of the treatment so that patients could evaluate their responses in light of the ultimate aesthetic effects of treatment as well as of their relatively fresh recollections of the treatment itself.

At the last follow-up assessment, patients were asked how satisfied they were with the laser treatments and what effects the improvement in appearance had had on their lives. On the basis of the theory that a patient's response to treatment may in part be determined by preexisting character dispositions, the research team wanted to find out whether any of the pretreatment personality measures could help predict subsequent patient satisfaction. In this regard, only one pretreatment personality measure, extroversion, was found to successfully predict posttreatment satisfaction. Interestingly, however, this measure was not found to significantly correlate with interim measures of satisfaction during treatment but only after it was completed. Apparently the more outgoing patients were better able to integrate the improvements in appearance that most patients obtained into their social and personal lives.

Several other factors were tested as predictors of patient satisfaction at the end of the follow-up period. One of these was the patient's sex, and in this regard, male and female patients were found to evaluate the effects of treatment about equally. The surface area of the PWS was one of the factors that did prove to be a significant predictor, in that patients who had larger PWSs tended to be more dissatisfied in the end, perhaps because their birthmark was more likely to fade unevenly. This source of dissatisfaction may be eliminated through improvements in the laser treatment. In the survey materials each patient filled out after the first laser session, the patient was asked how pleased he or she was with the overall manner of the physician and staff of the laser clinic. This initial rating proved to be strongly related to the satisfaction with the laser treatments patients felt at the end of the follow-up period; in fact, it proved to be a better predictor than any of the pretreatment personality measures. This finding once again underlines the importance of clinician-patient rapport to the success of treatment.

As noted earlier, all of the pretreatment psychological tests were administered again after the final treatment. None of the personality measures showed a significant improvement across this period, and each final measure was strongly correlated with the respective initial measure. This finding indicates that personality structure is unlikely to change greatly during adulthood and that it is more realistic to hope treatments will produce benefits by leading to improvements in the patient's coping mechanisms within an established personality structure.

Before the start of treatment and again after its completion, patients were asked to rate their degree of satisfaction with same-sex relationships, opposite-sex relationships, themselves as people, and life in general. Only satisfaction with opposite-sex relationships was found to improve significantly during the treatment period. Apparently this is the arena in which a blemish and its amelioration tend to carry the most weight.

At the time of the final treatment, 93% of the patients expressed slight, moderate, or great satisfaction at having taken part in the treatment program and only 7% expressed some degree of dissatisfaction. Many commented that, even if their PWS had not faded as fully as they had hoped, they were still pleased at having tried something new and different rather than sitting back and doing nothing. However, in the survey conducted 18 months after completion of the treatment, it was found that the percentage of patients satisfied with treatment had declined to 66%, with 16% dissatisfied and 17% neutral. Perhaps by then their pride in having been pioneer patients in a new treatment had diminished. After reviewing all the survey materials, including many lengthy written comments, the research team concluded that the laser treatment program, even when medically quite successful, was but one of many events in each patient's life, an event patients would ultimately use to the extent their existing resources for personal growth and self-fulfillment allowed.

CASE STUDIES OF LONG-TERM ADAPTATION TO LASER TREATMENT

Becker[38] studied the long-term adaptation of 19 patients to laser treatment who had begun argon laser treatment for their PWSs an average of 7.5 years before. Sixteen of these 19 subjects had taken part in the study conducted by Kalick and associates, and Becker approached them an average of 4 years after their final contact with Kalick and associates. Becker studied the patients' accounts of their social behavior throughout their lifetimes ("object relations") using semistructured interviews and paper-and-pencil measures. A standardized instrument developed by Blatt and associates (unpublished paper) was used to assess "object representations," which are essentially one's conceptions of the important people in one's life. Additionally, an independent professional photographer was asked to objectively rate the ultimate change in the PWSs on the basis of before and after color slides of the patients.

The sample consisted on 11 female and 8 male patients who had ranged in age from 14 to 55 years at the time of their first laser treatment; their average age at that time was 31 years. These patients represented a range of treatment regimens, from one patient who refused further treatment because of an unsuccessful test patch to two who each underwent 10 treatments. The average number of treatments was 5.6, and the success of treatment ranged from virtually complete lightening to scarring.

Patients were defined as having adapted well to the laser treatment to the extent that they met the following criteria: their facial defect had a relatively small effect on their personal and social functioning; there was minimal evidence that they saw the PWS as a central factor explaining others' behavior toward them; and they showed evidence of objectivity in evaluating the laser treatments, including the clinic staff and the treatment proper.

The patients who had better cosmetic outcomes were not found to necessarily be better adapted than those with a less favorable cosmetic result, indicating that it is not just the physical outcome that determines the adaptation process. Of 15 subjects judged from slides to have had good treatment results, nine were found to have adapted well and six were found to have adapted poorly. Of four subjects judged to have had poor results, three had adapted well and one had adapted poorly. The sample size is too small to allow for statistical analysis, however.

Among the patients who adapted well to the treatment, most classified their PWS as being more lightened than did the independent rater who compared pretreatment and posttreatment slides. They also reported that their PWS was less of a daily concern after treatment. Regardless of the physical results, these patients felt satisfaction at having made the effort to seek treatment.

We present in the following sections case materials on Becker's two counterintuitive subsamples: the patients showing limited results but good adaptation, and the patients showing good results but limited adaptation. We describe these two outcomes because they seem more in need of explanation than the outcomes in the two other subgroups.

Limited Result, Good Adaptation

An example of someone whose treatment was relatively unsuccessful in lightening her PWS but who was happy with the results is a patient we will call Karen. Her PWS was large, covering an irregular area from her forehead to under her chin. It was also moderately dark and mottled in texture and color. At the time of her initial interview she was 51 years old, married, and the mother of three children. She was employed as a high school science teacher.

As a child her parents had tried to help her to see her advantages in many aspects of life, and they had "downplayed" her PWS, often saying "it isn't that bad." She grew up in a neighborhood where everyone knew everyone else, and she felt accepted and protected. As she got older and left her neighborhood, she developed strategies for dealing with new people and making them and herself comfortable. For example, she cultivated an outgoing, friendly interpersonal style. She also began to regularly use an opaque makeup to conceal the PWS.

Karen believed that her birthmark had become lighter as the result of treatment and that this made it easier for her to conceal the PWS with makeup. By her own estimate she was 70% to 80% satisfied with the overall results. During treatment she took considerable scientific interest in the laser procedure and focused her attention on the change in appearance she felt was being accomplished. After treatment, she switched her concerns about her facial appearance from her PWS to her whole face and the signs of aging in her skin, which she could accept as a normal situation she could not change.

Another example of a patient who showed a good adjustment to both a severe PWS and a disappointing treatment result is a patient we will call Linda, who when interviewed was a single, 30-year-old bank executive. Her PWS was one of the most severe of those in the sample; it covered nearly the entire left side of her face and was a dark and irregular purple. Unfortunately, her laser treatment was relatively unsuccessful because of scarring and had to be discontinued.

As a child she had come to accept the PWS as a reasonably comfortable part of herself. She had developed a positive sense of self in an emotionally satisfying relationship with her parents. The interviewer felt her responses were proportionate to the normal vicissitudes of life. Her view of others reflected empathy for their needs and emotions rather than merely hinging on how they addressed her needs.

She saw herself as being more than average attractive and stated that she did not feel the PWS affected her overall attractiveness. As was generally true of the well-adjusted patients, she exuded a feeling of self-confidence and ease that overcame any discomfort on the part of the perceiver.

Her view of herself and others was sophisticated and cognitively complex. Despite the severity of her PWS, she never let it hold her back from making friends or entering social or business situations. Her friendships were vibrant and long lasting, many going back to early in her life. She felt that her PWS was rarely a key factor in deciding the nature of her relationships, but that this was determined by her overall personality. Although not married at 30, she felt that this was perhaps a price she had paid for her rise in the business world and that it was also partly due to chance. She was currently dating and felt satisfied with her life.

Linda's adaptation to the discontinuation of treatment was characteristic of much of her functioning: she found and focused on the positive aspects of the experience. She felt it had been incumbent on her to try laser treatment, and now that she knew its outcome for her she was freed of having to occupy herself with further concerns about it. She was thus better able to get on with her life.

Good Result, Limited Adaptation

A sizable minority of six patients did not adapt well to relatively good treatment results. Five judged their PWSs to be less lightened than did the independent rater. All six patients expressed mild to strong dissatisfaction with their participation in treatment and with the physical results.

During the initial interview these patients expressed extremely high expectations regarding both the physical improvement and the improvement in their lives as a result of treatment. The loneliness, alienation, and dissatisfaction that they continued to experience after treatment they attributed to a failure of the treatment. They tended to experience their PWSs in harsh, severe ways; they were more upset by them than other patients with birthmarks of comparable severity. Specifically, they perceived their PWSs as a central focus of their functioning, often attributing their lack of love, happiness, or success in personal or business relationships to other people's perception of their PWS. They were unable to compensate behaviorally or cognitively for what they lacked in their appearance.

Sarah is an example of someone whose treatment was relatively successful in lightening her PWS but who was unhappy with the results. At the time of being interviewed, she was 38 years old, unmarried, and living with her widowed mother. Like Karen, who was described earlier, she was employed as a high school teacher. However, Sarah's PWS was much lighter than Karen's and a quarter the size. It covered a roughly triangular area, starting below her right eye and extending to the upper corner of her mouth.

As a child and an adolescent Sarah did not like pursuing the activities she felt girls were expected to pursue. She felt all her problems "stemmed from the insecurity" of having a PWS and that throughout her life she needed "security against strangers." She noted that because she felt unattractive as the result of her PWS, instead of trying to make the most of her appearance, she "went the opposite extreme and said I don't care what I look like. I wore my hair long and straight, I wore glasses, I pretended that I was a super jock and I didn't care about guys and what I looked like and it didn't matter."

Sarah acknowledged that there was some lightening of her PWS after laser treatment. However, she still felt very unattractive and thought that when she met new people the only thing they looked at or were concerned with was her PWS. She had a hard time justifying her participation in the laser treatment, and in reviewing it she stressed the pain, inconvenience, and expense of the procedure rather than any resulting benefits.

Ronald is an example of a patient with a large birthmark who also adjusted poorly to the relatively successful results of laser treatment. At the time of his initial interview he was 34 years old and living with his mother. His PWS was extensive and dark; taking up a third of the right side of his face, it partly surrounded his eye and extended to his cheek and the side of his nose. Laser treatment had significantly lightened the PWS, which he ignored, focusing instead on slight scarring. He worked as a draftsman, a skill he had acquired after holding a variety of blue collar jobs. He had few close friends, and those he did have were from marginal groups such as motorcyclists and street people.

As was typical of the patients showing poor adjustment, Ronald had significant difficulty throughout the interview communicating his feelings and was largely unable to provide an organized account of his past. His affect was flat, except for some angry, sarcastic, and depressed qualities.

As a child, Ronald had had a distant and cold relationship with his father. He described it as "John Wayne like, no hugging allowed." Beginning in his earliest years and continuing into adulthood, he had had problems first with his parents and then with other authority figures. He continually felt "put upon because all everyone sees is, you know, the birthmark." His transition from childhood, through adolescence, and into adulthood was characterized by unhappiness and turmoil. For him the overriding factor in his social and emotional situation was his facial abnormality.

One of the most distinct features of the poorly adapted patients with PWSs was the cognitive role the PWS played as an organizer of mental representations of the self in social interaction. The poorly adapted patients dogmatically explained their life situations such that their PWS was a central rather than peripheral factor. Ronald claimed that his earliest memory was a traumatic one, in which his best friend told him he was ugly because of his PWS, and he asserted that his lifelong unhappiness was due to "people trying to make me unhappy [by], staring at me because I'm different." His assessment of the state of his life at the time of the posttreatment interview was unaltered despite a considerable lightening of his PWS.

Adaptation to Disfigurement and Treatment

A noteworthy finding from the retrospective review of the interview data was the persistence of patients' long-term adaptation, or maladaptation, to their PWS and the results of treatment. That is, patients who as children had had difficulty adapting to their PWS generally had difficulty adapting as teenagers and as adults. Conversely, those patients who appeared to have a good start in childhood generally continued to do well in adolescence and adulthood, and superimposed on this was a more subtle trend toward improvement. Most of the developmental changes that occurred in these patients were in the direction of greater health and adaptation.

Adolescence was the time all patients singled out as the most difficult developmental period of their lives. All described adolescence as a trying time in which they felt removed from the protection of childhood. What distinguished one patient from another was his or her ability to integrate, adapt to, and mature in response to the changes brought on by adolescence. Because of the effect of disfigurement on the maturational process already discussed, clearly the earlier in life laser treatment can be accomplished successfully, the greater the mental health benefits.

The laser treatment in these patients with PWSs posed a challenging developmental transition in itself. Having lived all their lives with their birthmark, they tended to regard the treatment in part as a loss of personal identity and history. For each patient in the study, the PWS was replete with personal symbolism and significance, having been in some measure an organizer of their experience of themselves in the world. After the laser treatments, the patients needed time to heal both physically and psychologically.

An example of temporary ambivalence to PWS amelioration is provided by a patient we will call Andrea. At the time of her retrospective interview she was a 26-year-old, single woman working in a professional capacity and pursuing an active social life. She acknowledged the effectiveness of laser treatment in lightening a relatively small PWS on her neck, but the price was that she "lost a part of my childhood identity." She had felt that her PWS had made her unique when she was little, although in adolescence it had caused her discomfort because it looked like a mark made during sex play. After successful treatment, it took her some time to comprehend that the PWS had been a symbol of her uniqueness, not the source of it. In her retrospective interview she was able to say that "now I'm very unique in my own way, but at the age of 17 I felt that I had lost something that was me; it was like losing a parent or something; it was part of me."

One question all patients were asked was "What is the positive side to having a PWS birthmark?" Most patients had been unable to find anything positive about the PWS they had had all their lives. It was only some of the better-adjusted patients such as Linda who were able to find something to be thankful for. She described how it had been an opportunity for her to make friendships "on a higher level than just a material one," and that, in coping with her birthmark, she had been able to develop empathy and to go beyond outward appearances to the true nature of relationships.

References

1. DiMatteo MR. A social-psychological analysis of physician-patient rapport: toward a science of the art of medicine. J Soc Issues 1979;35(1): 12–33.
2. Buller MK, Buller DB. Physician's communication style and patient satisfaction. J Health Soc Behav 1987;28:375–388.
3. Street RL. Communicative styles and adaptations in physician-patient consultations. Soc Sci Med 1992;34:1155–1163.
4. Kaplan RM. Health-related quality of life in patient decision making. J Soc Issues 1991;47(4):69–90.
5. Speedling EJ, Rose DN. Building an effective doctor-patient relationship: from patient satisfaction to patient participation. Soc Sci Med 1985; 21(2):115–120.
6. Kaplan SH, Greenfield S, Ware JE. Assessing the effects of physician-patient interactions on the outcomes of chronic disease. Med Care 1989; 27:S110–S127.
7. Egbert L, Battit G, Welch C, Bartlett M. Reduction of post-operative pain by encouragement and instruction of patients: a study of doctor-patient rapport. N Engl J Med 1964;270:825–827.
8. Seeman M, Seeman TE. Health behavior and personal autonomy: a longitudinal study of the sense of control in illness. J Health Soc Behav 1983;24:144–160.
9. Korsch BM, Gozzi EK, Francis V. Gaps in doctor-patient communication. I: Doctor-patient interaction and patient satisfaction. Pediatrics 1968; 42:855–871.
10. Lidz CW, Appelbaum PS, Meisel JD. Two models of implementing informed consent. Arch Intern Med 1988;148:1385–1389.
11. Green JA. Minimizing malpractice risks by role clarification: the confusing transition from tort to contract. Ann Intern Med 1988;109:234–241.
12. Cole NM. Informed consent: considerations in aesthetic and reconstructive surgery of the breast. Clin Plast Surg 1988;15:541–548.
13. Kyler-Hutchison P. Ethical reasoning and informed consent in occupational therapy. Am J Occup Ther 1988;42(5):283–287.
14. Wu WC, Pearlman RA. Consent in medical decision making: the role of communication. J Gen Intern Med 1988;3(Jan/Feb):9–14.
15. Byrne DJ, Napier A, Cuschieri A. How informed is signed consent? BMJ 1988;296:839–840.
16. Taub HA, Baker MT, Kline GE, Sturr JF. Comprehension of informed consent information by young-old through old-old volunteers. Exp Aging Res 1987;13(4):173–178.
17. Faden RR, Beauchamp TL. A history and theory of informed consent. New York: Oxford University Press, 1986.
18. Berscheid E, Walster E. Physical attractiveness. In: Berkowitz L, ed. Ad-

vances in experimental social psychology, Vol 7. New York: Academic Press, 1974;157–215.

19. Bull R, Rumsey N. The social psychology of facial appearance. New York: Springer-Verlag, 1988.

20. Kalick SM. Toward an interdisciplinary psychology of appearances. Psychiatry 1978;41:243–253.

21. Dion KK. Young children's stereotyping of facial attractiveness. Dev Psychol 1973;9:183–188.

22. Rumsey N, Bull R, Gahagan D. The effect of facial disfigurement on the proxemic behavior of the general public. J Appl Soc Psychol 1982;12:137–150.

23. Piliavin IM, Piliavin JA, Rodin J. Costs, diffusion, and the stigmatized victim. J Person Soc Psychol 1976;32:429–438.

24. Kleck RE, DeJong W. Physical disability, physical attractiveness, and social outcomes in children's small groups. Rehab Psychol 1983;28:79–91.

25. Richardson S. Age and sex differences in values toward physical handicaps. J Health Soc Behav 1970;11:207–214.

26. Belfer ML, Harrison AM, Murray JE. Body image and the process of reconstructive surgery. Am J Dis Child 1979;133:532–535.

27. Lauer E. The family. In: Macgregor FC, Abel TM, Bryt A, Lauer E, Weissman S. Facial deformities and plastic surgery. Springfield, IL: Thomas, 1953;103–129.

28. Arndt EM, Travis F, Lefebvre A, Niec A, Munro IR. Beauty and the eye of the beholder: social consequences and personal adjustments for facial patients. Br J Plast Surg 1986;39:81–84.

29. Barden RC, Ford ME, Wilhelm W, Rogers-Salyer M, Salyer KE. The physical attractiveness of facially deformed patients before and after craniofacial surgery. Plast Reconstr Surg 1988;82:229–235.

30. Lefebvre A, Barclay S. Psychosocial impact of craniofacial deformities before and after reconstructive surgery. Can J Psychiatry 1982;27:579–583.

31. Phillips J, Whitaker LA. The social effects of craniofacial deformity and its correction. Cleft Palate J 1979;16:7–15.

32. Pertschuk MJ, Whitaker LA. Psychosocial considerations in craniofacial deformity. Clin Plast Surg 1987;14:163–168.

33. Kalick SM. Laser treatment of port wine stains: observations concerning psychological outcome. In: Arndt KA, Noe JM, Rosen S, eds. Cutaneous laser therapy: principles and methods. New York: Wiley, 1983;215–229.

34. Kalick SM, Goldwyn RM, Noe JM. Social issues and body image concerns of port wine stain patients undergoing laser therapy. Lasers Surg Med 1981;1:205–213.

35. Edgerton MT, Jacobson WE, Meyer E. Surgical-psychiatric study of patients seeking plastic (cosmetic) surgery: ninety-eight consecutive patients with minimal deformity. Br J Plast Surg 1961;13:136–145.

36. Reich J. The surgery of appearance: psychological and related aspects. Med J Aust 1969;2:5–13.

37. Lanigan SW, Cotterill JA. Psychological disabilities amongst patients with port wine stains. Br J Dermatol 1989;121:209–215.

38. Becker MF. The role of object representations in the response of patients of the argon laser treatment of their port wine stains. Unpublished doctoral dissertation, Smith College School for Social Work, Northampton, Massachusetts, 1991.

19 ___ Hazards Associated with the Use of Lasers

Kenneth A. Arndt

When used properly and with adequate precautions, lasers are safe instruments. However, like other surgical tools, their use by those unaware of the hazards or untrained in their proper use can lead to substantial difficulties.[1] This chapter has therefore been prepared with the goal of describing these hazards and ways to prevent them. Following are the topics covered:

1. The magnitude of medical laser accidents
2. Proper use of the machinery and avoidance of inadvertent electric discharge
3. Environmental hazards and the problems of fire and explosion
4. Patient- and personnel-related hazards and eye safety
5. Hazards of the laser plume

The Magnitude of Medical Laser Accidents

Since the early 1980s, the U.S. Food and Drug Administration (FDA) has required that laser manufacturers and importers report information to them which might reasonably indicate that one of their devices may have caused or contributed to a death or serious injury or has malfunctioned. Such medical device injury and death data for 1985 to mid-1992 are provided in Table 19-1. More detailed information has also been provided by the FDA regarding all incidents reported to them from late 1984 to March 1989 (Tables 19-2 through 19-8), and this is useful for analyzing the hazards associated with laser surgery. However, this information does not represent a complete listing of laser surgery–related incidents, because during these years health care facilities were not bound by the reporting requirements and therefore submitted incident reports to the FDA only on a voluntary basis. Although most hospitals have notified manufacturers of laser malfunctions, and often of accidents, some health care facilities have seen no need to pass on such information. Because of the passage of the Safe Medical Devices Act of 1990, "user facilities" are required to report incidents in which a medical device may have

Table 19-1. Summary of injuries related to laser treatment: 1985–mid 1992

Year	No. of reports	No. of injuries	Location and comment
1985	6	3	Eye (3)
1986	10	7	Eye (5), tube fire (1), bronchus (1)
1987	8	5	Eye (3), bladder (1), hysterectomy (1*)
1988	14	9	Eye (2), burns (5), hysterectomy (2)
1989	18	10	Eye (2), burns (2), hysterectomy (2)
1990	36	16	Eye (1), burns (3), embolism (2) (3*)
1991	39	18	Eye (6), burns (6), embolism (1)
1992	5	5	Eye (4), burns (1)

*Death.
Source: Data from SS Charschan. Laser safety incident records illustrate deficiencies in reporting and training. J Laser App Fall, 1992;13–14.

been responsible for causing or contributing to the death of a patient or to a serious injury or illness. Hospitals must also submit to the FDA a semiannual summary of all device-related incidents. All of this results in the compilation of more detailed and complete information, and along with this the FDA has the authority to directly regulate most health care facilities.

Of the 134 incidents recorded in the 1984 to 1989 FDA material, 78 involved injury or death, 45 were considered serious, 26 were considered minor, and 7 resulted in death (see Table 19-3).[2] Most injuries involved either inappropriate exposure of the eye during ophthalmic procedures or accidental eye exposure in non-ophthalmic settings, totaling 42 (75%). The second most common injury was thermal burns, of which there were 19 (34%) (see Table 19-4). Many incidents involved malfunction of the laser, with several practitioners noting unexpected firing of the laser beam (see Table 19-5). In these situations, personnel were in a setting where exposure to the laser was unlikely, and therefore protective eyewear was not being worn.

Although lasers are extremely complex and highly sophisticated, they are still technologically in their youth. Although there are multiple safety systems built into all lasers, many of them redundant, these devices cannot be counted on to automatically protect the laser sur-

Table 19-2. Laser-related incidents reported to FDA during late 1984 to March 1989

Injury	No. of incidents	Percentage of incidents
Injury resulted	78	58
No injury resulted	56	42

Source: From FDA incident report a sobering reminder of laser perils. Clin Laser Monthly 1989;7:97–101. Reproduced with permission.

Table 19-3.   Breakdown of extent of laser-related injury

Extent of injury	No. of incidents	Percentage
Death	7	5
Serious	45	34
Minor	26	19
None	56	42

Source: From FDA incident report a sobering reminder of laser perils. Clin Laser Monthly 1989;7:97–101. Reproduced with permission.

geon and all those in the laser suite, because human error is too often a factor in the incidents that occur. For example, laser safety switches will not work if they are not engaged or they are ignored. Accidents have also occurred when, for example, surgeons have failed to put a laser in the standby mode, placed the articulated arm of a CO_2 laser on the patient's chest, or failed to ensure that all in the operating room were wearing appropriate eye protection.

It is the patient, however, who is at greatest risk from a laser-related accident (see Table 19-6), as pointed up by the fact that 75% of those injured were patients. Most incidents have occurred during a medical procedure (see Table 19-7), but it was rare that such incidents resulted from surgical error. Ten percent of those injured were medical team members. Most incidents occurred during ophthalmic procedures (28 [21%]), and only two (2%) were associated with the treatment of cutaneous lesions (see Table 19-8). The lasers most often involved in medical laser incidents are listed in Table 19-9.

The FDA classification of lasers, the hazards posed by each, and the control measures that come with the laser or to be observed with each are summarized in Table 19-10.

Two reports in which laser surgery was evaluated have been published since the latest FDA publication. A 1993 report was of a multi-center survey that reviewed the adverse reactions to laser surgery, the nature of malpractice suits filed by or on behalf of patients, and the compensation awarded, from among 94,872 laser surgery cases

Table 19-4.   Breakdown by type of laser-related incident

Type of injury	No. of incidents	Percentage
Inappropriate or excessive eye exposure	42	31
Burn	19	14
Airway fire	7	5
Other or undetermined	10	8
None	56	42

Source: From FDA incident report a sobering reminder of laser perils. Clin Laser Monthly 1989;7:97–101. Reproduced with permission.

Table 19-5.   Breakdown of laser-related incidents by cause

Potential cause	No. of incidents	Percentage
Laser malfunction	74	48
Lapse in safety precautions	16	10
Surgical error	8	5
Medical complication	14	9
Inconclusive/unknown	26	17
Maintenance deficiency	12	8
Not applicable	4	3
TOTAL	154	

Source: From FDA incident report a sobering reminder of laser perils. Clin Laser Monthly 1989;7:97–101. Reproduced with permission.

Table 19-6.   Breakdown of laser-related injuries by person injured

Person injured	No. of incidents	Percentage
Patient	56	72
Medical team member	8	10
Maintenance person	8	10
Other	6	8

Source: From FDA incident report a sobering reminder of laser perils. Clin Laser Monthly 1989;7:97–101. Reproduced with permission.

Table 19-7.   Breakdown of laser-related incidents by circumstances

Situation	No. of incidents	Percentage
During testing	90	67
During testing or maintenance	34	25
Unknown or not applicable	10	8

Source: From FDA incident report a sobering reminder of laser perils. Clin Laser Monthly 1989;7:97–101. Reproduced with permission.

Table 19-8.   Breakdown of laser-related incidents by specialty

Medical specialty	No. of incidents	Percentage
Ophthalmology	28	21
Obstetrics and gynecology	7	5
Otolaryngology/pulmonology	10	7
Urology	3	2
General surgery	3	2
Dermatology	2	2
Neurology	1	1
Not specified or not applicable	80	60

Source: From FDA incident report a sobering reminder of laser perils. Clin Laser Monthly 1989;7:97–101. Reproduced with permission.

Table 19-9. Breakdown of laser-related incidents by type of laser

Type of laser	No. of incidents	Percentage
CO_2	35	26
Nd:YAG	43	32
Argon	17	13
Argon dye	3	2
KTP	5	4
Argon/krypton	3	2
Contact Nd:YAG	5	4
Laser accessory	2	1
Unknown	21	16

Source: From FDA incident report a sobering reminder of laser perils. Clin Laser Monthly 1989;7:97–101. Reproduced with permission.

from 44 hospitals in 23 states in the United States dealt with over a 6-year period. Of those injured, 28 were patients (0.13%), and 13 of the injuries were major, 11 were burns, and 4 were other types of injuries. The authors concluded that laser surgery is safe and associated with a low risk of adverse reactions and malpractice claims if practiced in a hospital environment with a very good quality assurance system.[3] Rockwell[4] reviewed laser accidents recorded in a large data base, which had information on 272 such events occurring during 1964 to 1994. Eye injuries were the most common and constituted more than 73% of all incidents. Skin injuries accounted for 9.9%, and fire was involved in 7.3%. The CO_2 laser was responsible for 56% of the skin burns and was the laser most commonly involved in laser-produced fires. The Nd:YAG laser was responsible for 14.7% of skin injuries and was the laser next most commonly involved in laser-induced fires. Overall, the lasers most commonly involved in such incidents were the Nd:YAG laser (29.7%), the argon laser (20.5%), the CO_2 laser (12.8%), and dye lasers (9.9%). Technicians were the most frequently involved (21.3%) in the 272 events, followed by scientists (17.6%) and patients (12.9%). Physicians and nurses were involved in 25 of the incidents (8.4%).

Proper Use of Lasers and Avoidance of Inadvertent Electrical Discharge

To generate a coherent beam of light, laser systems use a high-voltage power supply, which necessitates the use of high-voltage connections to permit passage of the beam through plasma tubes. Charges on capacitors within the laser may exceed 1000 volts, and currents in discharge circuits may be as high as several thousand amperes. It is therefore essential for anyone using such high voltages to know the instrument well and to be able to prevent unintended electrical discharge.[5] Safety controls built directly into the medical lasers include

Table 19-10. Summary of laser characteristics by FDA class

FDA	Laser	Injury	Hazard	Control measures
Class I	Very low power laser systems that cannot emit radiation in excess of maximum permissible exposure levels	None	Safe to vision	Warning sign at access panel of laser products
Class II	Visible-light–emitting lasers that do not have enough power to injure a person accidentally but that may produce retinal injury if viewed directly for more than 0.25 second	Eye	Chronic if exposure is longer than 1000 seconds	Protective housing, signs: "CAUTION" and "DO NOT STARE DIRECTLY INTO THE BEAM"; indicator showing "LASER BEAM ON"
Class IIIa	Includes medium power lasers producing visible light that cannot cause injury if viewed directly with the unaided eye but may cause retinal damage if the energy is focused into the eye	Eye	Safe for brief viewing (less than 0.25 second); chronic if exposure is any longer	Engineering controls, protective eyewear, administrative controls, warning signs
Class IIIb	Includes medium power lasers that can cause accidental injury if viewed directly; intrabeam viewing of either direct or mirrorlike reflection of the beam is hazardous	Eye and skin	Not safe for brief viewing of direct beam or specular reflections	Engineering controls, protective eyewear, administrative controls, warning signs
Class IV	High power lasers that produce a hazardous direct beam or specular reflection and a hazardous diffuse reflection resulting in a significant skin hazard	Eye	Not safe for momentary viewing of direct or scattered radiation; fix hazard	Engineering controls, protective eyewear, administrative controls, warning signs

both enclosed and interlocked systems. These function to shield both the user and the patient from high-voltage sources. Interlock systems automatically shut off the power when the cover of the laser is removed. However, most lasers have override switches that permit the laser to be operated when the interlocks are open. Such switches are meant to be used only by specially trained maintenance personnel during servicing of the laser, and all high-voltage capacitors must be grounded when the personnel are working in power supply regions with these switches on. Additionally, it is necessary for personnel to use special insulated tools when aligning mirror systems in an area with a high electrical potential. It is also imperative for them to guard against inadvertent discharge of the laser beam during maintenance. Accidental deflection of the beam may, for example, result in serious injury to the eye.

Surveys evaluating laser-associated accidents have revealed that electrical accidents are much more frequent than injuries to the skin or eye caused by the laser radiation. Several instances of electrocution associated with laser use have been noted in the FDA report as well as in anecdotal case reports. At least five such deaths are known to have occurred as the result of carelessness while working around high-voltage laser power supplies. The growing list of fatalities occurring in people working on lasers, including seven between 1987 and 1991, further stresses the importance of electrical safety training for service personnel and others requiring access to laser power supplies.

Environmental Hazards and the Problems of Fire and Explosion

Accidents occurring in places where lasers are used are often due to the inadvertent discharge of the laser beam at an unintended light-absorbing compound or substance. Perhaps the most frequent type of laser accident is fire or explosion. Because laser light generates heat when absorbed, combustion is always a potential hazard. Lasers must never be used in the presence of explosive or flammable materials or an oxygen-enhanced anesthetic gas mixture.[6,7] This is pointed up by the case of a child who was undergoing treatment for a port-wine stain using a flashlamp-pumped, pulsed dye laser and who suffered hair and skin burns when the heat generated by the impact of the laser radiation on surface hair ignited the oxygen associated with oxygen insufflation during ketamine anesthesia.[8] The incendiary potential of this dye laser has been investigated by measuring the flammability of surgical materials and of hair in 21% to 100% oxygen and in nitrous oxide at fluences commonly used in laser therapy.[7] Hair was found to ignite easily in 100% oxygen but in room air only when struck repeatedly. Moistening the hair was noted to markedly decrease the potential for ignition. Gauze ignited in 100% oxygen, and green nasal cannula prongs were extremely flammable in this setting. Fire-retardant fabrics are available both for surgical drapes and gowns. A further problem is that some plastics and Teflon are not only combustible but they may also release toxic fumes when burning. Therefore it is essential to eliminate combustible explosive or potentially toxic materials from the treatment area to ensure a safe operation.[9] A recent article[9a] reviewed the literature on the ignition potential of the pulsed-dye laser and emphasized the risk of flash fires, particularly in patients receiving oxygen by face mask or nasal cannula.

It is equally important to be certain that the laser beam does not inadvertently discharge. Switches that must be engaged to operate medical lasers usually include a key, an on-off toggle switch, an enabling button, a beam shutter, and a hand or foot switch. In many systems, at least two activating switches need to be triggered for the beam to be discharged. To prevent someone from inadvertently activating the laser by accidentally stepping on a foot switch, foot pedals must have adequate protective guards so that the operator's foot must be placed inside the guard cavity to activate the machine.

Unintended discharge most frequently occurs near the patient, but the laser may be misfired in any direction. For this reason, the laser surgical suite must be totally enclosed and protected from unauthorized or unexpected entry. Proper safety features in a laser suite include a locked door; opaque, nonflammable shades for windows, which are sufficiently thick to absorb light from any of the lasers in use in the suite; and the posting of appropriate signs indicating that lasers are in use. All personnel in the laser treatment area are potentially at risk and must wear the same protective devices as the patient.

The principal thermal effects of laser exposure are related to several factors; these are the absorption and scattering coefficients of tissue at the particular laser wavelength; the irradiance or radiant exposure of the laser beam; the duration of the exposure and the pulse repetition rate; the extent of the local blood flow; and the size of the area irradiated. The levels of visible and infrared radiation necessary to injure the skin are quite high, in that at least several watts per square centimeter are usually required to cause thermal injury. The threshold of injury also depends on the duration of exposure, the area of skin affected, and the wavelength. The irradiance required to produce injury increases as the exposure duration decreases, starting at exposures of less than 0.5 seconds. The thresholds for skin injury associated with the use of high-energy pulsed lasers generally range from approximately 0.2 to 0.4 J/cm^2 (for Q-switched ruby lasers), depending on the pigmentation of the skin. The thresholds for injury associated with continuous-wave lasers are always greater than 1 W/cm^2 and are highly dependent on the duration of exposure.

Laser-associated hazards and the protection necessary to ensure safe use vary with the type of laser used. As noted earlier, the CO_2 and Nd:YAG lasers pose a higher risk of fire, because they are often used at higher powers and have a much broader absorbance spectrum than visible-light lasers. Argon, dye, and other continuous-wave lasers are associated with a lower risk of fire stemming from the inadvertent absorption of the laser light. Tunable dye lasers, however, are not only associated with fire hazards but also with exposure to toxic fumes released by the solvents used.

Patient- and Personnel-Related Hazards and Ocular Hazards

OCULAR HAZARDS

Ocular injuries are the most serious of those encountered in laser use. The eye may be exposed either directly to the laser beam or indirectly to a reflected beam. Both can be equally damaging. Unlike the light emitted from a light bulb, laser light is of extremely high intensity. For example, a small, relatively low power CO_2 laser can generate intensities on the order of 10^5 W/cm², and this is related primarily to the ability to tightly focus laser light to a small-diameter beam. As a result, laser irradiation of the eye can cause serious damage. It has been estimated that one to two laser-related eye accidents occur each week in the United States.

Ultraviolet (UV) light in the UVC wavelengths (200–315 nm) and to some extent in the UVB wavelengths (315–400 nm) is absorbed in the cornea, and excessive exposure of the eye may produce photophobia, with redness and tearing, splitting of the corneal surface cell layer (exfoliation), and stromal haze. This represents the syndrome of photokeratitis, or Welder's flash, that develops after damage to the outer epithelial cell layer of the cornea. This most often occurs after short-term exposures to light in the UVB and UVC regions.

UV light in the 315- to 400-nm range is absorbed by the lens and may contribute to cataract formation. However, because the cornea, lens, and ocular media are largely transparent, light in the visible (400–780 nm) and near-infrared (780–1400 nm) portions of the electromagnetic spectrum is transmitted through the media with little loss and focused on a retinal spot that is 10 to 20 μm in diameter. This happens because the cornea and the lens focus the light so that the radiation incident on the cornea is increased approximately 100,000 times at the retina. Under normal circumstances, only about 5% of the incident radiation is used for vision. The rest of the absorbed energy is converted into heat, and if this is above threshold, it can cause an irreversible burn.

CO_2 laser radiation is absorbed by water. When light at this wavelength (10,600 nm), which is in the infrared portion of the spectrum, impacts the eye, it is absorbed in the cornea and the degree of corneal damage that occurs depends on the duration of exposure. To protect the eye from such damage, wraparound glasses must be worn by all in the laser room from the time the laser is activated until it is turned off, and not simply when the actual treatment is taking place.

The most serious retinal injury occurs in the macula, resulting in blindness that can develop after an exposure so short it will not have been visible. Because such focusing can cause intensities high enough to damage the retina, light in the 400- to 1400-nm region is particularly hazardous to the eye. For example, the blue-green radiation of the argon laser and the yellow radiation of the 577- to 585-nm tunable dye lasers are well absorbed by hemoglobin in the retinal vessels and by melanin in the retinal pigment epithelium and thus can cause retinal burns, even if the patient is not staring directly into the beam. An additional concern is that phototoxic and photosensitizing drugs, either taken internally or applied to the skin, can potentiate the effects of lasers operating in this spectrum, and this is a danger that pertains both to patients and to personnel in the laser suite.

The eyewear to be worn by all working around lasers should be adequately absorptive at the wavelength or spectral range in which the laser is being used, protect against maximum irradiance (W/cm^2) for at least 5 seconds, optimize visual transmittance for both day and night vision, be available with prescription lenses or fit over prescription glasses, be resistant to impact, be comfortable, and not bleach with time (AO standards). There are many manufacturers who produce goggles in several designs for use with any of the lasers.

Any plastic lens provides adequate protection during use of the CO_2 laser. However, polycarbonate fibers have been shown to be the most resistant to burn-through and safety lenses made of this material are the ones of choice.[10] Lenses in the complementary color of the colored laser light are used to absorb the incident beam. These are usually orange for the argon laser; they may be a bluish hue or red for the 577- to 585-nm dye laser; deep blue or green for the ruby laser; and light gray or dark green for the Nd:YAG laser. For patients undergoing the treatment of lesions close to the eye, the globe can be shielded with intraocular eye shields composed of metal or acrylic, which are placed against the globe behind the eyelids on top of the anesthetized cornea. However, laser light of certain wavelengths or heat resulting from laser impact can penetrate through plastic or other eye shields, so care should be taken to ensure that shields made of the proper material are used. An ophthalmic ointment or protective lubricant is applied inside the eye shield cup. Heavily moistened pads should be placed over the eyes of patients undergoing CO_2 laser treatment. Other shielding materials, including dark absorptive, soft cloths such as felt, may be used in patients undergoing treatment using other lasers. Because eye shields and surgical instruments with reflective surfaces can reflect laser light to operating room personnel, care must be taken to prevent this.[11]

CUTANEOUS HAZARDS

Care must also be taken to irradiate only those areas that are intended to be irradiated and to prevent the inadvertent irradiation of adjacent skin, clothing, or other personal effects. Cutaneous exposure may result in thermal burns, ranging in severity from mild reddening, to blisters, to charring, and to ulceration. To prevent other risks in or near the operative field, the area should simply be kept clear of flammable items such as dry gauze and of surgical instruments with bright, reflective surfaces. Laser instruments with an ebonized finish may be purchased to eliminate the risk of spectral reflection.

Very short wavelength radiation in the 100- and 200-nm region, such as that emitted by excimer lasers, causes molecular bonds to break and for this reason may be mutagenic. Slightly longer wavelengths, in the UVB light range (315–400 nm), may induce sunburn and increase pigmentation. Longer-wavelength UV light, visible light, and infrared light may all induce thermal injury and photocoagulation. Long-wavelength UV light penetrates deeply into the skin, and very short wavelength light is absorbed superficially. For example, light from an excimer laser in the short UV spectrum can penetrate only partially through a single cell in the stratum corneum, but visible light in the red region can reach several millimeters into the dermis.

Hazards of the Laser Plume

CHARACTERISTICS OF AEROSOLS AND LASER SMOKE

As tissue is heated by a CO_2 laser, water, which is the absorbing chromophore, reaches 100°F (37.7°C) and vaporizes to steam. Smoke from the destroyed tissue, which is well known to be extremely malodorous, leaves the operative surface in the form of the laser plume. The amount of laser smoke produced varies greatly with the tissue being irradiated, the laser being used, the amount of lasing being performed, the surgeon's technique, and the type of procedure. Most laser smoke is controlled through mechanical smoke evacuator systems.

For many years, however, clinicians and researchers were concerned that the smoke and its accompanying moisture-laden particulate matter may act as a vector for disease. There was particular concern about the possible spread of cancer cells to other sites or to operators through inhalation of the plume.[12] Until the past few years, however, the composition of laser smoke had not been well studied. In one such study, Nezhat and colleagues[13] examined plume samples from women undergoing CO_2 laser laparoscopic treatment. The samples were collected and analyzed for the aerodynamic size range of any particles in the plume and by microscopy to determine their configuration. Although previous studies had shown the existence of morphologically intact cells as well as cell parts in the plume from various tissues irradiated with CO_2 and Nd:YAG lasers, these investigators found the collected particles to be round and homogeneous, with a physical diameter equivalent to their aerodynamic diameter. No sign of char was present. The median aerodynamic diameter was 0.31 μm and ranged from 0.1 to 0.8 μm. No intact bacteria or cell-sized particles were found in the plume. However, another potential hazard became evident: the laser plume particles were in the size range referred to as *lung-damaging dust* (0.5–5.0 μm). Particles of this size, which include those from coal, cotton, and grain, can penetrate to the alveoli and cause serious pulmonary disease. In addition, although it seemed unlikely that intact bacteria could be inspired, the possibility of a virus "hitching a ride" on or within a particle was a concern. Of further note, the laser smoke particles were found to be approximately 16 times smaller than the pore size of common surgical masks. The need to develop and use adequate equipment protective against aerosols thus quite suddenly became clear in 1987 and 1988, when these pioneering studies were carried out.

As tissue becomes aerosolized, it goes from being blood or tissue fluid to spatter, to spray, and then to an aerosol, the latter being defined as consisting of particles less than 10 μm in diameter. Aerosolized particles are produced either by rotary instruments, such as abrasive wheels and dermabraders, or by lasers or electrocautery devices. Only those produced by the latter two means, however, are heated. Size is the most important characteristic of airborne particulate matter, and the hazards posed by aerosolized particles are related directly to their size. Their size also correlates directly with the inspirability, filterability, settling velocity, and distribution of airborne particles. The size and number of particles further relate directly to the load of infectious agents and the viability of particle-borne agents. In addition, the size of particulate matter may decrease up to tenfold in air by evaporation and may also expand by an equal amount when dry particulate matter enters a humid environment such as the lungs. Large particles settle rapidly. If a particle exceeds 50 μm in diameter, it drops through the air quickly and cannot enter the lungs or respiratory mucosa but it can affect the skin or conjunctivae. If the particle is less than 10 μm in diameter, it can penetrate the nasopharynx; if it is less than 7 μm in diameter, it may penetrate to the alveoli. There is little deposition in the lungs of particles less than 0.6 μm. Particles less than 0.8 cm produced both by laser and dermabrasion procedures settle at a rate of 0.0025 cm/sec (9 cm/hr).[14] Particles of increasingly smaller diameters settle much more slowly; for example, a particle 10 times smaller settles a hundred times slower, and such material may therefore become suspended in the air of an operative suite for an indefinite time.

Nezhat's study confirmed the findings from previous investigators, which had shown that, in the absence of efficient smoke evacuation, the laser irradiation of 1 g of tissue results in a pollution level seventeen times the Japanese safety standard.[15] The latter in vitro studies revealed that most particles generated by the laser range from 0.1 to 2.0 μm in diameter, the same size as the particles in cigarette smoke or other lung-damaging dusts. Further, smoke generated during laser or electrocautery treatment of canine tongue was found to be mutagenic when exposed to various strains of *Salmonella typhimurium*.[16] The mutagenic effect of electrocautery smoke was more pronounced than that of laser plume and was equivalent to the smoke from three to six cigarettes.

Baggish and colleagues[17,18] studied the effect of laser smoke on the lungs of rats. In the first of two studies,[17] they found that the long-term inhalation of smoke generated by CO_2 lasers results in severe pulmonary damage, including congested interstitial pneumonia, bronchiolitis, and emphysema. These findings were not substantially unlike those observed in the context of exposure to other types of particulate material. In a follow-up study,[18] the effect of passing laser plume through smoke evacuation filters was also evaluated. In this study, rats were exposed to CO_2 laser exhaust passed through standard filters rated to filter particles as small as 0.5 μm in diameter. Pulmonary lesions developed in the animals that were identical to but less severe than those that formed in animals inhaling unfiltered vapor. However, the lungs of rats protected by ultralow-penetration air filters, which trap particles as small as 0.1 μm, were identical to those of control animals not exposed to laser exhaust. No pathologic changes whatsoever developed in these animals. Wenig and colleagues[19] confirmed these results in a study of rats exposed to Nd:YAG laser and electrocautery exhaust passed through smoke evacuation filters.

The chemicals contained in the laser plume may also be hazardous. Because the plasma formed during the interaction of laser radiation with materials has been estimated to reach a temperature as high as 10,000°K, it has been hypothesized that chemicals formed by pyrolizing protein and lipid may also be formed in the plasma. This was borne out by studies of the plume released from beef liver irradiated with CO_2 and Nd:YAG lasers, in which small but significant quantities of several toxic and carcinogenic chemicals were found.[20,21] These included benzene, polycyclic aromatic hydrocarbons, acrolein, and formaldehyde. Without the proper evacuation of smoke and chemical byproducts, the vaporization of more than 3 g of tissue would produce enough acrolein and hydrocarbons in one square meter of air to exceed the OSHA limits for these chemicals. In a study[22] evaluating the hazard of smoke production to patients undergoing endoscopic surgery, the methemoglobin levels in a group of patients undergoing operations in which smoke-generating devices were used were compared with those in a control group not exposed to smoke. A positive correlation was found between exposure to smoke generated by laser or electrosurgical devices and the circulating methemoglobin levels. Although the smoke material is usually absorbed via the respiratory tract, this study showed that the collection of smoke material in the closed space of the peritoneal cavity leads to enough absorption of toxic chemicals to induce the systemic changes.

PRESENCE OF BIOLOGIC MATERIAL IN THE LASER PLUME

Is Viable Material Present in the Laser Plume?

Studies analyzing the presence of viable cells or infectious material after CO_2 laser irradiation initially have yielded varying results. Some investigators were unable to find viable tissue in airborne particles collected during CO_2 laser vaporization of canine tongue,[23] and others have found no metabolic activity in laser plume after papovavirus irradiation.[24] In addition, CO_2 laser vaporization of mouse melanoma cells was found to produce no viable tissue fragments,[25] nor were viable organisms found in the plume created by the CO_2 laser irradiation of skin seeded with bacteria.[26] On the other hand, the plume and splatter from the CO_2 laser treatment of tattoos and basal cell epitheliomas were found to contain intact erythrocytes and keratinocytes,[27] and the CO_2 laser vaporization of postmortem skin injected with bacterial spores was found to produce a plume containing viable infectious particles when irradiated at low levels of radiation (less than 500 W/cm²), a level similar to one that might be used for the treatment of tattoos, warts, and cutaneous tumors.[28] Other investigators had demonstrated viable *Escherichia coli* and *Staphylococcus aureus* after CO_2 irradiation of agar tubes simulating the vaginal vault,[29] and biologically active material has been shown to be transported from the surface of the liver or the gelatin and agar targets into the depth of the material during laser cutting with the CO_2 and erbium:YAG (2940-nm) lasers.[30] The latter investigators hypothesized that the contraction and condensation of hot-water vapor draws material into such simulated wounds, and bacteria thus transported have been shown to survive the shock of transport. Viable bacteriophage has been identified in the plume created during argon and CO_2 laser irradiation of an agar substrate containing high titers of this virus and was found to be contained in particles large enough to settle out within 100 mm of the beam impact site, in one instance showing a median aerodynamic diameter and a mass median aerodynamic diameter of 23 and 55 μm, respectively.[31] The appearance of viable virus in such plume particles is extremely rare, however.[32]

PAPILLOMAVIRUS IN LASER PLUME

Garden and colleagues[33] studied the laser plume produced by the CO_2 laser during the vaporization of papillomavirus-infected verrucae for the presence of viral DNA. In their study, four bovine fibropapillomas and seven plantar warts were exposed to varying CO_2 laser power densities and energy fluences similar to those used in clinical laser surgical procedures. Intact bovine papillomavirus DNA was identified in the plume produced by the laser at all power densities and energy fluences used. Intact human papillomavirus DNA was present in the vapor from two of the seven patients with plantar warts. Sawchuck and associates[34] studied the vapor released during the treatment of human and bovine warts to further define the presence of papillomavirus and test whether the wearing of surgical masks reduced exposure. Half of each wart was treated with the CO_2 laser and the other half with electrocoagulation. Of the plantar warts treated, five of eight of the laser-generated plumes and four of the seven electrocoagulation-induced plumes were found to contain human papillomavirus DNA. In addition, greater amounts of DNA were recovered from the laser-induced plume than from the electrocoagulation-induced one. Infectious bovine papillomavirus was present in the plume from all bovine warts treated with either modality. Surprisingly, a 3M surgical mask was found to be capable of removing virtually all papillomavirus present in the plume, strongly implying that such masks do protect the clinician from inhalation exposure to viruses the size of papillomavirus (55 nm in diameter). The results indicate that the particles in laser plume may be trapped by a charged microfiber, which serves as an electrostatic filter and is present as a middle web in these masks. Abramson and colleagues[35] subsequently evaluated the plume from laser-treated laryngeal papillomas for the presence of human papillomavirus DNA. No DNA was found except in those instances in which there had been direct contact of the suction tip with the papilloma tissue during surgery, in keeping with the findings of Kashima and associates.[36] Garden and Bakus[37] collected the plume from bovine papillomavirus irradiated with the CO_2 laser in pulsed and continuous-wave modes and reinoculated this material into cows. This was successful in inducing tumors, proving that the virus liberated during CO_2 laser surgery is not only viable but also capable of transmitting disease.

Have clinicians been shown to acquire warts from laser surgery? To answer this question, Lobraico and colleagues[38] distributed a questionnaire to a multispecialty group of physicians and nurses involved in laser surgery. Of 824 people who responded, 26 had possibly acquired verrucae in this way, for an overall incidence of 3.2%. The highest incidence of such acquired lesions was observed in dermatologists, with verrucae developing in 17 of 112 (15.2%) and constituting 65.4% (17 of 26) of the total number of acquired lesions. Fifteen of these lesions were on the hands and two were on the face.

Hallmo and Naess[39] described the case of a laser surgeon who presented with laryngeal papillomatosis. The in situ DNA hybridization of tissue from these tumors revealed HPV DNA types 6 and 11 in this surgeon, who had performed laser therapy in patients with anogenital condylomas. However, a study in which a large group of CO_2 laser surgeons was compared with an equally large group of population-based control subjects with warts showed that, when these lesions are grouped together without regard to anatomic site, CO_2 laser surgeons are no more likely to acquire warts than people in the general population. However, the types of papillomavirus causing genital warts appeared to have a predilection for infecting the mucosa of the upper airway, and it was concluded from this that laser plume containing HPV types 6 and 11 may represent more of a hazard to surgeons than plume containing other types of papillomavirus.[40]

The contamination of medical personnel with human papillomavirus DNA has been investigated using polymerase chain reaction (PCR) techniques. The results of this study, which was carried out under routine operating room conditions, showed that there is a definite risk of operating room personnel being contaminated during both CO_2 laser surgery and electrocoagulation treatment. It was also found that the risk of preoperative contamination from virus already in the atmosphere is higher after laser procedures than after electrocoagulation, probably related to the increased persistence of HPV DNA–containing aerosols during laser surgery. HPV DNA was found on surfaces as far as 2 meters away from the treatment field, but this was not the case for rooms in which electrocoagulation was performed.[41]

HEPATITIS B VIRUS AND HUMAN IMMUNODEFICIENCY VIRUS

Infection with hepatitis B virus (HBV) or human immunodeficiency virus (HIV) represents a serious potential hazard. Of the two, infection with HBV is the greater hazard, because this virus can remain viable for up to a week at room temperature, serum contains up to 10^9 viral particles per milliliter of serum and is infectious in dilutions up to 10^8, and HBV can be transmitted by the respiratory and conjunctival route. The hepatitis B Dane particle, with a diameter of 42 nm, could in theory penetrate a surgical mask. In contrast, the concentration of HIV in serum is much lower. Only 10 to 50 particles are present per milliliter of serum, and no association between infection and exposure to low numbers of particles has been noted. In addition, the virus remains infectious at room temperature for only 3 days. HIV, with a diameter of 100 nm, is also less likely to penetrate a surgical mask, and HIV-infected cells, if intact, would be trapped within surgical masks. Baggish and colleagues[42] have shown, however, that HIV is present in laser smoke. These investigators determined this by infecting cells with one HIV copy per cell, an infectious load much higher than that in an infected patient, in which case there would be one viral copy per 10,000 cells. All cells present in Petri dishes were vaporized with a continuous-wave CO_2 laser at 20 W until they were totally gone. The smoke was evacuated using a vacuum apparatus connected to the culture media with Sylastic tubing. This tubing was then cut into multiple segments. Alternate segments were tested for evidence of virus using PCR or cultured for P24 protein. Alternate slices 1, 3, 5, 7, and 9, which were tested using PCR, were all found to contain the virus, and HIV was present in material cultured from the alternate even-numbered segments up to day 14, after which the amount of virus decreased and disappeared by day 28. HIV could not be identified in the culture material, however—the virus appeared to be cultured only from within the tubing. This study showed that HIV DNA and nucleic acid are present in laser smoke, but that the virus appears to be damaged by the laser. This emphasizes the fact that the vacuum tubing used during laser surgery must be considered hazardous and disposed of appropriately and, more importantly, that laser surgery and other common forms of surgery, such as electrosurgery, that generate tissue smoke must be considered potentially hazardous procedures. The potential risk of HIV transmission to health care workers exposed to aerosols generated during the care of HIV-infected patients was further shown by the findings of Johnson and Robinson,[43] who cultured viable HIV-1 from the aerosols and vapors generated by surgical power implements when known HIV-1 inoculated blood was bubbled through sterile viral culture media. Of note, however, viable virus was not cultured from the plume generated during electrocautery.

Starr and colleagues[44] studied the viability of the simian immunodeficiency virus (SIV) after CO_2 laser irradiation. This virus has been found to be considerably homologous to HIV, and sensitive culture techniques are available for its growth. After the culture medium containing concentrated SIV was irradiated at variable radiances, the plume was collected and cultured. All cultures were negative for the virus over an 8-week period, indicating that SIV is not viable in laser plume after CO_2 laser irradiation.

On the basis of the findings from all studies, it appears that the risk of operators acquiring viral infection from laser plume is real but unlikely.[45] The amount of infectious material in laser plume is actually low, and naked viral DNA, which can indeed be found in plume on some occasions, does not readily infect cultured cells.

SAFE USE OF LASERS

The risk of infection in operators can be minimized through the use of appropriate safety precautions. For example, a high-volume smoke evacuation system must be used and the tip of the laser suction should be placed within 1 to 2 cm from the treatment site. It has been shown that the smoke generated by continuous-wave lasers is completely controlled when the vacuum nozzle is located 2 inches (5 cm) or less from the tissue.[46] Ultra-low penetrating air filters (ULPA) rated for 0.1-μm–sized particles with 99.9999% efficiency should also be used. This filter can capture HBV, which is 0.042 μm in diameter; human papillomavirus, which is 0.18 μm in diameter; and HIV, which is 0.18 μm in diameter. It can also capture the "carrier" particles (0.1–0.8 μm) on which they travel. The wearing of properly fitted and tied laser surgical masks can greatly reduce the risk of respiratory exposure to viral and other infectious agents. Protective eyewear and gloves are also necessary. However, disposable or sterilized surgical gowns or clothing do not adequately protect the skin against the low concentrations of chemicals and the amount of plume expected, even if adequate evacuation methods are taken.

The use of ultra-short–pulse lasers, such as any Q-switched device, is associated with even greater potential risks. Severe eye damage and blindness may result from exposure to a single pulse; therefore the wearing of wavelength-specific wraparound goggles is mandatory. Impact of the beam on the skin results in considerable tissue splatter that contains viable cells. In addition, the velocity of the miniexplosion within the skin and of the spread of tissue fragments exceeds the speed of sound and escapes collection by smoke evacuation units. For this reason, splatter guards must be used on the laser handpiece to prevent the dispersion of splatter. It is also mandatory for all personnel to wear gloves and gowns during the use of Q-switched lasers.

Guidelines for the safe use of lasers in health care facilities are outlined in the recently revised American National Standards Institute document ANSI Z136.3-1996 (American National Standard for Safe Use of Lasers in Health Care Facilities). This booklet and other laser safety guides and information are available through the Laser Institute of America, 12424 Research Parkway, Suite 125, Orlando, Florida 32826 (407-380-1553, fax 407-380-5588).

References

1. Sliney DH. Laser safety. Lasers Surg Med 1995;16:215–225.
2. FDA incident report a sobering reminder of laser perils. Clin Laser Monthly 1989;7:97–108, 1S–4S.
3. O'Leesky K, Wirth C, Joffe ST. What is the risk of laser surgery? A multicenter study. J Clin Laser Med Surg 1993;11(6):305–308.
4. Rockwell RJ Jr. Laser accidents: reviewing thirty years of incidents—what are the concerns—old and new? J Laser Appl 1994;6:203–211.
5. Varanelli AG. Electrical hazards associated with lasers. J Laser Appl 1995;7:62–64.
6. Arnold JE, Allphin AL. Effect of extraluminal oxygen on carbon dioxide laser ignition of endotracheal tubes. Arch Otolaryngol Head Neck Surg 1992;118:722–724.
7. Epstein RH, Brummett RR Jr, Lask GD. Incendiary potential of the flash-lamp pumped 585 nm tunable dye laser. Anesth Analg 1990;71:171–175.
8. Lowe NJ, Burgess P, Bordon H. Flash pump dye laser fire during general anesthesia oxygenation: case report. J Clin Laser Med Surg 1990;April:39–21.
9. Bean AK, Ceilley RI. Reducing fire risks of the flashlamp pumped 585-nm pulse dye laser. J Dermatol Surg Oncol 1994;20:221–224.
9a. Fretkin S, Beeson WH, Hanke CW. Ignition potential of the 585-nm pulsed-dye laser. Dermatol Surg 1996;22:699–702.
10. Sliney DH, Sparks SD, Wood RL Jr. The protective characteristics of polycarbonate lenses against CO_2 laser radiation. J Laser Appl 1993;5:49–52.

11. Wood RL Jr, Sliney DH, Basye RA. Laser reflections from surgical instruments. Lasers Surg Med 1992;12:675–678.
12. Voorhies RM, Lavyne MH, Strait TA, Shapiro WR. Does the CO_2 laser spread viable brain-tumor cells outside the surgical field? J Neurosurg 1984;60:819.
13. Nezhat C, Winer WK, Nezhat F et al. Physical properties of aerosols produced by dermabrasion. Arch Dermatol 1989;125:1637–1643.
14. Wentzell JM, Robinson JK, Wentzell JM et al. Physical properties of aerosols produced by dermabrasion. Arch Dermatol 1989;125:1637–1643.
15. Fisher WR. Laser smoke in the operating room. Biomed Technol Today 1987;Nov/Dec:191–195.
16. Tomita Y, Mihasi S, Nagata K et al. Mutagenicity of smoke condensates induced by CO_2 laser irradiation and electrocauterization. Mutat Res 1981;89:145–149.
17. Baggish MS, Elbakry M. The effects of laser smoke on the lungs of rats. Am J Obstet Gynecol 1987;156:1260–1265.
18. Baggish MS, Baltoyannis P, Sze E. Protection of the rat lung from the harmful effects of laser smoke. Lasers Surg Med 1988;8:248–253.
19. Wenig BL, Stenson KA, Wenig BM, Tracy D. Effects of plume produced by the Nd:YAG laser and electrocautery on the respiratory system. Lasers Surg Med 1993;13:242–245.
20. Kokosa JM, Eugene J. Chemical composition of laser-tissue interaction smoke plume. J Laser Appl 1989;July:59–63.
21. Kokosa JM. Hazardous chemicals produced by laser materials processing. J Laser Appl 1994;6:195–201.
22. Ott D. Smoke production and smoke reduction in endoscopic surgery: preliminary report. Endosc Surg 1993;1:230–232.
23. Mihashi S, Jako GJ, Incze J et al. Laser surgery in otolaryngology: interaction of CO_2 laser and soft tissue. Ann NY Acad Sci 1975;267:263–294.
24. Belina JH, Stjernholm RL, Kurpel JE. Analysis of plume emissions after papovavirus irradiation with the carbon dioxide laser. J Reprod Med 1982;27:268.
25. Oosterhuis JW, Verschveren RCJ, Eibergen R, Eibergen R, Oldohoff J. The viability of cells in the waste products of CO_2 laser evaporation Cloudman mouse melanomas. Cancer 1982;49:61.
26. Mullarky MB, Norris CW, Goldberg ID. The efficacy of the CO_2 laser in sterilization of skin seeded with bacteria: survival at the skin surface and in the plume emissions. Laryngoscope 1985;95:186.
27. Matthews J, Newsom SWB, Walker NPJ. Aerobiology of irradiation with the carbon dioxide laser. J Hosp Infect 1985;6:230–233.
28. Walker NPJ, Matthews J, Newsom SWB. Possible hazards from irradiation with the carbon dioxide laser. Lasers Surg Med 1986;6:84–86.
29. Byrne PO, Sisson PR, Oliver PD, Ingham HR. Carbon dioxide laser irradiation of bacterial targets *in vitro*. J Hosp Infect 1987;9:265–273.
30. Frenz M, Mathezloic F, Stoffel MHS et al. Transport of biologically active material in laser cutting. Lasers Surg Med 1988;8:562–566.
31. Matchette LS, Faaland RW, Royston DD, Ediger MN. In vitro production of viable bacteriophage in carbon dioxide and argon laser plumes. Lasers Surg Med 1991;11:380–384.
32. Matchette LS, Vergella TJ, Faaland RW. Viable bacteriophage in CO_2 laser plume: aerodynamic size distribution. Lasers Surg Med 1993;13:18–22.

33. Garden JM, O'Banion K, Shelnitz LS et al. Papillomavirus in the vapor of carbon dioxide laser–treated verrucae. JAMA 1988;259:1199–1202.

34. Sawchuck WS, Wever PJ, Lowy DR, Dzubow LM. Infectious papillomavirus is the vapor of warts treated with carbon dioxide laser or electrocoagulation: detection and protection. J Am Acad Dermatol 1989; 21:41–49.

35. Abramson AL, DiLorenzo TP, Steinberg BM. Is papillomavirus detectable in the plume of laser-treated laryngeal papilloma? Arch Otolaryngol Head Neck Surg 1990;116:604–607.

36. Kashima A, Kessis B, Moutes P, Shah K. Polymerase chain reaction identification of human papillomavirus DNA in CO_2 laser plume from recurrent respiratory papillomatosis. Otolaryngology 1991;104:191–195.

37. Garden JM, Bakus AD. Health safety issues of laser generated plume. Lasers Surg Med 1993(suppl.);5.

38. Lobraico RV, Schifano MJ, Brader KR. A retrospective study on the hazards of the carbon dioxide laser plume. J Laser Appl 1988;Fall:6–8.

39. Hallmo P, Naess O. Laryngeal papillomatosis with human papillomavirus DNA contracted by a laser surgeon. Eur Arch Otorhinolaryngol 1991;248:425–427.

40. Gloster HM Jr, Roenigk RK. Risk of acquiring human papillomavirus from the plume produced by the carbon dioxide laser in the treatment of warts. J Am Acad Dermatol 1995;32:436–441.

41. Bergbrant IM, Sameulsson L, Olofsson S, Jonassen F, Ricksten A. Polymerase chain reaction for monitoring human papillomavirus contamination of medical personnel during treatment of genital warts with CO_2 laser and electrocoagulation. Acta Derm Venereol (Stockh) 1994;74: 393–395.

42. Baggish MS, Poesz B, Jorot D, Williamson P, Refai A. Presence of immunodeficiency virus DNA in laser smoke. Lasers Surg Med 1991;4:197–203.

43. Johnson GK, Robinson WS. Human immunodeficiency virus-1 (HIV-1) in the vapors of surgical power instruments. J Med Virol 1991;33:47–50.

44. Starr JC, Kilmer SL, Wheeland RG. Analysis of the carbon dioxide laser plume for simian immunodeficiency virus. J Dermatol Surg Oncol 1992; 18:297–300.

45. Sawchuck WS, Felton RP. Infectious potential of aerosolized particles. Arch Dermatol 1989;125:1089–1092.

46. Smith JP, Moss CE, Bryant CJ, Fleeger AK. Evaluation of a smoke evacuator used for laser surgery. Lasers Surg Med 1989;9:276–281.

20 —— Strategic Planning and Establishment of a Laser Surgical Unit in an Office Practice and in a Hospital

Elizabeth I. McBurney
Richard O. Gregory

An Office-Based Laser Surgical Practice

Health care is increasingly being provided in an accessible outpatient setting to achieve lower costs and better care and to be more convenient for both patients and physicians. Most cutaneous laser surgical procedures can be performed in this modern environment and fall under the aegis of ambulatory surgery, which is surgery that does not require the patient to stay overnight in the hospital.

Cutaneous laser surgery can be performed in one of several outpatient settings: an outpatient surgical suite in a hospital, an ambulatory surgery center separate from the hospital, or a physician's office. Laser surgical procedures performed in an office setting are generally more cost-effective to the patient than procedures performed in a hospital or an ambulatory surgery center.[1] Most such procedures can be performed with the patient under local or no anesthesia and take a brief operating time (15–45 minutes).

To establish an office laser unit, the physician must be prepared and educated in seven major areas (Table 20-1).[2] Purchase or rental of the laser is only one aspect. The physician must also select the appropriate unit, or units, for his or her practice; ensure the proper training and education of all involved with the equipment; inform and instruct patients of the risks, benefits, and nature of laser surgery; design appropriate handouts and consent forms; become familiar with reimbursement Current Procedural Terminology (CPT) laser codes[3]; design and ensure the ongoing safety and quality management of equipment, facility, and staff; and establish a public awareness campaign. If the physician gives proper attention to all of these aspects, he or she will have a safe, cost-effective office laser unit and patients will be educated and have realistic expectations regarding laser surgery.

RATIONALE FOR OFFICE LASER UNIT

Office-based laser surgery serves the patient and physician well, without compromising the patient's safety and welfare. The safety record

Table 20-1.   Major considerations for establishment of office laser unit

1. Equipment and office surgical facility requirements
2. Physician and staff education and training
3. Record documentation
4. Patient education and preparation
5. Safety and quality assurance program
6. Economic reimbursement
7. Public awareness

for such procedures is well documented,[1] and the low morbidity associated with outpatient surgery is attributed to careful selection of both the patients undergoing the procedures and the type of procedures performed in this setting. Other advantages to surgery performed in an office environment are that the same staff is available to support the physician, and the staff can be trained exclusively in the physician's technique and the types of patients he or she treats.

Having a laser in an office setting offers several advantages to the patient and the physician. The patient is familiar with the office and staff and does not have to fill out new information forms. There is also no additional charge for use of an operating room. In addition, the physician does not have to leave the office, the equipment is available throughout the day, and the physician does not have to conform to a hospital surgery schedule.

There are, however, also several disadvantages to an office-based laser unit. A primary disadvantage is the cost of the laser and the service contract, if the physician decides to purchase the laser. The price of some of the new laser systems can be particularly onerous for the laser practitioner in a solo private practice. To circumvent this problem the laser can be rented, and there are many medical laser rental companies that can bring the laser to the office on a regular schedule. The laser rental fees are also reasonable. A second disadvantage is the lack of availability of general anesthesia, unless special arrangements are made. In addition, if complications arise during surgery, there are no hospital backup facilities available. Last, performing surgery in the office may actually be more costly to the physician, because the amount realized from fees once the increased overhead factor is taken into account may actually be decreased. Further, currently Medicare does not allow additional fees for the operating room space and laser equipment used in office settings, as it does for hospitals.

EQUIPMENT AND OFFICE SURGICAL FACILITY REQUIREMENTS

One of the first things a physician must consider when setting up an office laser surgical unit is which type of laser to purchase or rent:

CO_2, argon, flashlamp-pumped dye, argon pumped dye, KTP, Q-switched, Nd:YAG, ruby, alexandrite, or others. The choice depends on the physician's specialty, the costs, and the types of lesions that can be treated. The list of current established vendors and manufacturers is updated annually in the *Medical Laser Buyer's Guide* (Table 20-2).

The CO_2 laser is the one most frequently used in an office setting, because of its comparatively low price and the wide variety of lesions that can be treated with it. This laser has an excellent track record, in that there are few maintenance problems and little to no on-site preparations necessary for installation of the equipment. Further, some currently available units are quite compact and portable.

There are several factors to consider when purchasing a laser (Table 20-3). One of these is the price. However, when a laser vendor quotes a price for a unit, the buyer should ask what the price specifically includes. For example, does it include handpieces for use in special procedures or a smoke evacuator? An initially attractive offer may not prove to be competitive once all that the price does or does not include is considered.

The potential physician/purchaser should also be cognizant of physical on-site requirements for the laser unit being considered for purchase. For example, most Nd:YAG and argon lasers require special electrical connections and unusual plumbing setups. The temperature of the cooling water can be critical, and this may require the installation of a cooler. Some laser units and smoke evacuators generate considerable noise. Such units can be placed in an adjoining room and connected to the surgical suite to minimize the problems with sound pollution, but this can necessitate an additional construction expense. Also, some laser units, such as the KTP/YAG laser, produce considerable heat during use and additional room cooling may be necessary.

Most lasers are offered with a lease or purchase contract option. In negotiating the contract, the physician should inquire about the cost

---

Table 20-2.   Resources for the laser center

American Society for Laser Medicine and Surgery, 2404 Stewart Sq, Waussau, WI   54401.

American National Standards Institute, Inc., 1430 Broadway, New York, NY   10018.

Laser Institute of America, 12424 Research Pkwy, Orlando, FL   32826; tel: 1-800-34LASER or 1-407-380-1553.

Medical Laser Buyer's Guide, Laser Focus/Penn Well Publications, 1 Technology Park Dr, P.O. Box 989, Westford, MA   01886; tel: 1-508-392-2117. Cost of annual guide is $85.

International Society of Cosmetic Laser Surgery, 401 North Michigan Ave, Chicago, IL   60611-4287.

American Board of Laser Surgery, Inc., 2722 W. Oklahoma Ave, Suite 202, Milwaukee, WI   53215; tel: 1-414-653-1066.

Table 20-3.   Factors to consider when purchasing a laser

1. Cost
2. Physical on-site requirements for installation
3. Lease/purchase availability
4. Warranty
5. Maintenance/service contract
6. Service availability
7. Delivery time
8. Manufacturer's reputation
9. FDA approval
10. Education: preceptorship, in-service training courses
11. Size of laser
12. Portability of laser
13. Laser parameters: wavelength, variable spot sizes, power capability, pulsed versus continuous-wave delivery, handpiece
14. Smoke evacuator system

of buying the unit at the end of the contract and also about the possibility of upgrading to a better, more versatile unit should one come available during the contract life.

The warranty offered by a laser vendor can vary but usually extends for 1 to 2 years. The physician purchasing the unit should clearly understand what is included in the warranty, such as whether it includes the full cost of tube replacement in an argon laser, the cost of maintenance and service, and the cost of annual routine checks.

After the warranty expires, the physician/purchaser must then consider whether to purchase a maintenance service contract. This is a hidden cost often overlooked by the purchaser, and such contracts can vary from $1,500 to $15,000, depending on the type of laser. After expiration of the warranty, some physicians do not buy service contracts for the small, low-voltage CO_2 lasers, because of the few maintenance problems associated with these lasers. Laser companies may offer different levels of service contracts. For example, in an argon laser maintenance agreement, the lower-priced basic contract may include all labor and travel expenses and all needed parts, with the exception of the laser tube, and the more expensive, full-service contract may include tube replacement in addition to labor and travel. Preventive maintenance visits may cost the owner an additional fee.

The warranty and maintenance service contracts are useless unless the service experts provided by the manufacturer can be available soon to evaluate and repair the laser. This is one of the reasons to purchase a laser from an established manufacturer. Although on-site diagnosis of the problem is usually made within 24 to 72 hours, there is often a delay of a few days to weeks while receipt of the replacement part is awaited, necessitating a second trip by the technician and prolonging the "down" time for the laser. The newer light-weight, portable CO_2 lasers offer a real advantage in this regard, because they can be packed into a suitcase-like container and shipped to the laser manufacturer for repair. Some companies make a replacement laser available to the physician until the repairs are completed.

An additional expense of the dye laser is replacement of the dye components. Their cost can add considerably to overhead.

Potential purchasers should request the names of other customers to find out about their experience with the company regarding the delivery time, service availability, and any technical problems. The potential purchaser should also ask the manufacturer how long the laser has been on the market, the number sold, and the problems encountered. Over time, many laser companies have gone out of business. It is therefore important to deal with one that has been in business awhile and has a very good record.

Lasers are generally delivered promptly after they are purchased. In the case of foreign-made lasers, there is the manufacturer and the United States distributor, and they are separate entities. It is important to understand the responsibility of each.

The U.S. Food and Drug Administration (FDA) regulates the status of medical lasers for specific applications. Most lasers have been approved for many clinical applications, but those still under investigation require specific protocols. Therefore, the physician should be aware whether the laser procedures he or she is planning to perform with a particular laser are FDA approved or still under investigation.

Most laser vendors offer a wide range of educational opportunities for the physician and staff. These can include a preceptorship, an in-service program conducted on site by the laser company representative after the laser has been delivered, and courses sponsored by the manufacturer. The potential purchaser should take advantage of all available educational opportunities. Some smaller laser companies do not offer their own programs but may give the purchaser a stipend to pay for attendance at a course or to do a preceptorship.

The physical size of the laser can be a definite factor in an office, because office space is frequently limited. Pictures of the laser unit can be deceiving. It is therefore important to make sure in advance that the unit can be accommodated in the office space available, remembering also that additional equipment such as smoke evacuators may need to be accommodated. The purchaser should buy a laser that fulfills all the laser medical requirements of his or her practice and takes up the least amount of space. The place where the laser is stored should also be considered. For example, it should not be a place where it could be hit by other equipment or personnel nor should it be in an area of extreme temperatures.

The portability of the laser may be important to a physician with more than one office or with a new laser to be shared by two or more physicians in different locations. Some CO_2 and argon lasers can be lifted by an able-bodied person and transported in a car or van, making them relatively portable. However, the physician should check to see whether the warranty and service maintenance contract cover units transported to different locations.

In considering different lasers of a particular type, the physician also needs to explore the following aspects: wattage capabilities, variable spot size, sealed tube technology (relevant to CO_2 lasers), pulsed versus the continuous delivery of energy, sapphire tips (Nd:YAG), and wavelength. The physician/purchaser can be educated as to what his or her particular needs will be in terms of the power, spot size, and timed delivery through attendance at courses and preceptorships. It is also important for the physician/purchaser of lasers to realize that the technology is continuously developing and that the most updated information may well be obtained at one of the laser society conferences or at a laser vendor's conference, and not in print.

The physician should ask the laser vendor to bring the laser to the office, where he or she can take the opportunity to use the equipment for several days. This hands-on time can keep the physician from making a costly mistake, such as purchasing a laser with too little output wattage for the procedures to be done.

Adjuvant equipment is as necessary as the laser proper. This includes protective eye shields or glasses, laser safety signs for the door, smoke evacuation systems, room deodorizers, appropriate surgical masks and equipment, fire extinguishers, and a radio/cassette player with earphones for the patient (Table 20-4).

Protective eyewear is a necessity. One should purchase eye shields or glasses of the appropriate optical density to protect the eyes from the wavelength of the laser used. Half glasses and contact lens are not acceptable and are not safe. Intraocular or scleral eye shields are particularly necessary for the patient being treated for eyelid lesions.[4] Another option for patients undergoing periorbital laser surgery is to cover their eyelashes with vaseline and have an assistant hold moist oval gauze pads over their eyes.

The laser safety door sign can be obtained from the laser vendor. It is useful to frame the sign, and it should be placed on the outside of the door to the surgery room whenever laser surgery is being performed. This is a highly visible alert and helps prevent the inadvertent entry of personnel into the room when the laser is in operation. Another precaution is to hang eye goggles on the door next to the laser sign, so that people who enter the surgical area will be instantly reminded to put the goggles on beforehand. Hospital and ambula-

Table 20-4.   Adjuvant equipment

1. Protective eye shields or glasses
2. Laser safety door sign
3. Smoke evacuation systems
4. Appropriate surgical masks and instruments
5. Room deodorizers
6. Fire extinguisher
7. Radio or cassette player with earphones for patient

tory surgery centers often have interlock systems that automatically put the laser on standby when someone enters the room.

It is of vital importance to use a high-flow suction smoke evacuation system wherever a laser plume is generated, including an office laser practice. As noted in the previous chapter, there is a continuing concern over the infectivity of the plume to patients, staff, and physicians,[5-7] and new research has confirmed that disease can be transmitted by laser plume particles.[8] Some CO_2 lasers have built-in smoke evacuators, but this is the exception. A separate unit must usually be purchased and maintained, and these units vary in price from $1,200 to $2,500. Filters, tubing, and service contracts after the warranty expires represent added expenses. There are no bargains in this area, and an efficient smoke evacuation system is an absolute necessity for an office laser practice. Vendors of smoke evacuation systems are also listed in the *Medical Laser Buyer's Guide*.

It is important for all present in the laser surgery area to wear appropriate surgical masks during laser surgery. It has been shown, however, that the commonly used surgical masks do not effectively filter the laser plume particles, which average around 0.3 μm in diameter.[6] Specialized masks have been developed that are made of material dense enough to filter out particles as small as 0.3 μm. There are at least six commercial brands of laser masks currently on the market. Another way to diminish the hazards posed by the laser plume is to have all in the surgical room wear two or three regular surgical masks in layers.

The surgical tools used with the CO_2 laser should be blackened or anodized to prevent accidental reflection of the laser beam. Studies have shown that there is a definite risk of ocular injury resulting from the reflection of the CO_2 laser beam off of stainless steel instruments,[2] and potentially acute damage can be drastically diminished if anodized instruments are used. The physician/purchaser should therefore have currently used instruments anodized for use in laser procedures. Some laser surgeons continue to use nonanodized stainless steel instruments for these procedures. If this is done, all personnel and patients must wear glass or plastic wraparound eye protection to prevent ocular damage.

A fire extinguisher in the surgical room where a laser is in use is a must, because it is possible for this laser beam energy to ignite drapes, sponges, and clothing. A secondary measure is to have a basin full of water and wet towels readily available on the surgical tray. If a fire is caught early, the staff may be able to smother it with wet towels or pull the burning object away from the patient and immerse it in a bucket of water or douse the entire area with water. A fire plan and fire drills also are suggested to prepare the staff for potential emergencies.

Several of the newer Q-switched lasers generate considerable tissue backsplatter when the laser light impacts the tissue. The physician/surgeon should be aware of this backsplatter and take appropriate precautions to prevent it, either through the wearing of a plastic shield or by placing synthetic dressings over the surgical site.

There should also be a radio or cassette player with earphones for the patient to wear to help mask the noise from the smoke evacuator and laser equipment. Patients vary in their anxiety, and music can help calm them.

The surgical table, tray, and lighting used are basically the same as those used in any routine outpatient surgical site.[1] However, the number of reflective surfaces should be kept to an absolute minimum, and all flammable chemicals and materials should be removed. Any windows in the laser surgical office must also be draped when the laser is in use.

PHYSICIAN AND STAFF EDUCATION AND TRAINING

Physician and staff education and training are an important part of the establishment of an outpatient laser surgery unit. To help physicians meet this requirement, the American Society for Laser Medicine and Surgery has established guidelines specifying the qualifications physicians who wish to perform the laser surgery should have.[10] However, physicians should consider these only minimal requirements. Staff members can be trained by the physician. In-service training can be provided by the laser manufacturer at the time of delivery of the laser equipment, and other instruction can be obtained through attendance at laser courses.

Membership in the American Society for Laser Medicine and Surgery is also suggested. This society holds an annual meeting that includes sections in each specialty as well as general plenary sessions. Membership dues include subscriptions to the quarterly journal and monthly newsletter, with specialty literature survey, published by the society. The International Society of Cosmetic Laser Surgery is a section of the American Academy of Cosmetic Surgery that also holds an annual meeting and workshop.

Although not yet recognized by the American Board of Medical Specialties, the American Board of Laser Surgery was organized to promulgate standards of competence and training for those who perform laser surgery. The examination is held annually and consists of a written examination followed by an oral examination administered by a physician in the specialty of the examinee.

SAFETY AND QUALITY ASSURANCE

It is essential for all physicians performing outpatient laser surgery to establish safety procedures, because emergencies do occur. As part of this effort the physician and staff should go down a checklist before beginning a laser procedure. This list should include making sure that all in the room are wearing the correct eye protection and appropriate masks, that the sign warning that laser surgery is in progress is on the outside of the door to the room, that the windows are draped, that the surgical field has been appropriately prepared, and that fire precautions have been taken. When a laser with variable wavelength capabilities (i.e., copper vapor) is to be used, it is essential that appropriate eye protection be available for each wavelength.[11]

The formulation of national standards and regulations concerning laser surgery is guided by the American National Standards Institute (ANSI), which is a nongovernmental organization of experts who determine appropriate laser standards for various fields. These standards are designed for users of lasers and are used by Occupational Safety and Health Administration (OSHA) and other national and state organizations in developing guidelines for laser hazard control. The Laser Institute of America is the secretariat of the ANSI Z136 series of laser safety standards, and copies of the guidelines can be obtained from it. The institute also offers laser safety training courses and additional publications on safety concepts. Surgeons should also be aware of state and local regulations and requirements pertaining to laser surgical procedures.

A quality assurance program should be set up to monitor important aspects of the care provided on an ongoing basis. This involves the ongoing collection of certain data and their periodic evaluation to identify actual or potential problems adversely affecting patient outcomes. For example, data regarding postoperative infection or intraoperative laser burns could be reviewed. After this, policies could be examined and altered as appropriate and reevaluated at a later date to determine objectively whether the corrective measures have achieved and sustained the desired results. At least two physicians should be involved in such quality assurance activities to provide peer-based reviews. Appropriate records of quality assurance activities are maintained by staff members.

RECORDS AND DOCUMENTATION

It is vital for the physician to complete a laser operative report for each patient treated, and it is useful to have a preprinted report for this purpose, thus ensuring complete data recording. The uses of such reports are several. Medically it is a record that can be reviewed to assess the success or lack of success of procedures. Legally it is a complete account of the operation for the patient's records.

A laser surgical log is also helpful. This should list the date, patient's name, diagnosis, procedure, duration of the procedure, and the laser used. The log can be divided into sections according to the type of laser used and each section subdivided according to the diagnosis. This log enables the physician to review his or her work and to document his or her laser surgical experience, should the need arise to have such a record for the purpose of applying for hospital surgical privileges or for legal reasons.

There should also be surgical and photograph consent forms available for the patient to sign before the laser surgery. The same guidelines for all surgical consent forms should be followed. In some states, one form is used for all types of surgery. The laser surgery consent form should include a statement to the effect that alternative therapies and the potential for hypertrophic or keloid scarring, for the recurrence of warts or other lesions, for residual pigmentation after tattoo removal, and for infection have been discussed with the patient.

PATIENT EDUCATION AND PREPARATION

Just as the physician and staff must be educated regarding laser surgery, so also must the patient be instructed, because many patients have unrealistic and inaccurate expectations of laser surgery in terms of the pain, curative potential, and equipment dangers. This need for patient education is pointed up by the fact that occasionally patients undergoing electrocautery treatment erroneously think they are undergoing laser treatment. Patient handouts are therefore invaluable.

Information sheets on different conditions can be sent to the patient before the initial visit. These should contain information on the various ways to treat a particular condition, details of the treatment using a laser, the potential side effects of such treatment, the healing time, and the cost. Color photographs of preoperative and postoperative lesions treated with the laser should also be shown to the patient at the initial visit. This should include both good results and undesirable ones, such as hypertrophic scarring and residual pigmentation after tattoo removal. Such color and black-and-white pictures can be found in several published laser surgery books,[12–15] or 5 × 7–inch photographs of the physician's own patients can be used, but only if permission for use of the photographs for this purpose has been given by the patient.

If the physician is using his or her own photographs, they can be arranged in a permanent book. At the beginning of this book, the physician can list his or her qualifications for doing laser surgery and the relevant training received, followed by the preoperative and postoperative photographs of various conditions. Videotapes are expensive to produce, but many laser manufacturers have such tapes available. This visual education can be an important adjunct in preparing the patient.

Written postoperative instructions should also be prepared for patient use. These should include a clear description of the physician's preferred treatment and regimen, a phone number to call in case of emergency, and a place to fill in the date and time of the follow-up appointment. It is also quite helpful for the patient if this sheet of instructions has a list at the top of all items he or she will need at home for postoperative care (e.g., cleaner, surgical dressing, tape, scissors, antibiotic ointment).

ECONOMIC REIMBURSEMENT

Unfortunately, few CPT codes have been established pertaining to laser surgery, especially cutaneous laser surgery. Such codes are added and deleted each year, and the physician should closely check the relevant codes in the most current CPT book.[3] The most recently added CPT codes are 17106 to 17108, and these are for the laser treatment of vascular proliferating lesions.

A "medical necessity" letter can also be sent to the insurance company or third-party payor before the laser surgery to obtain, if possible, their agreement to pay for the procedure. An accompanying photograph of the patient can be useful, especially if multiple procedures are anticipated (e.g., treatment of port-wine stains [PWSs] with the yellow light laser).[16]

The treatment of PWSs and other vascular lesions is not uniformly accepted by all third-party payors as being medically necessary. To help convince such payors of the medical necessity of the treatment of vascular hamartomas, the physician can send a letter to the insurance company containing details of the natural history of the particular patient's PWS; emphasizing the potential for soft-tissue hypertrophy, and for the formation of nodules or pyogenic granulomas as well as the psychological effects of such lesions; describing the procedure commonly used by specialists for the correction and removal of birth defects; and stressing the fact that the success of laser treatment is well documented in the literature. Photocopies of recent medical articles can be included with the letter.[16–18]

PUBLIC AWARENESS AND EDUCATION

After a physician has established an office laser surgery unit, he or she needs to make physician colleagues and potential patients aware of his or her skills and of the outpatient laser unit. This can be accomplished in several ways.

For example, the physician can make presentations to community and professional organizations, using clinical slides to illustrate the success of such procedures. This will educate both the public and the physician's colleagues to the way a laser works and the indications for such treatment. It would also be helpful for him or her to write articles describing laser treatment for professional journals, newspapers, and magazines. These efforts will also serve to promote his or her skills. In addition, physicians should inform nursing homes of their laser capabilities, because of the fact that cutaneous laser surgery, especially that done using the CO_2 laser, can be performed in patients receiving anticoagulants.

A physician can also add a tasteful, discreet line regarding the fact that he or she is now performing skin laser surgery to his or her letterhead, professional cards, and listing in the telephone yellow pages. Information on cutaneous laser surgery should also be put in the reception area for patients to read while waiting for appointments.

Summary

To establish a successful office laser surgery unit, the physician should purchase a safe, functional laser and adjuvant equipment, acquire the necessary skills, set up proper documentation procedures, distribute appropriate patient information brochures, and properly educate staff, patients, and the public.

Hospital-Based Laser Surgical Unit

Strategic Planning of Hospital Laser Center

There are many differences between establishing an office-based laser surgical practice and starting up a hospital laser center. However, the latter can also vary considerably, in that it could simply involve the purchase of a single laser for a community hospital or it could involve a concerted effort on the part of a referral hospital to position itself as a major provider of laser surgical treatment. No matter what the objectives are, however, the principles outlined in this section apply to the establishment of any hospital-based laser program.

First of all, the hospital or institution should ensure that the laser center fits in with its mission. In the future, almost every hospital will have at least one or more lasers. Currently, however, too frequently hospitals are motivated to start laser centers by the urge to be competitive, in response to aggressive marketing by laser companies, or by a well-meaning but misguided staff physician who sees an opportunity to advance his practice using the universal appeal of laser technology as his lure. Certainly the goal of every health care institution should be the delivery of excellent but cost-effective health care to its patients. If, however, the demanding and somewhat risky prospect of starting a laser center does not fit in with the mission of the institution, the hospital should reexamine its need for a laser center.

Nearly every specialty has identified some use for the laser among the conditions it treats. Ophthalmology was the first specialty to make use of the laser, and even this specialty continues to witness the advancement and refinement of laser techniques and technology. However, the use of lasers in many other specialties, such as orthopedics, is still in its infancy. The laser has also been responsible for redefining areas of expertise in many fields of medicine. General surgery is unique, however, in having adopted the laser for very few uses; at the same time, it is rapidly losing patients to other specialties such as gastroenterology because these specialties have added the laser to their armamentarium.

The strategic planning necessary to establish a comprehensive laser center is a complex process drawing on the expertise of many different people in the hospital environment. Physicians in various specialties with laser experience who are likely to use the laser should be included in the planning, and realistic expectations in terms of the types and number of uses for the laser within these various specialties must be used as a basis for assessing the need. Hospital administrators are involved in planning the financing of the laser acquisition and the administration of the laser center, as well as in the long-range planning of future building programs and laser acquisitions. Operating room nursing staff and the staff of other clinics within the hospital where the laser is likely to be used should also be included in this planning process. Members of the biomedical engineering staff must assess the present resources of the hospital and the future needs of the laser center.

A market analysis should be undertaken to determine the type and quantity of laser services needed within the area serviced by the hospital. Demographic studies of the population served are also needed, including the number of people, the age of the population, and the unique characteristics of the population served. For example, an older population living in Florida would very likely have need for a laser to treat cutaneous carcinomas, whereas a pediatric hospital would likely need a different laser for treating vascular birthmarks. Referral centers may establish a center for particular laser specialties to treat patients referred by surrounding community hospitals. In fact, there are hospitals, most notably in Japan, dedicated solely to the laser treatment of patients. The market analysis should, in addition, determine the incidence of those disorders likely to be treated by laser within the particular population served. Such statistics may be misleading, however, in indicating the potential revenue to be gained in the treatment of some disorders, because insurance companies may view some treatments as cosmetic and consequently refuse to pay for them. Because it is often the patient who then pays for such procedures, this would have the effect of reducing use of the laser center.

Insurance coverage by third-party payors must be taken into consideration when doing a market analysis for a laser center. However, commercial insurance companies vary considerably in their coverage of the costs of laser procedures, and the Diagnostic Related Group (DRG) payment system used by Medicare has further complicated the payment picture. Indeed, a comparison of hypothetical laser treatments with conventional treatments has shown that the DRG system may favor use of the laser treatments because some of these procedures can be done on an outpatient rather than an inpatient basis, thereby increasing the profit margin of the hospital.[21] It is expected, however, that DRG reimbursement will be reduced as statistics regarding the cost-effectiveness of these procedures accumulate.

From a cost-effectiveness point of view, it is possible that a sufficiently large laser treatment caseload could cause a decrease in the bed census in a hospital by shortening the number of inpatient days necessary to treat a patient with a particular disorder. Conversely, there is a certain synergy associated with new techniques, which leads to the additional use of other hospital services, such as radiologic and laboratory services because of the new patients attracted by the laser center. Because of the lengthy time involved in the development of a laser service, however, only conservative estimates of the financial benefits of a laser center should be used in the market analysis. In fact, most hospital laser centers are a financial drain on the hospital for many months before they become self-sustaining.

Finally, as alluded to earlier, there are two very poor reasons for a hospital to start up a laser center. The first is known as the "high tech halo effect," and it is when a hospital does so to demonstrate its progressiveness. The second is a desire to compete with other hospitals, either in response to pressure from the hospitals or from its medical staff. Too frequently this results in the purchase of an expensive laser that then gathers dust in the corner of a hospital room and the fading of the dream of a busy laser center. There is also a considerable tendency to try to expand the indications for using a particular laser once the hospital is heavily invested in a laser center. In this instance, it becomes a laser looking for a clinical application.

As a final aspect of the market analysis, enough data should be gathered regarding the caseload for the hospital to assess the type and number of cases likely to be done per year as well as the likely reimbursement for each case. A cadre of dedicated physicians who are likely to sustain an interest in the laser center during its growing phase should also be identified at this time. Although they do not need to constitute a majority of the medical staff, nevertheless, those few physicians who are likely to be using the lasers should be strongly committed to the development of the laser center during the early phases of the program.

The next strategic planning phase is an assessment of the appropriate regulations concerning a laser center. Many of the early rules and regulations pertaining to laser usage within the medical environment were derived from the *American National Standard for the Safe Use of Lasers* publication Z136.01-1980, but this publication has now been superseded by the *American National Standard for Laser Safety in the Healthcare Environment* (ANSI Z136.3), which is available from the Laser Institute of America. Although these are currently nonbinding standards, many federal and state regulatory agencies will be adopting these standards, which will then give them the force of the law. These standards include detailed guidelines concerning the administration of safety programs, the credentialing process, the training of laser personnel, and other aspects critical to the operation of a laser center. Although many states have no specific laser regulations at present, the Conference of Radiation Control Directors formulated and published in 1983 their suggested guidelines for state legislatures contemplating laser regulations.[22] OSHA has also published its *Occupational Health and Environmental Controls; Nonionizing Radiation* (Code of Federal Regulations Title 29, Chapter 17, Part 1926.43).* Additionally, the planning committee should be aware of local and state codes regarding specific requirements for operating rooms or health care institutions that have a bearing on the laser center. For example, the need for special electrical circuitry in the operating room where laser procedures are to be performed may necessitate significant alterations in the physical environment, and these alterations may need to conform to building codes. The just-named publications may also dictate the incorporation of certain safety features, necessitating further significant alterations in the facilities where the laser will be used. Included in this might be door safety interlocks, which are devices that automatically turn off the laser if a person should inadvertently enter the room where the laser is being used. Appropriate safety warning lights, signs, and protective coatings for windows of laser facilities must also be considered during the planning phase of the laser facility.

Although not directly applicable to the establishment of a laser center, the Joint Commission on Accreditation of Healthcare Organizations is becoming increasingly involved in overseeing the administration of laser programs, particularly from the standpoint of quality assurance.

Finally, an extensive building renovation or expenditure of funds for a new project in a health care institution may require that the hospital obtain a certificate of need, as dictated by state and local statutes.

Additional assistance in this planning and analysis may be obtained from the laser companies. However, because of their natural bias their recommendations should be viewed conservatively. Private laser consultants are also available who can assist in the planning and implementation of a laser center program. More recently, commercial enterprises have come available that can assist in the market analysis and implementation as well as in the long-term administration, maintenance, and promotion of a laser center. These services can be very valuable and indeed can make the difference between the success and failure of a laser center. On the down side, these services are also very expensive, and this would create an additional drain on the income of the laser center. Likewise, the recommendations made by outside laser consultants or laser services should be reviewed by the hospital board to make sure they fit in with the mission of the hospital as well as to make sure they do not in some way compromise the hospital's reputation.

---

*Pfister J, Kneedler JA. A guide to lasers in the OR. Aurora, CO: Educational Design Editorial Consultants, 1983.

SELECTING A LASER

The process of selecting a laser for a hospital laser facility is somewhat more complex than that involved in the purchase of a laser for an office, because the wants and needs of many people have to be considered. Those in certain specialties who will likely use the laser most should have the greatest voice in the selection of the laser, but those in other specialties who may also use the laser should never be totally excluded from the process.

A general call should therefore go out to the medical and dental staff of the facility planning to open a laser center. Many of the staff have probably had the opportunity to use the laser or at least been instructed in the use of the laser at their various specialty meetings. However, sometimes these types of presentations focus on the "cutting edge" of laser technology that may not be available to the average practitioner for some time, either because it is pending the approval of the FDA or a refinement of the techniques. Thus, the information gathered from the medical staff should be checked against that in the literature on the particular applications and lasers. Consultants once again can be useful in determining the type, size, and perhaps even the specific manufacturer of the lasers to be purchased. Another source of information is the American Society for Laser Medicine and Surgery, which has an individual section chairman from each of the medical specialties who can be useful in providing information that can guide the decision.

As discussed elsewhere in this book, the three lasers most commonly used have been the CO_2, argon, and Nd:YAG lasers. Therefore much of the literature has dealt with these three lasers, and indeed many procedures have been developed with them in mind. In addition, most laser courses teach the use of these three lasers. A further reason for their popularity is that, with improvements in technology, they have become the most reliable of the lasers available.

Although these three lasers are the mainstay of most laser centers, problems associated with the use of these lasers in various procedures have prompted efforts to develop new laser instruments, but not always with success. For instance, despite years of research, an acceptable fiberoptic delivery system for the CO_2 laser has yet to be developed. Therefore, surgeons wishing to use the CO_2 laser in a tight location or through an endoscope continue to be plagued with problems stemming from the lack of such a delivery system. For this reason, the Nd:YAG laser, which has contact tips that cause it to function similarly to the CO_2 laser, is replacing the CO_2 for some uses.

The CO_2 laser has many optional features which must be carefully considered. The wattage output of the laser can vary from less than 20 W to more than 100 W. In general, neurosurgeons prefer a high-powered CO_2 laser, whereas cutaneous procedures can be done using a 20-W or less CO_2 laser. Most other uses require 20 to 40 W of power. However, the higher the power, the more costly the instrument; therefore, one must temper the desire to have the highest-power laser available with the cost of the instrument. Because the higher-wattage CO_2 lasers are infrequently used, the planning committee should assess the actual need for a higher-powered instrument before spending the several thousands of dollars extra for a laser capable of the additional wattage.

Another feature of the CO_2 laser that might be included is the so-called superpulsed mode. Although the beam appears to be continuous, this laser emits very high, very short spikes of power, with latent periods between the spikes that allow the tissue to cool between the spikes. This has the effect of causing less thermal damage to the surrounding tissue, and thus this feature is used primarily for cutting tissue, with minimal thermal damage to the surrounding tissue.[23] However, it is also a quite costly feature, and therefore the expense has to be weighed against the disadvantage of the greater surrounding tissue damage inflicted by the continuous-wave lasers. Recently, the development of an ultrapulsed CO_2 laser has further advanced cosmetic laser surgery.[26–28]

Likewise, although the argon laser has been the workhorse of physicians treating superficial vascular lesions, it is not selective for the vascular tissue and therefore it causes damage to surrounding normal tissue. It is now being replaced for many applications by one of the new yellow-light lasers, which may produce better results, especially in young children with superficial vascular lesions.[24]

The argon laser is primarily a coagulating laser and has found considerable use in ophthalmology, plastic surgery, and dermatology. More recently, it has found use in urology and gynecology, where its coagulation abilities have been of particular use in the treatment of a variety of lesions, including endometriosis and bladder tumors. Most argon lasers used for the treatment of cutaneous lesions generate less than 10 W of power; however, their use for intraabdominal procedures may require up to 20 W of power. Unlike the CO_2 laser power, the argon laser power can be delivered by means of a fiberoptic delivery system.

Many attachments are required to enable the most efficient use of a laser by a variety of specialties. In general, otolaryngologists and gynecologists require certain microscopic and endoscopic attachments, which may not be available with every CO_2 laser on the market. Although these attachments add considerable cost to the laser purchase price, in most instances, this additional cost is justified by the additional uses to which the laser can be put.

The CO_2 laser and other lasers have become more efficient over time, and thus the electrical power requirements have been reduced, such that many of these lasers can now be plugged into a standard outlet. Unusual power requirements, of course, can necessitate additional on-site preparation costs and limit the versatility and mobility of the laser. Cooling requirements have also decreased over time, such that many lasers which formerly required water-cooling systems

laser, including an anesthesiologist, but also members of the hospital administration, biomedical engineering department, and nursing staff, as well as other hospital staff considered essential to ensuring the success of the laser center.

One of the responsibilities of the hospital laser committee is to organize both the physical arrangement and administration of the laser center. With regard to the latter, policies and procedures that pertain to the operation of the laser center should be written and incorporated into the hospital policies and procedures. In addition, the laser committee is responsible for the safety of the hospital personnel and patients during use of the laser. To this end, a laser safety officer who has specific training in laser safety should be appointed by the committee and serve as a member of the committee. This person should also have the authority to restrict the use of the lasers or indeed to stop a laser procedure if a safety violation or hazard becomes apparent.

Nursing personnel should be included in the training given hospital personnel, and this should include both nurses who will work in the laser operating room or the laser center and those on the nursing service who will care for the patients preoperatively. Preoperative patient education is frequently necessary to allay the fears of the patient, who may have many misconceptions regarding laser treatment. Laser nurses should also be designated who are responsible for making sure that the laser is available and trained to make sure it is working safely. They should also be responsible for making sure that other instruments that may be needed during the laser procedure are available, that the laser is turned on and checked for alignment, and so on, before the patient is brought to the operating room. Laser checklists are available from the laser manufacturers for this purpose.

Thorough records of the laser procedures performed in the laser center are necessary. These should include the patient's name and hospital number, the name of the laser surgeon, the name of the procedure, the preoperative checklist filled in for the particular procedure as well as the laser parameters used, and a list of the accessories used. The laser parameters should include the wattage, pulse duration, spot size, and total energy used during the various phases of the operation. These records should be kept on file in the laser area and are later combined with the maintenance and malfunction records for the lasers and included in the comprehensive report presented during the hospital laser committee meetings.

Biomedical engineering personnel of the hospital who are responsible for performing minor maintenance on the lasers should also be members of the laser committee. Specific training courses are available for such biomedical engineering personnel.

Usually the nursing service of the laser center or operating room is responsible for scheduling use of the instrument. This is essential to avoid scheduling conflicts. When a laser procedure is scheduled, the scheduling person should also check the credentials list to make sure the physician scheduling the laser procedure is qualified to use that particular laser for that procedure.

The hospital laser committee is responsible for credentialing physicians to use the lasers.[10] This is covered in the hospital policies and procedures (see also Chap. 21). Usually physicians applying for laser privileges complete an application which lists the lasers they are applying for privileges to use as well as the laser procedures they are planning to perform. Certificates of training from laser training courses or from the physicians' residency training directors documenting their training and use of the laser should be reviewed by the laser committee as part of this credentialing process. In addition, the practitioner's department head should be asked for an endorsement of the applicant to ensure he or she is in good standing in the department.

Specific training requirements for laser certification should be written into the hospital laser policies and procedures, and laser practitioners should undergo periodic recertification to ensure they are current in their knowledge of and ability to perform laser procedures.

After receiving the requisite application and documentation, the laser committee should review this material and make recommendations to the hospital's credentialing committee regarding the acceptability of the applicant. The hospital operating room committee may wish to review the credentials of nonsurgical physicians who desire to use a laser in the operating suite to make sure they are adequately trained in operating room procedures.

The procedures done, maintenance required, training requirements, and the like should be reviewed at the periodic meetings of the hospital laser committee in an effort to keep the laser procedures safe and up-to-date. Proposed laser purchases or laser needs are also reviewed at these meetings and the recommendations generated passed along to the hospital administration. Applications for laser privileges are reviewed and forwarded to the hospital credentials committee and executive committee for action. Members of the various medical specialties using the laser might present periodic updates of the current status of laser usage in their specialty and future trends.

Copies of the hospital policies and procedures relating to laser use should be kept current and made readily accessible in the laser center and operating room. In addition, appropriate rules, regulations, and publications relating to laser procedures should be available not only in the laser center, but in the hospital library as well. The library should also maintain a section of books and periodicals relating to laser medicine. Publications regarding laser use are published by the American Society for Laser Medicine and Surgery, the Laser Institute of America, and the American National Standards Institute.*

The laser committee should also regularly review the policies and procedures as well as the costs of using the laser. As can be deduced

*American National Standards, Inc., 1430 Broadway, New York, NY 10018.

from the foregoing discussion, there are many costs to using lasers that need to be included in the charge to the patient or third-party payors.

THE PRESENT AND FUTURE TRENDS

Because the lasers used in medicine are in a state of constant flux, it is difficult, if not impossible, to keep current in the field. Those administering a laser program and who are making decisions regarding such matters as equipment, techniques, and safety should attend meetings where they can be informed regarding current practices and future trends in laser medicine. Although a moderate number of specialty courses, seminars, and meetings are offered by various organizations, schools, and manufacturers, probably the best way to acquire this information is by attending the annual meeting of the American Society for Laser Medicine and Surgery. Excellent general sessions and exhibits of laser equipment are held at this meeting of clinicians, administrators, research and development people, laser manufacturers, and government regulators. Information ranging from the theoretical, to the basic science, to practical clinical applications—what's good and what's not—is also available there. Attendance at this meeting is therefore nearly mandatory for those wishing to remain current in laser medicine.

Lasers are now starting to be used for dental and orthopedic procedures which would form part of a hospital-based laser program. They are also finding new uses for lasers in specialties where they are already an established tool.

Orthopedics is one of the specialties in which the use of lasers is growing rapidly. For example, the holmium laser is being used endoscopically to correct intraarticular disorders, and this procedure is associated with a further reduction in the already reduced morbidity associated with arthroscopic techniques. Endoscopic spinal disk surgery, although controversial at present, continues to be refined and may prove to be an efficient way to manage these difficult-to-treat problems. The laser's ability to remove bone fixation cement as well as to dissect tissue has also found application in orthopedic laser surgery.

Urologists, although long users of lasers, are now using the laser for lithotripsy and other techniques. Laser transurethral prostatic ablation is an example of an exciting and rapidly growing urologic application.

Ophthalmologists continue to improve techniques of radial keratotomy using the excimer laser as well as to refine other long-established procedures.

General surgeons are using the Nd:YAG laser in the contact mode for such procedures as endoscopic cholecystectomy and bowel resections. After an initial surge of enthusiasm for lasers, there was a waning of interest in lasers, only to be followed by a reemergence of interest as the limitations of electrocautery in these procedures became evident.

Plastic surgeons and dermatologists are finding increased hospital-based uses for the laser. One of these uses is the excision of vascular tumors. Because the laser promotes circulation to tissue, in comparison with electrocautery techniques, lasers are being used to dissect tissue and raise flaps for such purposes as mastectomy reconstruction. The use of new and existing lasers for the treatment of superficial skin lesions continues to expand. For instance, superficial vascular lesions may now be treated using the argon laser, the pulsed dye laser, the copper vapor laser, the Q-switched Nd:YAG laser, the copper bromide laser, or the krypton laser, as well as others. Tattoos and pigmented lesions can be removed with some of these lasers, as well as with the Q-switched ruby and alexandrite lasers. The proliferation of lasers in these fields further demands that a person remain current regarding the techniques and equipment.

Probably the hottest area of laser medicine at present is cosmetic CO_2 laser surgery. This has been made possible by the introduction of extremely high powered, short-pulsed CO_2 lasers that can ablate skin and reduce wrinkles and scars.[26,27] The use of lasers for blepharoplasty, hair transplantation, and other invasive techniques has also been growing.[26] This tidal wave of enthusiasm has led to the introduction of many lasers allegedly designed for rejuvenation procedures. Because some of the claims made for such lasers may be unfounded, the purchaser should thoroughly research the sales proposal as well as the literature before purchasing such a machine.

The overwhelming advantage to the therapist using lasers for cosmetic surgery is that it is almost all fee-for-service and thus the hassles of insurance and managed care are eliminated. An advantage as well as a disadvantage to the health care facility is that many of the procedures are accomplished on an outpatient basis with the patients under local anesthesia.

One of the concerns regarding those who want to enter the lucrative field of cosmetic laser surgery is the fact that many have little training that enables them to deal with the care and complications. The facility must therefore prevent the increasing liability risk posed by such a situation by closely supervising the operation of such a laser center. Institutions providing such training should also screen applicants for the laser courses to ensure that all have the basic training consistent with the laser application, such as training in dermatology or plastic surgery in those desiring training in laser resurfacing procedures.

Because many physicians entering the laser field cannot afford the expensive equipment necessary to start up a laser practice, this presents an opportunity for a facility to set up a cosmetic laser facility where many physicians can work. However, it should be borne in mind that as these practitioners build their own practices, they will likely eventually establish their own laser centers.

Maintaining a state-of-the-art laser facility can be very expensive, but new leasing and rental programs have come available that allow hospitals and clinicians to share the expense of remaining up-to-date. Further as lasers become more compact and rugged, it will be possible to transport them readily and for them to be shared by many different facilities through a variety of innovative programs. For example, hospitals will be able to form cooperatives for sharing lasers on a time-share basis. Leasing programs are also available in many areas that allow many practitioners to use the same lasers. Frequently these programs include training and technical assistance as well as maintenance of the equipment. As the economics of medicine continue to change, such programs that involve the use of lasers and other high-tech equipment will assume increasing importance.

Finally, the horizons of laser medicine are expanding with the advent of new techniques. Photodynamic therapy (PDT) is one such technique that is being used for the treatment of many types of cancer. It involves the administration of a drug-dye that is absorbed by specific laser wavelengths, causing the cancer to necrose with little damage to surrounding tissue. This technique has many advantages over other therapies, although it also has several limitations. After many years of testing, the use of PDT in the management of certain gastrointestinal and pulmonary tumors is pending FDA approval; other applications of PDT for the management of bladder, skin, and other cancers will follow rapidly.

Laser angioplasty for the treatment of arterial occlusions continues to be a fertile field of experimentation, as does use of the laser to accomplish the sutureless fusion or welding of tissue.

Summary

The task of starting a hospital laser center is challenging and exciting. Though some laser procedures will undoubtedly be done in regional referral centers, practically every hospital or outpatient center will have one or more lasers for a variety of tasks as the laser assumes a greater role in medicine.

References

1. Bennett RG. Fundamentals of cutaneous surgery. St. Louis: Mosby, 1988;181–193.
2. McBurney EI. Strategic planning and establishment of a laser unit in an office surgical practice. Am J Cosmetic Surg 1993;9:213–218.
3. Coy JA, Fanta CM, Kirschner CG, McNamara MR, Pirrucello FW, AMA Editorial Staff. Physicians' current procedural terminology. Chicago: American Medical Association, 1993.
4. Wheeland RG, Bailin PL, Ratz JL et al. Use of scleral eyeshields for periorbital laser surgery. J Dermatol Surg Oncol 1987;13:156–158.

5. Garden JM, O'Banion MK, Shelnitz LS et al. Papilloma virus in the vapor of carbon dioxide laser–treated verrucae. JAMA 1988;259:1199–1202.
6. Nezht C, Winer WIK, Nezht F et al. Smoke from laser surgery: is there a health hazard? Lasers Surg Med 1987;7:376–382.
7. Baggish MS, Poiesz BJ et al. Presence of human immunodeficiency virus DNA in laser smoke. Lasers Surg Med 1991;11:197–203.
8. American Health Consultants. New research confirms laser plume can transmit disease. Clin Laser Monthly 1993;11:81–84.
9. Friedman R, Saleeby ER, Rubin MG et al. Safety parameters for avoiding acute ocular damage from the reflected CO_2 laser (10.6 µm) laser beam. J Am Acad Dermatol 1987;17:815–818.
10. American Society for Laser Medicine and Surgery. Standards of practice for use of lasers in medicine and surgery. Clin Laser Monthly 1984;2:59.
11. Lundergan D. Practical laser safety. In: Dixon JA, ed. Surgical application of lasers, 2nd ed. Chicago: Year Book, 1987;79–94.
12. Wheeland RG. Lasers in skin disease. New York: Thieme, 1988.
13. Kaplan I, Giler S. CO_2 laser surgery. Berlin: Springer-Verlag, 1984.
14. Olbricht SM, Arndt K. Lasers in cutaneous surgery. In: Fuller TA, ed. Surgical lasers: a clinical guide. New York: Macmillan, 1987;113–135.
15. Dover JS, Arndt KA, Geronemus RG et al. Illustrated cutaneous laser surgery: a practitioner's guide. Norwalk, CT: Appleton & Lange, 1990.
16. Geronemus RG, Ashinoff R. The medical necessity of evaluation and treatment of port-wine stains. J Dermatol Surg Oncol 1991;17:76–79.
17. Tan OT, Sherwood K, Gilchrest BA. Treatment of children with port-wine stains using the flashlamp-pulsed tunable dye laser. N Engl J Med 1989;320:416–421.
18. Ashinoff R, Geronemus R. Capillary hemangiomas and treatment with the flashlamp-pumped dye laser. Arch Dermatol 1991;127:202–205.
19. Morelli JG, Tan OT, Weston WL. Treatment of ulcerated hemangiomas with the pulsed tunable dye laser. Am J Dis Child 1991;145:1062–1064.
20. Garden JM, Bakus AD, Paller AS. Treatment of cutaneous hemangiomas by the flashlamp-pumped pulsed dye laser: prospective analysis. J Pediatr 1992;120:555–560.
21. Mackety CJ. Perioperative laser nursing: a practical guide. Thorosare, NJ: Charles B. Slack, 1984.
22. Lundergun DK, Rockwell RJ. ANSI medical laser standards. Clin Laser Monthly 1984;2:99–100.
23. Hobbs ER, Bailin PL, Wheeland RG, Ratz JL. Superpulsed lasers: minimizing thermal damage with short duration, high irradiance pulses. J Dermatol Surg Oncol 1987;13:955–964.
24. Tan O, Gilchrest B. Laser therapy for selected cutaneous vascular lesions in the pediatric population: a review. Pediatrics 1988;82:652–662.
25. Joffe SN, Oguro Y, eds. Advances in Nd:YAG laser surgery. New York: Springer-Verlag, 1987.
26. Weinstein C. Ultrapulse carbon dioxide laser removal of periocular wrinkles in association with laser blepharoplasty. J Clin Laser Med Surg 1994;12(4):205–209.
27. Waldorf HA, Kauvar ANB, Geronemus RG. Skin resurfacing of fine to deep rhytides using a char-free carbon dioxide laser in 47 patients. Dermatol Surg 1995;21:940–946.
28. Gregory RO, Baker S. Laser blepharoplasty. Aesthetic Surg Quarterly 1995(summer).

21 ____ Education and Credentialing in Laser Surgery

Judith I. Pfister

The primary purpose of a laser education and credentialing program is safety—to ensure that all physicians and staff members who work with or around lasers have sufficient education and thereby ensure that patients and personnel are protected from injury. This chapter examines the educational needs of health care personnel who work with lasers or in environments where the laser is used. The educational needs of practicing physicians are highlighted, but the laser education for residents, anesthesiologists, laser safety officers, and nurses and other technical personnel is also covered. Laser safety education and operational training on specific laser devices are explored, as well as the need for education in the fundamentals of laser physics. The issue of laser credentialing is examined in depth, and a sample laser credentialing policy is provided that can be adapted to suit individual institutional settings.

Laser Education

It is customary in many health care facilities to form a separate, permanent task-oriented laser committee. One of the responsibilities of this committee is to work with the education/training/inservice department to ensure that appropriate education is provided for all personnel who will be working with lasers.

COMPONENTS OF LASER EDUCATION

In addition to system-specific information, laser education courses must include the concepts, principles, and facts necessary for a generalized understanding of all laser systems. Topics that should be covered in a comprehensive laser education program include the following:

- The physics of electromagnetic energy
- The tissue effects of laser energy

- Operational aspects of the lasers and accessory devices
- Laser safety
- Clinical applications
- Legal and regulatory requirements

Too often, however, such courses focus strictly on operational and safety considerations, leaving participants without a fundamental understanding of what they are doing and why.

The Physics of Electromagnetic Energy

It is important that health care personnel understand the physics of the electromagnetic spectrum and wavelength energy. Used improperly, lasers can cause severe injury to patients or staff. Without some knowledge of the way in which wavelength energy actually is created and works, personnel may not respond appropriately in the face of unforeseen events. The possibility of accidents may be increased, and the quality of patient care and treatment may be compromised.

The first objective of laser education should be to provide learners with the concepts, principles, and facts necessary for a generalized understanding of all laser systems.[1] The provision of such comprehensive background information should have the effect of enhancing the quality of patient care, preventing accidents, ensuring compliance with policies and procedures, and facilitating the delivery of appropriate care and the proper maintenance of equipment.

Tissue Effects of Laser Energy

Lasers are capable of producing biophysical tissue effects previously unseen with conventional medical devices, and it is important that health care professionals who work with lasers understand these effects. Laser energy interacts with biologic tissue through absorption, reflection, transmission, or scattering. However, only when it is absorbed does the energy exert an effect on tissue. The penetration, or depth of radiation, of different laser wavelengths varies according to the ratio of absorption. The absorption of laser energy by biologic tissue generally results in the thermal effects of either coagulation (photocoagulation/hemostasis or necrosis) or vaporization (tissue evaporation). In some instances, laser energy causes photochemical, photodynamic, or photodisruptive effects.

The biophysical reaction of tissues to lasing varies according to the type of tissue, the laser wavelength, the modality used, and the power settings chosen. Laser parameters that affect tissue response are spot size, the duration of application, and operational wave mode (continuous wave versus pulsed waves). Characteristics of tissue that in turn influence the effects of laser energy include the thermal conductivity of the tissue, reflectivity and internal scattering losses, the degree of nonhomogeneity of tissue components, and the amount of the circulating blood supply.

Operational Aspects

Operational training on specific laser systems is usually readily available to health care institutions. Most laser companies provide inservice education on the use of their equipment at the time it is delivered and installed. It is important that the hospital in turn ensure the attendance of all appropriate personnel, including physicians, nurses, and technicians, at these training sessions.

Operational training should include demonstrations and return demonstrations on the operational use of the laser, the draping of patients, the use and care of accessories, and the proper use of and operation of smoke evacuation systems. Power and plumbing requirements for the individual laser system should also be covered. The purpose and use of various delivery systems available for the specific laser being introduced into use should also be a focus of discussion.

Laser Safety

The American National Standards Institute (ANSI) has put together a list of the specific content that should be covered in a laser safety education program for different health care personnel, including physicians and laser technical support staff, health care support staff, laser safety officers (LSOs), and medical laser service personnel.

ANSI requires that laser safety programs providing a complete understanding of the requirements of a safe laser environment be established for all health care personnel using class 4 health care laser systems and for personnel responsible for caring for patients during such procedures (e.g., anesthesia personnel, nursing staff). ANSI also requires that laser safety training be provided for the technical support personnel responsible for preoperative and postoperative laser system checkout and for those responsible for monitoring the system during surgery (e.g., laser technicians, nurses, or clinical engineers).[2]

ANSI recommends that this laser safety training focus on ensuring safety during the surgical procedure and on preventing the potential hazards associated with the surgical use of lasers. Where possible, training aids, manuals, and audiovisual materials should be used.

Nurses, operating room (OR) technicians, and surgeons must know all aspects of patient safety as it relates to lasers. Eye injuries, tissue burns, fires, smoke inhalation, the formation of emboli, and electrocution are also possible hazards. Laser safety education must include learner objectives for each of these topics, and the educational process must ensure that the objectives are met by each attendee.

Clinical Applications

New medical and surgical applications of lasers are continually being discovered. Any laser education course should include an explanation of the advantages of lasers in procedures appropriate to the learners' specialties as well as illustrations of the use of lasers in such procedures. One of the most effective ways to teach physicians and support staff a specific clinical application is to show them a slide presentation, followed by a videotape of the actual procedure. Because physicians are responsible for the energy application, physicians should teach physicians the actual skills needed in applying the beam. In addition, the faculty member teaching a course on laser applications must have had enough experience in actual applications so as to be able to teach not only all the skills needed to use the technology to best advantage but also the way to use it safely. Hands-on skill laboratories are almost mandatory for teaching these skills.

Legal and Regulatory Requirements

Every physician, nurse, institution, and manufacturer involved with the medical application of laser devices must understand the attendant legal and ethical responsibilities. Pertinent legal issues include potential liability for injury to patients or staff, the need for informed consent, the use of lasers in investigational procedures, and compliance with institutional policies and procedures, as discussed in the following paragraphs:

- If use of the laser results in injury to patients or staff, responsibility for damages may be assigned to the person, or persons, causing the injury, to the manufacturer, or to the institution, or to a combination of these. If an injury results from laser malfunction, the manufacturer is responsible—but only if the laser is used according to the manufacturer's recommendations, used for intended applications, and has not been altered in design or damaged.
- Informed consent is critical. The patient must know what is to take place, what is expected, what complications are possible, and what alternative treatments are available. He or she must give written consent to be treated accordingly.
- Specific approvals, protocols, and case-by-case documentation are required to use lasers for procedures that the U.S. Food and Drug Administration (FDA) considers investigational.
- If the laser education program is based at the participants' home institution, it is appropriate to include in the program a discussion of the institutional policies and procedures that apply to laser use. Such policies and procedures typically cover laser maintenance, use, safety, the educational preparation and credentialing of users, the role of the laser safety committee, scheduling considerations, and documentation requirements for laser surgical procedures.

It is also important for health care personnel to be aware of federal regulations and voluntary guidelines that affect the medical use of lasers, including those promulgated by the:

- U.S. Food and Drug Administration, which regulates the manufacture and investigational uses of health care laser systems.
- Occupational Safety and Health Administration, which provides safety codes for manufacturers and users of lasers.
- American National Standards Institute, which classifies lasers according to their ability to cause biologic damage and has published voluntary standards for laser safety.
- Association of Operating Room Nurses, which has issued a series of four recommended safety practices pertaining to the use of lasers in the operating room.

LASER EDUCATION NEEDS OF SPECIFIC LEARNER GROUPS

To be effective, laser education programs must be appropriate for the group targeted. Obviously the needs of a practicing surgeon, for example, differ from those of a postoperative unit nurse. Physicians, anesthesiologists, residents, LSOs, nurses, and laser service personnel all have specific educational needs and requirements. Furthermore, all new employees, regardless of their background and area of specialization, must also receive training in the specific equipment used and the policies of the institution.

Physicians

The laser educational needs of physicians who have already completed their medical training can best be met through continuing medical educational programs, laser center seminars, in-hospital in-service presentations offered in conjunction with laser manufacturers, and preceptorships. Continuing medical education programs should provide background information on laser physics and tissue effects, specific clinical applications of the laser in the physician's specialty, and an opportunity for hands-on experience with return demonstrations.

ANSI has recommended that the following topics be included in the laser safety courses for physicians, nurses, and laser technical support staff (e.g., clinical engineers, laser technicians):

- The biologic effects of laser radiation and the potential hazards associated with laser use, including eye and skin injuries caused by exposure to direct and reflected beams; fire hazards; hazards and concerns about laser-produced fumes and particulate matter; and other associated hazards (e.g., high-pressure gas, anesthesia).
- Laser safety standards; practical measures to ensure the safe use of the laser for medical purposes, including laser eye protection (types and proper selection); methods to eliminate explosion hazards; methods of smoke evacuation; methods to reduce fire hazards; ways to reduce reflected beam hazards; and standard operating procedures for medical laser use.

Anesthesiologists

Although many anesthesiologists have never administered anesthesia to patients undergoing laser treatments, virtually all are aware of the danger of endotracheal fires during such procedures. To reduce the risk of this potentially catastrophic event, any anesthesiologist who participates in, or anticipates participating in, laser procedures should attend a 2- to 4-hour laser safety workshop. The workshop could be given by another anesthesiologist in the community, a laser consultant, or a trained representative of a manufacturer of lasers or laser-resistant endotracheal tubes. Such a program should include a brief introduction to lasers and laser physics and a discussion of safety regulations as well as the institutional policies and procedures that pertain to laser use. Appropriate hands-on experiences might include the preparation of endotracheal tubes for laryngeal surgery and the testing of the effects of the laser beam on various types of endotracheal tubes. The workshop should leave a vivid impression on the anesthesiologist of the risks of laser surgery.

At one hospital, anesthesiologists assigned to work on otolaryngology procedures must attend a 4-hour anesthesia workshop that covers the risks of anesthesia associated with each ENT technique. This workshop includes demonstrations of endotracheal tube fires.[3]

Residents

Medical schools are now incorporating education in laser treatments into many residency programs, particularly the gynecology and ophthalmology programs. The content of the laser education offered to residents should be similar to that offered to practicing physicians.

Laser Safety Officers

In most institutions, the laser committee appoints a person, usually a physician or a nurse manager, to serve as the LSO. The LSO is responsible for evaluating and monitoring laser safety hazards and often has the authority to stop a laser operation if safe practices are not being followed. Although the ANSI standards do not mention this consideration, LSOs must have a working schedule that permits them to be present during laser surgical procedures.

ANSI has recommended that the training programs for LSOs should include the same information on practical procedures and equipment included in medical and technical staff. In addition, the education of LSOs should provide a basic understanding of the local, state, and federal regulations, as well as the practices recommended by ANSI.[4]

ANSI also recommends that the following specific topics be included in a laser safety education program for LSOs:

- Basic laser concepts
- Biologic effects

- Effects on the eye and skin
- Laser hazards
- Hazards analysis and laser standards
- Hazard classifications
- Laser controls in the medical environment
- Safe practices and programs in the medical environment
- Medical surveillance
- Anesthesia problems
- Local, state, and federal regulations
- Practices recommended by ANSI[4]

Nurses and Support Staff

Laser education is also important for nursing and support staff, including unit nurses working in postoperative care units, the operating room, or day surgery; postanesthesia nurses; and personnel involved with laser treatment in the eye clinic, cardiopulmonary laboratory, and gastroenterology laboratory. Educational programs must give specific information on each type and model of laser, as well as information on specific procedures and patient care needs.[5]

The content of a hospital-wide educational program on lasers for unit nurses should include an introduction to lasers and basic laser physics, the clinical applications of lasers in various specialties, safety considerations, and preoperative, intraoperative, and postoperative nursing roles, including assessing the patient, identifying potential problems and formulating nursing diagnoses, planning care, performing nursing activities and patient teaching, and evaluating patient outcomes. OR nurses need to receive intensive education and hands-on training in laser use, whereas OR personnel who will not be directly involved with the laser may only need an introductory course or overview that provides a basic understanding of lasers and the policies that govern their use.

Patients who undergo laser surgical procedures typically experience less swelling and edema, tissue trauma, bleeding, and pain than patients who undergo comparable conventional surgical procedures. These differences have implications for the nursing care rendered in postoperative units. For instance, laser surgery patients may need less pain medication and their length of stay may be shorter. Postanesthesia nurses also need to know the expected physiologic responses of the patient to laser surgery, the complications that may occur, and what to do should they occur. They should also know the outcomes to expect in patients undergoing laser procedures. An example of a possible postoperative complication is bleeding, which may not be observable or go undetected because of the fact that laser surgery is associated with less bleeding. They will also have to monitor the pain level in the patient, which may be less immediately after a laser procedure than after a conventional procedure but be increased later in the recovery period.

ANSI recommends that laser safety courses for nurses and technicians include the following subject matter:

- The laser beam: what it is and what it can do, eye and skin hazards, and other laser hazards.
- The dangers posed by laser surgery, including exposure to reflected beams, and smoke, explosions, and fire.
- Methods and procedures to ensure safety, including the boundary of the nominal hazard zone, laser area warning signs, entryway controls, the wearing of personal protective equipment (e.g., eyewear, flame-retardant gowns), control of unauthorized personnel to prevent access to the laser, safety techniques, use of surgical drapes in laser surgery procedures, and proper laser system controls (e.g., foot switch). Details of the standard operating procedures for the OR should also be covered.

It is important that nurses attend courses that have been designed by and for nurses. Nurses who attend physician training programs may be disappointed to find out that nursing considerations are not covered. Courses that are designed specifically for nurses should focus on the role of the nurse during laser therapy.[4]

Laser Equipment Service Personnel

The personnel who service laser equipment need both didactic training and hands-on experience, including specialized operational training offered by the manufacturer. ANSI recommends that laser service and repair personnel, whether in-house technical staff or contractor personnel, participate in a laser safety course that emphasizes total safety during service procedures, not just for the service personnel themselves but also for uninvolved persons who may be in the general area where a laser is being worked on.

Programs designed for service personnel should highlight the special precautions that need to be taken during high-hazard periods when portions of the laser's protective housing are removed, because the potential for eye damage is much greater at such times. Service personnel must also be knowledgeable about the potential electrical and fire hazards, as well as the possible risk of injury as the result of eye and skin exposure to direct and reflected laser beams. They should also be instructed in the general precautions that need to be taken in operating rooms and other clinical areas.

ANSI specifically recommends that the following topics be included in a laser safety course for service and repair personnel:

- Operational characteristics of lasers, including optical pathways in the laser systems and the electrical circuits involved.
- Laser bioeffects, including ocular and skin effects; the potential for fire, explosion, and electrical shock; and the effects of laser-induced fumes and particles.

- Methods for the safe use of lasers, including eye protection, the prevention of electrical shocks, the evacuation of smoke and fumes, warning signs, door interlocks, and general rules of safety applicable to a medical environment.[4]

New Employee Orientation

Any new employee who will be working in a laser treatment area needs to go through a formal orientation program, regardless of the person's previous experience and expertise. Such orientation sessions should cover the clinical applications of the laser in each specialty, patient needs relative to treatment plans, and the wavelength of choice, as well as all institutional laser policies and procedures pertaining to the use of lasers, including safety rules.

Steps in Developing a Laser Education Program

The design of a laser education program varies with the intended audience and the scope of the material to be presented. Regardless of the content, however, there are certain logical steps to be followed in the design phase of an educational program, beginning with a needs assessment and ending with documentation of the strengths and weaknesses of the program. The steps to be followed include:

- Determining the educational needs
- Defining the purpose and objectives
- Selecting the program content
- Considering the logistics
- Selecting faculty
- Choosing teaching methods and learning activities
- Presenting the material
- Evaluating the program
- Providing recognition of attendance
- Documenting content and outcomes

The specific details regarding these steps are given in the following sections.

DETERMINING THE EDUCATIONAL NEEDS

The first step in designing any educational program is to define the background and needs of the audience. This information helps determine the particular content of the program and the type of learning activities that should be incorporated.

The purpose of a needs assessment is to identify the target group's overall educational needs as well as the needs of individual members. It also identifies the needs of the organization, including standards of care, the philosophy and goals of the laser program, institutional policies and procedures, and the requirements of in-house resources, such as the laser safety committee.

There are a variety of ways to determine the learning needs of the prospective audience. These include questionnaires, a literature review, observation of skills, job analyses, interviews with prospective attendees, performance appraisals, identification of expected competencies, informal feedback, and staff meetings. It is important to determine not just what the staff wants to know but also what they know in terms of such basic but less-understood areas as laser physics, tissue response, and the expected outcomes of laser surgery. Some consideration must also be given to the learners' psychological needs. For example, one group may be overly concerned about safety principles, whereas another is relatively unconcerned about this area. Summaries of course evaluations specifying additional information that was needed in the course will guide the nature of future changes in course design.

DEFINING THE PURPOSE AND OBJECTIVES

During the design of a laser education program, it is important to define exactly what the program is trying to accomplish. A purpose statement provides a starting point from which to develop the content and activities of the program. It should reflect the educator's philosophy on teaching and should further the program's goals or objectives. It should also describe the level of learning (basic, intermediate, or advanced) at which participants in the program begin and end and who should be the intended audience. An example of such a statement might be:

Program Scope and Purpose
The purpose of this full-day workshop is to provide general and specific knowledge regarding medical and surgical laser applications. The intended audience is professional nurses responsible for perioperative patient care and those in related fields.

Basic physics and functions will be reviewed, and safety precautions and the advantages of these procedures from the standpoint of patient outcome will be discussed. The role and activities of nurses have been altered with the advent of new technology, and the broadening applications of lasers to patient care are further proof of this. Attendees will be able to identify those changes that directly affect nursing activities.

The next important step is to develop program objectives—specific learner outcomes achieved by the educational activity. The objectives are summed up by the mnemonic RUMBA. That is, they should be *r*easonable, *u*nderstandable, *m*easurable, *b*ehavioral, and *a*ttainable; they should also be appropriate to the knowledge level of the attendees and the course content.

Verbs such as "list," "describe," "demonstrate," or "differentiate" should be used in objectives to identify what attendees should be able to do at the end of the activity. These words are also more tangible, in the sense that they identify the means to "measure" the attendee's knowledge. Objectives should also be simply stated so that participants will know exactly what is expected of them before they begin. The person, or persons, developing the course objectives should keep in mind that the objectives should:

- Focus on the learner's, not the instructor's, behavior.
- Specify exactly what the learner will be able to do at the end of the program.
- Be limited to one-learner behavior.
- Consider the cognitive, psychomotor, and affective domains of behavior.

Once they are clearly defined, the objectives can serve as a basis for the development of criteria to evaluate the learner's level of learning and to assess the overall program.[5]

SELECTING THE PROGRAM CONTENT

The more clearly the purpose and objectives are stated, the easier it is to then select the program content. This is done simply by detailing the information and skills participants will need to have to meet their identified learning needs.

If outside teaching resources are being used, however, it is important to distinguish operational- and safety-oriented inservice programs from comprehensive continuing education programs that include such subjects as patient care considerations, physician-nurse responsibilities, and problem-solving. The latter programs go into more depth regarding laser applications and safety issues.

CONSIDERING THE LOGISTICS

Once the course content has been determined, the date and location of the program can be determined. Laser education may be provided on site, or it may be provided at other facilities or educational institutions, such as postgraduate programs or laser centers. Because of their convenience, on-site courses seem to reach the maximal number of people prepared to work with the lasers. Nevertheless, off-site specialty laser courses and medical and nursing laser seminars are becoming a more common form of continuing education.

The physical environment is an important aspect of the learning process. It should be quiet and away from distractions. The best setting for the teaching of didactic content, such as physics, applications, and safety, is probably a classroom that has the appropriate audiovisual equipment available. Classroom-style seating, with desks or tables on which participants can write or set materials, is usually best. Adequate working space is important, too, especially for a group of relative strangers.

For hands-on sessions, personnel may be most comfortable working in their own environment, such as in the room where the laser will actually be used. Frequently, because of the environmental specifications of the laser, such as plumbing or electricity, such teaching has to take place in a specific location.

The time of day and the day of the week on which the course is held must also be considered. If participants are tired, they will not be able to focus on the material presented, so it is best to schedule the program as early in the day as possible. It may also be helpful to schedule it on the days of the week when the workload is lightest, so the staff can give their full attention to the course content. Most laser courses last for 1 to 3 days, depending on the content.

SELECTING FACULTY

The first place to look for appropriate people to teach a laser education course is right within the organization, where there may be qualified people on the staff, such as the postanesthesia staff educator, the operating room instructor, the laser safety officer, or the laser coordinator.

If no such people are identified, it may be appropriate to consider bringing in outside consultants or other health care providers in the community who have laser treatment experience. Local or regional postgraduate programs and laser centers often have experts in their fields who conduct courses and seminars. It may also be advantageous for laser facilities in the community or region to join efforts in this regard.

Some hospitals offer educational seminars or workshops in conjunction with laser distributors and manufacturers. Manufacturer-sponsored programs may be less expensive or may even be provided free of charge as part of the laser purchase agreement. However, programs provided by manufacturers and distributors may not cover patient care aspects of laser therapy. Manufacturers best teach the mechanical aspects of the laser devices. Specific patient needs, outcomes, and treatments are best learned from those with clinical experience. Therefore physicians should teach the procedural aspects and nurses should teach the nursing aspects.

If speakers are hired from outside the organization, their topics must be determined in advance to minimize the duplication of information.

CHOOSING TEACHING METHODS AND LEARNING ACTIVITIES

The design of a learning activity must include a description of the teaching methods that will be used. Although it is important to follow the general principles of adult education and learning, teaching methods need not be limited to traditional lecture or didactic presentations. Lectures are more interesting if augmented with videocassettes, films, slides, demonstrations, simulated situations, and case presentations.

It is important to remember that different people have different learning styles. They may learn best by inquiry, instruction, performance, observation, conceptualization, or a combination of these methods. Most health care professionals, however, prefer the performance mode of learning. Hands-on work or experiments can help participants learn both skills and concepts. Eggs, grapefruit, oranges, tomatoes, chicken, and steak have all been used to help learners appreciate the laser's power and capabilities. Such hands-on laser exercises can also help to alleviate some of the anticipatory anxieties people planning to work with lasers experience.[5]

References, bibliographies, and recommended reading lists should also be provided to students. Medical and nursing journals provide current and specific information on laser procedures, the nursing care for patients undergoing such procedures, and the uses to which lasers are being put in various medical specialties. Learners should be encouraged to read such publications and to stay current regarding new information that can be applied within their facilities.

PRESENTING THE MATERIAL

Didactic Sessions

Didactic sessions should start with a discussion of basic laser physics and end with a description of postoperative follow-up. Each speaker should be limited in the time he or she speaks, and these limits must be enforced. A discussion period should be provided so that attendees can ask questions or relate specific experiences that need to be discussed. Time must also be allotted for introductions, breaks, and lunch periods.

Laboratory Experiences

If laser equipment and supplies must be brought in for hands-on exercises, vendor participation can be helpful. Equipment or supply needs, the delivery address, the setup time, and disassembly information should be specified and confirmed in writing with the vendor. If the laser has special electrical or water requirements, these details must also be dealt with in advance.

On the day of the course, all equipment and supplies should be set up in advance. Laboratory stations must be functional before the participants arrive.

A limited number of students should participate in laboratory experiences, preferably less than six at each station. Exercises should be outlined in writing so that the instructors and participants can refer to them for guidance.

Learners can better understand the properties of wavelengths by applying them to various food items, which simulates their particular effect on tissue. By varying power levels and exposure times, learners can also appreciate the effects of various power densities and radiant exposures. The power density can be altered by varying the spot size, wattage, and duration of exposure. The pigment-specific properties of the argon or Nd:YAG laser can be illustrated by using white chicken meat in which small bits of dark liver have been implanted or a piece of slightly wet white paper with black ink on it. Egg white is a good learning model for appreciating beam depth penetration. The protein of the white coagulates and chars after the impact of the thermal beam. If the egg white is in a shallow clear cup, the learner can place the cup at eye level to view the effect of each beam impact. A cow's cervix reacts similarly to human cervical tissue during Nd:YAG laser conization and can be pinned to a cork board to simulate the positioning appropriate for beam application.

If live animals are used to demonstrate the response of living tissue to different wavelengths, all state and federal regulations must be adhered to. Regulations of the U.S. Department of Agriculture must be strictly enforced, and animals must be procured through approved vendors. The animals must be anesthetized and controlled by a qualified veterinarian.[6] The Animal Welfare Act governs uses of animal learning models.

EVALUATING THE PROGRAM

The objectives that were defined during the program development phase should also be used to evaluate each student's level of learning and to demonstrate the effectiveness of the educational program. Evaluations can take the form of written pretests and posttests, oral tests, clinical presentations, or return demonstrations. The results provide feedback on the amount of material the students have learned, and they also indicate the effectiveness of the program as a whole, including the teaching methods and the appropriateness of content.

It is also important to have all participants evaluate their experience. They should be asked to evaluate the program's speakers, its content, the appropriateness of the objectives, and the methodology used in the laboratory experiences.

Evaluations should be summarized and reviewed by the person, or persons, responsible for coordinating the course. This documents participants' views of the strengths and weaknesses of the course. Any weaknesses noted can then be rectified before the course is offered again, thereby ensuring that the course better meets subsequent participants' needs.

PROVIDING RECOGNITION OF ATTENDANCE

At a minimum, all participants should be given a certificate of attendance as proof of their educational experience. To give the program more credibility, the course should be approved by the appropriate accrediting body. Health care professionals may be more apt to attend such an accredited course, because continuing education is required by many states and certification programs.[6]

Laser nursing courses should also offer continuing education units from an accredited approval body. A nursing contact hour is equal to 50 minutes of continuing education, not including lunches, breaks, welcome statements, and registration times. Physician laser courses should offer continuing medical education units or other recognized approval units. The Accreditation Council for Continuing Medical Education is the recognized accrediting body for surgeons.

DOCUMENTING CONTENT AND OUTCOMES

A summary should be written after the course is over that goes into detail regarding its overall achievements, strengths, and weaknesses. Expenses and revenues should be noted to provide a financial picture and, if the findings are encouraging, to help justify offering another course.

Laser education can be a rewarding experience for the institution and for the people involved. Being recognized as a laser education resource helps to promote the leadership of the hospital in the area of laser technology. Physicians and patients both are attracted to facilities that are recognized as pacesetters in innovative, high-technology fields such as laser surgery.

Credentialing

It is not enough that the personnel involved in laser procedures participate in appropriate educational activities. Given the unusual hazards to patients and personnel posed by the use of lasers and the potential legal and financial liabilities involved, health care institutions in which lasers are used also have a responsibility to maintain and document a formal laser surgery credentialing process. The principal rationales for this are to ensure quality of care and safety—to protect both patients and personnel from accidental injury related to laser user.

Credentialing is also important for the legal protection of the facility, its surgeons, and other personnel involved in laser procedures. Numerous court cases have confirmed the fact that a hospital owes its patients a duty of due care in the selection of its medical staff and in the granting of specialized surgical privileges. This principle has also been applied to reapplications for clinical privileges,[7] in that a hospital can be held accountable if it knows or should have known that a physician was unqualified for clinical privileges or was incompetent to practice medicine in accordance with the required standard of care.

Credentialing guidelines must be clinically sound without being unreasonably restrictive. Issues such as disturbing local referral patterns and competition must be avoided; credentialing should not be used as a means to protect a select few who want to keep the laser and facility to themselves. Furthermore, credentialing mechanisms should not be cumbersome and time-consuming, because this can thwart utilization.

It is important to distinguish "credentialing" and "certification." Credentialing is first and foremost an effort to ensure the provision of safe and competent patient care. It is an internal activity of a hospital or other institutions, which grants credentials to people who meet certain criteria, thereby allowing them to perform specific functions. Certification, on the other hand, is an external activity of state licensing boards and of professional associations, societies, organizations, and boards, who typically test an applicant and award certification in their specialty.

At the present time, there are no national, state, or local certification guidelines to help hospitals, insurance carriers, or other institutions decide who is qualified to perform medical procedures involving lasers. Individual health care institutions must therefore establish their own guidelines defining the requirements for education and experience for physicians and other personnel who wish to use this new technology.

NATIONAL CREDENTIALING GUIDELINES

Suggested standards of practice for the use of lasers in medicine and surgery were devised by the American Society of Laser Medicine and Surgery (ASLMS), the major multispecialty laser surgical organization in the United States. Their guidelines, which are reproduced in Table 21-1,[6] define the formal academic training and clinical preceptorship requirements and other important elements of the laser credentialing process. However, they represent only the minimal requirements for those wishing to perform laser surgery. It must also be remembered that these are only guidelines and should be regarded as such by physicians and other health care professionals who are working to establish a compatible credentialing mechanism.

The American Board of Laser Medicine and Surgery also planned to develop a credentialing examination, but it is doubtful that such an examination could cross the numerous specialty lines involved. The need for a national multispecialty certification board for laser users is also questionable, because, like any new surgical instrument, lasers are gradually becoming an accepted tool in the appropriate specialties. As this happens, education in the use of lasers is being

Table 21-1.   Recommended guidelines from the Nursing Division of the American Society of Laser Medicine and Surgery

Hospital privileges are, and must remain, the responsibility of the hospital governing board. Those requesting privileges to use a laser shall meet all the standards of the hospital with regard to board certification, board eligibility, special training, ethical character, good standing, judgment, indications for laser application, etc.

In addition, the following laser training and experience is recommended:

1. The applicant shall review the pertinent literature and audiovisual aids and shall attend training courses devoted to teaching of laser principles and safety. These courses shall include basic laser physics, laser tissue interaction, discussions of the clinical specialty field, and hands-on experience with lasers. Such courses should entail a minimum of 8 to 10 hours.

2. The individual shall consult with an experienced operator in the specialty area involved. Such consultation may consist of several brief visits or a more prolonged stay, with a minimum of 6 to 8 hours of observation and hands-on involvement. It is essential that the individual observe and document actual clinical application of the laser in the outpatient or hospital setting, as appropriate to the procedures in which the training is conducted.

3. In lieu of the above, the applicant may present a letter from the Program Director of an accredited residency in which laser utilization is part of the experience obtained.

   Individuals in training are urged to obtain laser experience as part of their residency. This must include a minimum of 6 to 8 hours of observation and hands-on involvement.

4. The applicant shall perform only those procedures which he or she is capable of accomplishing by conventional means, and initially should perform only simple procedures.

5. The applicant shall establish a means to work closely with biomedical engineering personnel.

Source: From Ball K. Lasers: the perioperative challenge, ed 2. St. Louis: Mosby, 1995;409–414.

incorporated into residency programs, with the result that questions regarding laser technology will be included in the certifying examinations given by the respective boards that oversee the certification of physicians in the various specialties and subspecialties. In the years to come, all newly certified physicians will have been trained in and tested on the use of lasers as it pertains to their particular specialty. CME courses in the use of lasers are proliferating for physicians already in practice. Specialty boards can play an important role in the training of both residents and practicing physicians by standardizing the credentialing process, and they can do this by setting guidelines for residency training, continuing medical education, course content, and laser safety, treating the laser as a specialized surgical tool whose use should be regulated in the same way as other earlier technologies.

In the meantime, the responsibility for the credentialing of laser surgeons and support personnel belongs with individual health care institutions. This is not to say that there are no formal requirements that govern the use of lasers in health care settings. For example, ANSI[4] requires that health care facilities and private practitioners establish and maintain an adequate program for the control of laser hazards, including limiting the number of personnel who enter the hazard zone to those who have an adequate knowledge of safe procedures and control measures appropriate to the function of each. ANSI suggests that many health care facilities have found it convenient to incorporate laser user authority into the credentialing procedures connected with granting privileges. The ANSI standards incorporate the ASLMS standards only by reference, not as a requirement.

DEVELOPING INSTITUTIONAL CREDENTIALING GUIDELINES

If the responsibility for developing laser credentialing mechanisms is to be left to individual health care institutions, at least for the time being, there are certain factors that must be considered, beginning with deciding who will develop the credentialing guidelines.

In most states, the ultimate responsibility for credentialing surgeons rests with the institution's governing board. This responsibility is frequently delegated to a department chairman, who asks the hospital's credentialing committee to assist him or her; the surgical committee, the laser committee, the medical staff, or a hospital-wide safety committee may also be involved.

Hospital privileges in traditional specialties are typically awarded or withheld on the basis of the physician's formal education; whether he or she has received specialty board certification; findings from a review of the previous procedures performed by the person and the associated morbidity and mortality; his or her membership in selected surgical organizations; the "track record" of the surgeon, if he or she has practiced at another hospital; and character references. Board certification alone is insufficient; credentials committees have learned the hard way about the need to investigate all of these areas.[8]

The process followed in determining whether a surgeon is qualified to receive privileges to perform laser surgical procedures should follow the same pattern as that used for surgeons seeking approval to perform traditional procedures, with the exception that the laser clinical director and frequently the LSO or the laser advisory committee should also advise or make recommendations to the credentials committee.[8] In many cases, laser credentialing criteria are developed jointly by the laser committee and the credentialing committee.

STEPS IN THE CREDENTIALING PROCESS

Credentialing criteria vary by institution, depending on the types of lasers used and the hospital's laser surgery case mix. Usually the physician must be credentialed for each wavelength he or she wishes to use. Criteria for physician credentialing usually include the following:

1. The physician must already have staff privileges in the specialty in which he or she plans to use the laser.
2. The physician must provide documentation of his or her educational preparation in the use of each laser for which privileges are requested.
3. The physician must be precepted by an accepted expert who has privileges in the laser procedure for which credentialing is requested and has observed a specified minimum number of procedures.
4. The physician must demonstrate continued competence in the use of the laser, through annual or biennial (every 2 years) reviews.

Staff Privileges

Approval to use lasers for treatment is considered an extension of the physician's existing privileges. Before requesting laser credentialing therefore, applicants should first be board certified, already have staff privileges in their specialty area, and be trained and have proven abilities in both the laser and standard techniques.

Not all physicians applying for laser privileges are surgeons, because physicians in various medical subspecialties (e.g., pulmonary specialists, gastroenterologists, cardiologists, and radiologists) are now performing endoscopic procedures that have traditionally been considered surgical in nature. These innovations have all resulted from advances in medical instrumentation, including the laser, which have made it possible for such medical specialists to perform relatively noninvasive procedures previously performed surgically. If an endoscopic procedure is to be performed with a laser and the person who will use the laser is properly trained, then he or she should be given privileges to perform the laser procedure, regardless of his or her basic education. Therefore, credentialing criteria need to apply not only to surgeons but also to such medical subspecialists.

Educational Background

Physicians who request laser credentialing must provide documentation of their attendance at a laser education course that includes both lecture and hands-on experience using human or other living tissue. The content of such a course should include laser theory, safety considerations, and clinical applications specific to the physician's specialty.

ASLMS suggests that such a course should minimally be 8 to 10 hours long; however, many hospitals require that the courses be 14 to 16 hours long. It has been suggested that at least half of that time be spent performing supervised hands-on work on laboratory animals.[9] Such hands-on experience is invaluable, as shown by the fact that the morbidity associated with laser procedures performed by a total of 300 surgeons who over a 3-year period participated in a hands-on CO_2 laser course in otolaryngology was less than that associated with comparable laser procedures performed by a random group of surgeons who had not received such training. Very little research has been done to determine the number of hours in a course needed to ensure competency in learning. However, in actuality, learning is not time related; instead it is the amount of exposure and experience offered in a course that determine whether the learner accomplishes the objectives.

As already noted, course work may also be completed in a residency or fellowship program that includes the techniques of laser therapy in the curriculum. Many new physicians have acquired enough experience during their residency programs to qualify them for credentialing. Such laser experience and education may be substituted for attendance at a laser course, with letters from the directors of residency programs describing the applicant's experience and education serving as the documentation.

Preceptorship

After attending a laser workshop, the applicant usually is required to complete a preceptorship. This involves having the applicant spend a certain amount of time with an experienced laser physician who is certified to use the laser for the application in question and having that person oversee one or more procedures performed by the applicant to document his or her safe and appropriate use of the laser. It is usually necessary for the applicant to complete a designated number of specific laser procedures using a specific type of laser and wavelength.

During the startup period of a laser program, however, a preceptorship may be difficult to procure. In this situation, it may be best to bring in an outside laser expert to work with each physician. Alternatively, if during the startup of such a program there is no one on staff who is credentialed to use the laser, the preceptorship requirement may be adjusted at the recommendation of the laser committee.

Ossoff contends that a preceptorship may not be required for each procedure a person wishes to perform if he or she is board certified, has adequate education, and can perform the same procedures without the laser.

In some cases, physicians are required to go through a 3- to 6-month probationary period before they are considered to have the necessary experience and expertise in the performance of laser procedures, the management of intraoperative complications, postoperative care, and follow-up. At the conclusion of the probationary period, the physician may then appear before the laser committee to explain or defend his or her work.[1]

Continued Competence

An annual or biennial credentialing review is important to document the physician's continued use of and proficiency in the laser. Such reviews should include an analysis of the physician's caseload of specific laser procedures as well as a critical review of patient outcomes and the complications that occurred. Recredentialing should not be automatic.

Many facilities review the actual numbers of laser procedures that individual physicians perform each year. Because laser use requires skill, a physician who has not used the laser for a long time may need to attend a refresher course to ensure his or her safe and effective use of this technology. If the number of cases performed is unusually low (sometimes defined as less than three laser procedures per year), the physician may be asked to describe how he or she is staying current with the ever-changing laser technology. If there is a question as to the physician's continued proficiency, he or she may be required to work in a laser laboratory, staffed by the LSO, to review and practice laser applications using the various wavelengths. Sometimes this credentialing review will reveal that a physician is using the laser at another hospital, and if so, it is important to know why.

REVIEW OF CREDENTIALING APPLICATIONS

The credentialing process can become cumbersome if it is not organized and monitored properly. A member of the laser committee should be responsible for expediting the process, with the objective of getting each physician through the credentialing process as rapidly and efficiently as possible. After the physician has met the educational requirements and completed the requisite preceptorships, the physician's laser credentialing request is usually reviewed by the specialty department and then submitted for the approval or disapproval of an executive committee or board of trustees. Approvals or denials should be communicated in writing to the applicant.

If the application is approved, copies of the approval should also be sent to the appropriate parties (e.g., the operating room director or medical staff office). If the hospital board has any doubts about the privileges requested, they should ask the laser committee or the appropriate clinical department to reexamine the application and offer more complete documentation or support for their recommendation. It is not unusual for the board to require additional education or preceptorships or to require mandatory consultations and monitoring by a professional colleague on a probationary basis.

If the application is denied, a reason must be provided and recommendations made for ways to obtain privileges. It is important that any health care facility base their actions (both favorable and unfavorable) on the need to ensure high-quality patient care. Preserving the market share and eliminating competition (i.e., preventing a competent and qualified physician from treating patients to protect the patient base or other physicians' incomes) is anticompetitive conduct and is a violation of antitrust laws.

A mechanism for appeal must be provided for physicians who are denied laser credentials or who are granted them on a temporary or provisional basis. In such instances, the physician must be given an opportunity to argue the decision and to provide additional documentation, as appropriate.

Credentialing Supervision

A laser credentials book may be kept in the OR for the OR supervisor or his or her designee to check the credentials of physicians scheduled to perform laser procedures. Any doubts about privileges must be eliminated before the laser treatment is started.

Credentialing of Residents

The laser committee must also deal with the need for residents to become credentialed in the use of lasers. Some facilities require that residents attend a laser education course or view videotapes that specifically address laser safety and applications before assisting with laser procedures.[6] Residents should also meet with the LSO to review the operation of the specific laser to be used clinically and be allowed time to practice with the laser system in a laboratory setting.

A staff member who is credentialed in the laser application in question should always supervise through direct observation laser use by residents. The attending physician is ultimately responsible for the safe and appropriate operation of the laser during the procedure in which the resident participates, and should the physician leave the resident alone to perform the lasing, he or she must be immediately available in case any problems arise.

Credentialing of Nurses and Other Support Staff

A nurse skilled in working with a laser can free up the physician to concentrate on the surgery proper, while he or she operates the laser; therefore, in addition to physician credentialing, some facilities also formally credential nurses and other technical support personnel. Such credentialing is limited to people who have demonstrated a sound knowledge of laser principles, hazards, and safety precautions. The criteria used for such people are similar to those used for physicians and are usually established and overseen by the laser committee, in conjunction with the LSO and the supervisor of the area in which the laser is used. These criteria include the following:

- Documented evidence of attendance at an approved laser course, ideally including hands-on experience. Educational experience should relate to the specific wavelength as well as the brand and model of laser used.
- Experience with and demonstrated proficiency in the operation of the specific laser, or lasers, and ancillary equipment for which the person will be responsible, obtained through a preceptorship with an experienced nurse who has had laser education and experience.
- Knowledge and understanding of the institutional laser policies and procedures.
- Knowledge of the clinical and safety aspects of the particular procedures and types of lasers the person will be responsible for, focusing especially on the nursing responsibilities.

The last three criteria might be fulfilled through a structured preceptorship program.

Sample Credentialing Policy

The following is a sample of a generic laser credentialing policy that can be adapted as necessary by laser committees wishing to establish credentialing policies and procedures for their institutions. The policy proposed follows the recommendations of ANSI and ASLMS.

SAMPLE LASER CREDENTIALING POLICY AND PROCEDURES

Objectives

To establish a written policy stating the requirements for physicians who wish to use lasers in the treatment and diagnosis of their patients. It should specify the education and experience needed to receive these credentials.

Purpose

To adopt a policy whereby physicians are required to obtain the necessary education, experience, and credentials in laser procedures and to establish standards that must be met by all physicians before they can proceed to use lasers to treat patients.

Requirements for Laser Credentialing
(full and provisional privileges)

The physician applicant wishing to perform laser procedures that have been approved by the FDA must:

1. Be a member of the medical staff with privileges for, and demonstrated competence in, performing the same treatments by conventional means, as approved by the appropriate specialty department. Those seeking laser privileges shall meet all of the standards of the institution with regard to board eligibility or certification, special education, ethical character, and good standing.

2. Provide documentation of his or her educational experiences in the use of each laser for which privileges are requested. These experiences include:
   a. An accredited course in theory and application specific to the physician's specialty, including hands-on experience using human or living tissue. Such a course should be a minimum of 8 to 10 hours (ASLMS recommendation), and the content should include basic laser physics, laser-tissue interactions, the clinical applications of the laser in the specialty field, and hands-on experience with lasers, as well as any other content specified by the specialty department. Such courses must be approved by the Accreditation Council for Continuing Medical Education of the American Medical Association.
   b. A residency or fellowship program in which the techniques of laser therapy are a part of the curriculum. A letter from the residency program chairman will serve to document the physician's educational background.

3. Receive operational inservice instructions on the specific lasers at the hospital for which he or she is seeking privileges.

4. Be precepted by an active member of his or her department who has laser privileges. The minimum number of observed procedures is two. It is essential that the person see and document his or her clinical applications of the laser in the outpatient or hospital setting, as appropriate to the procedure, or procedures, involved.

   OR

   Provide documentation of a preceptorship by a person recognized as an expert in this field.

5. Demonstrate continued competence in the use of the laser. Privileges to use each laser will be reviewed by the laser committee every 2 years. An important element in the renewal of privileges will be evidence of continuing education and frequency of use sufficient to maintain skills. Requirements will vary with the discipline.

6. The credentialing process must be repeated for each type of laser for which privileges are requested.

These credentialing requirements may be expanded upon by individual departments, which may wish to further define the required laser education and preceptorship requirements.

Approval Procedure

1. Physicians seeking laser privileges will obtain a laser privilege application form from the laser committee or medical staff office. The physician will complete the form and attach documentation showing that the departmental criteria for privileges have been met. This information and form shall be returned to the laser committee.
2. The laser committee will review applications monthly and approve or deny applications.
   a. Denials will be communicated in writing to the applicant with a rationale for the decision and recommendations for additional education and/or a preceptorship. The applicant has the right to appeal the decision and provide additional documentation to the laser committee.
   b. Approvals will be communicated in writing to the applicant, with notices sent to appropriate parties as well. Notices of approval should be sent to the department chairman, medical staff office, and director of the appropriate treatment service in which the physician primarily practices, such as the operating room, digestive disease service, or eye clinic.
3. A permanent copy of all approval letters will be kept on file with each applicant's application form and documentation. The minutes of the laser committee will list the names of approved candidates.
4. The medical staff office will keep a copy of the approval letter as part of the physician's hospital file.
5. A list of physicians who have been granted laser privileges will be kept at each operating room suite. A similar list should be available to personnel in the admitting office. The laser authorization list should be kept current and reviewed every 3 months.
6. The laser committee should review the laser privileges, guidelines, and policies at least every 2 years. The laser privileges of each physician are subject to review at least every 2 years.

Special Provisions

Residents

1. Senior residents will be allowed to use laser equipment as a clinical tool during ENT, gynecologic, and other specialty service procedures only under the supervision of a certified attending physician.
2. A current list of senior residents authorized to use laser equipment under staff supervision should be available to the laser committee at all times.

3. Residents interested in assisting during a laser procedure must review laser material specified in the library, view specified videotapes, make an appointment with the laser staff to review the equipment, and fire the laser at an inanimate object.

4. Physicians working to perform procedures that are considered investigational by the FDA must meet additional requirements. The physician who introduces the procedure into the hospital must complete the appropriate forms and submit them to the FDA, the manufacturer, and the institutional review board. The protocol for each procedure must be approved by this board. Once the originating physician has received approval, he or she becomes the principal investigator. Any additional physicians wishing to perform the same procedure using the same laser are required to work through this principal investigator. Reports on any investigational procedures performed must be filed with the FDA on a case-by-case basis.

References

1. Apfelberg DB, ed. Evaluation and installation of surgical laser systems. New York: Springer-Verlag, 1987.
2. American National Standards Institute. American national standards for the safe use of lasers in health care facilities (ANSI Z136; January 1993). Toledo, OH: Laser Institute of America, 1993.
3. Ossoff R. Solving the credentialing riddle: tips to ensure user competency. In Breedlove B, Schwartz D, eds. Clinical lasers: expert strategies for practical and profitable management. Atlanta: American Health Consultants, 1985;261–268.
4. American National Standards Institute. American National Standards for the Safe Use of Lasers in Health Care Facilities. ANSI Z136; February 3, 1996. Toledo, OH: Laser Institute of America, 1996.
5. Pfister JI et al. The nursing spectrum of lasers, 2nd ed. Denver: Education Design, 1996.
6. Ball K. Lasers: the perioperative challenge, ed 2. St. Louis: Mosby, 1995.
7. Blaes SM, Knight GE. Effective physician credentialing: properly monitoring medical staff can protect hospitals from liability. Health Progress 1990;71:60–65.
8. Dixon JA. Surgical application of lasers, 2nd ed. Chicago: Year Book Medical Publishers.
9. Ossoff RH. The credentialing riddle: with no national certification in lasers, how do you ensure your physicians and staff are adequately trained and fully competent? In Proceedings of the American Society of Laser Medicine and Surgery, 1992, pp. 62A–62D.

Subject Index

Page numbers followed by an f *indicate figures; page numbers followed by a* t *indicate tables.*